Primary Care Occupational Therapy

Sue Dahl-Popolizio • Katie Smith
Mackenzie Day • Sherry Muir • William Manard
Editors

Primary Care Occupational Therapy

A Quick Reference Guide

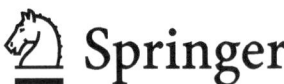 Springer

Editors
Sue Dahl-Popolizio
AT Still University
Mesa, AZ, USA

Arizona State University
Phoenix, AZ, USA

Mackenzie Day
Corte Madera, CA, USA

William Manard
SCL Health
Broomfield, CO, USA

Katie Smith
Revolutionary Alignment, LLC
Detroit, MI, USA

Sherry Muir
University of Arkansas at
Fayetteville/UAMS
Fayetteville, AR, USA

ISBN 978-3-031-20881-2   ISBN 978-3-031-20882-9   (eBook)
https://doi.org/10.1007/978-3-031-20882-9

This Springer imprint is published by the registered company Springer Nature Switzerland AG
The registered company address is: Gewerbestrasse 11, 6330 Cham, Switzerland

User Guide

Throughout this text, the authors will be using the following abbreviations, to maximize brevity of the overall text.

Most Commonly Used Abbreviations Throughout the Text:

ADL	Activities of Daily Living
CDC	Centers for Disease Control and Prevention
CPT	Common Procedural Terminology codes (billing codes used in practice)
EHR	Electronic Health Record
HTN	Hypertension
IADL	Instrumental Activities of Daily Living
ICD-10	International Classification of Diseases
OT	Occupational Therapy
OTP	Occupational Therapy Practitioner
PC	Primary Care
PCP	Primary Care Provider

Abbreviations Specific to Musculoskeletal Issues:

CMC	Carpometacarpal joint
DIP	Distal interphalangeal joint
FMC	Fine motor coordination
GMC	Gross motor coordination
IP	Interphalangeal joint (can be either PIP or DIP or both)
MCP	Metacarpal phalangeal joint
PIP	Proximal interphalangeal joint
ROM	Range of motion (A/AA/PROM active/active assist/passive ROM, respectively)

Additional Terms:

The use of the term 'client' versus 'patient' was determined by the authors of each chapter. The term chosen is used consistently within the chapter. This reflects the use of both terms based on the preference or industry standard of the setting in general or the practice site.

Additional Note Regarding Resources:

The authors have provided assessments, patient handouts, and other resources whenever possible. When they could not provide the actual resource, they provided links to the online resource whenever possible for ease of access for the reader. The reader is responsible for obtaining any necessary permissions for use. As links can break over time, the authors have included the name of the resource so the reader can find it online.

Social Networking:

For connection with OTPs and other professionals who are passionate about the topic of PC OT and related progressive concepts of prevention and health promotion, please visit https://www.facebook.com/groups/323579324877922/

Contents

Part I
General Topics for Primary Care Occupational Therapy

Chapter 1
Introduction

William Manard

When I was in medical school, knowing how therapies integrated into my practice was clearly defined by my instructors. If a patient had a lower extremity or back complaint, you sent them to physical therapy (PT); if a patient had an upper extremity complaint, you sent them to OT. This simple algorithm helped a forming physician understand what therapists did without engaging with them to determine exactly how they participated in patient care. Although I had some interactions that made this appear less than complete, this was the framework with which I entered into postgraduate training.

During residency training, I discovered that these divisions were not always so clear; I also learned that perhaps there were broader services that differing therapists could provide. This is when I first learned that, although physical therapists often performed assessments prior to discharge for adaptive equipment, OTPs often had a broader view on overall patient safety at home, including the impact of cognitive impairment on potential readmission or appropriate level of care. At this point, I started reconsidering my initial learning, which positioned me for my next experience.

I was fortunate to work in a Program of All-Inclusive Care for the Elderly (PACE) as my first position after residency. In this setting, we were able to provide holistic services, across the entire continuum of care, for a population of frail elderly persons. Freed from reimbursement considerations, each professional on the care team was able to provide any services within their experience and licensure. Because of this, I first learned the full extent of services that OTPs could provide our patients in a PC setting. I didn't have to use simplistic algorithms to determine potential home safety or potential issues with motor vehicle operation (simply because my services would be reimbursed); I could instead rely on my professional colleague to

W. Manard (✉)
SCL Health, Broomfield, CO, USA
e-mail: bill.manard@sclhealth.org

© Springer Nature Switzerland AG 2023
S. Dahl-Popolizio et al. (eds.), *Primary Care Occupational Therapy*,
https://doi.org/10.1007/978-3-031-20882-9_1

complete a more comprehensive evaluation and provide recommendations for patients and families in a more robust fashion than I could ever hope to do. With each member of the care team able to provide any services within their skill set, patients and families received more comprehensive primary care (PC) and were generally more satisfied with care versus that provided in a more traditional PC setting.

Upon moving into a more academic setting, I again had an opportunity not offered to many PCPs. As part of a patient-centered medical home transformation project, we were able to offer non-traditional services, including workplace and home ergonomic evaluations, behavioral health services, and integrated holistic person-centered care, again without direct concern to existing payment structures. In this environment, I again increased my appreciation for the services that OTPs could offer our patients in the PC setting, as I gained a greater understanding of the cognitive services available to help our patients struggling with behavioral health issues. Again, although other professionals, including myself, could provide some of these services, the holistic approach of OT seemed a natural fit for the holistic nature of family medicine, and this experience has made me an advocate for expanding the role of OT in PC, including enhancing our reimbursement structure to support these services.

This need for additional professionals to enhance services to our communities has an even more acute importance at this time. Professional and popular media are replete with stories of shortages of PCPs, both currently and, more worrisome, as our current population ages. In a 2020 study commissioned for the American Association of Medical Colleges (AAMC) [1], it was estimated that by 2023, there will be a shortage of PCPs between 21,400 and 55,200. This potential shortage is accelerated by increasing age of existing PCPs, and it could be exacerbated if payment structures were improved to remove barriers to care for historically underserved persons.

The COVID-19 pandemic may have worsened this potential shortage, and these fears are being presented in recent news stories. As an example, a survey published in the Washington Post in 2021 reported that a significant fraction of physicians who ceased or reduced providing care during the pandemic do not anticipate returning to their prior level of practice, for those who return to practice at all [2]. This will likely make it more difficult to receive PC for all segments of the population in the future.

Because of the broad array of services that OTPs are able to provide to our communities, I am happy to introduce this practical guide to the provision of these services in the PC setting. As OTPs become more integrated members of the PC team, the value of the care we provide people will continue to increase. Additionally, by increasing the number of professionals in the care of our patients, the workforce strains that are anticipated in the coming years will be somewhat blunted; this will help allay some of the concerns described above. Beyond all of this, providing a broad array of services in our communities, especially in the setting of the patient's medical home, will help improve the overall health of our communities and make our society a more holistically healthy place in which we all live.

Thank you to my colleagues for preparing this important guide to help our fraternity better understand how to integrate their valuable services into community PC practice. Thank you to those who read this and apply its principles to your own practice. Finally, thank you for taking this newly developed knowledge and applying not just to patient care but to also advocate for broadening the integration of OT services in the provision of PC within our communities.

References

1. The complexities of physician supply and demand: projections from 2018 to 2033. https://www.aamc.org/system/files/2020-06/stratcomm-aamc-physician-workforce-projections-june-2020.pdf. Accessed 23 Oct 2021.
2. Wan W. Burned out by the pandemic, 3 in 10 health-care workers consider leaving the profession. https://www.washingtonpost.com/health/2021/04/22/health-workers-covid-quit/. Accessed 23 Oct 2021.

Chapter 2
Overview of Occupational Therapy in Primary Care

Katie Smith, Sue Dahl-Popolizio, Lydia Royeen, and Brenda Koverman

Introduction

In the United States, primary care (PC) is gaining recognition as the key setting where patients can receive accessible and integrated care to address the majority of their healthcare needs in one setting [1]. With the integration of preventative services and behavioral health into PC practices, the focus of PC is shifting from a reactive approach to illness and disease, to a more proactive approach that empowers and engages the patient as an active participant in their healthcare and overall health and wellness. This approach includes a care spectrum ranging from preventative strategies to acute and chronic condition management, with a population-focused approach to care, and an awareness of underlying or comorbid behavioral health issues, available resources, cultural customs, and all other social determinants of health [1, 2]. This approach to PC provides an opportunity for early detection of acute illnesses and chronic disease onsets, chronic disease management, a triage system for connecting patients to specialty resources as needed, and a focus on increasing patient self-management of health and wellness [1, 3–5]. This approach encourages active patient involvement and planning and reduces the

K. Smith (✉)
Revolutionary Alignment, LLC, Detroit, MI, USA
www.RevolutionaryAlignment.com

S. Dahl-Popolizio
Arizona State University, Phoenix, AZ, USA

AT Still University, Mesa, AZ, USA
e-mail: Sue.Dahlpopolizio@asu.edu; sdahlpopolizio@atsu.edu

L. Royeen
Texas Woman's University, Dallas, TX, USA

B. Koverman
Rush University Medical Center, Chicago, IL, USA

© Springer Nature Switzerland AG 2023
S. Dahl-Popolizio et al. (eds.), *Primary Care Occupational Therapy*,
https://doi.org/10.1007/978-3-031-20882-9_2

dependence on emergency rooms and hospitalizations for conditions that can be proactively managed by the patient and their primary care team.

In 2010, the passage of the Affordable Care Act provided more Americans with insurance coverage to increase access to PC services. This influx of patients into PC resulted in an increased shortage of PCPs and provided an opportunity to rethink our approach to PC [3–5]. As a result, the concept of an interprofessional team approach has gained popularity to offload work from the PCP, while meeting the needs of the patient population in PC through the more holistic provision of services from prevention, to acute illness, and chronic condition management of individual patients, and patient populations [3]. With an interprofessional team, each provider practices at the top of their license, using the skills most unique to their profession [4]. This approach improves job satisfaction and can also reduce provider burnout due to overwork or the requirement to complete tasks that do not require the provider's unique skills or interests. Burnout is a growing concern among PC practices [3, 7]. The specific professionals comprising these interprofessional teams vary across PC practices. Considering the whole person approach to care of the OT profession and their broad training in medical and behavioral health conditions, the integration of OT into the PC setting is a natural fit [8, 9]. With their lens of treating all issues within the context of the patient's habits, roles, and routines, OTPs can maximize the patient's experience with care and offload patient visits from the PCP that do not require the PCP's skill set, but do require behavioral or behavioral health intervention [3, 4, 7–9]. This can reduce PCP burnout, reduce healthcare costs, improve health outcomes, and meet public health goals while demonstrating how OT functions as a member of the PC team [7, 8]. With their patient-empowering approach, having an OTP available on a PC team is an opportunity for OTPs to have a positive impact on the lives of patients, populations, other team members, and also the overall management of health and health care.

Defining PC

As defined by The Institute of Medicine [1, 5], PC "is the provision of integrated, accessible health care services by clinicians who are accountable for addressing the large majority of personal health care needs, developing a sustained partnership with patients, and practicing in the context of family and community." The increasingly interprofessional team of clinicians who deliver services in a PC context may include PCPs, behavioral health providers, medical assistants, pharmacists, social workers, and more [3]. A team-based approach occurs when at least two healthcare professionals collaborate with each other, patients, and their caregivers, to achieve shared goals while striving to provide high-quality care [10]. An effective team-based approach includes clear roles, effective communication, shared goals, mutual trust, and measurable processes and outcomes [10].

PC is an umbrella term that includes many different practice types, such as family practice, internal medicine, pediatrics, and more [7]. The specifics of OT practice within a PC setting depends on the specific focus of the clinic, the physical and operational requirements of the setting, and the conditions commonly seen in the specific PC clinic. See the ***Conditions Addressed by Occupational Therapy in Primary Care*** section for condition-specific considerations for PC OT practice. There are a variety of business organizational arrangements that can all be considered PC. Ideally, PC settings have all clinicians on the interprofessional team operating within the same physical clinic [5, 7]. This arrangement is optimal for increasing patient engagement with interprofessional services and in supporting clinician communication. If sharing a physical clinic location is not possible, PCP referrals to an offsite OTP may still be considered PC OT, as the key quality of team-based integrated PC is the overall collaborative approach to care with effective communication among providers and a plan of care that includes and empowers the patient.

OT Theory in PC

OT is a whole-person oriented profession, and OT training addresses the biomechanical, psychological, social, spiritual, and environmental factors that are directly applicable to addressing the broad needs of the diverse population that comes to a PC site for care [5]. OTPs are skilled in addressing physical dysfunction, and also behavioral and mental health issues. OTPs work with individuals across the lifespan to maximize function and participation [6, 8] and improve health outcomes. The preventative focus of PC is well aligned with OT philosophy that supports patients in independence and self-efficacy with managing their health and engaging in self-determined, value-driven tasks that bring meaning to their lives. The population-focused approach of PC is also reflective of OT values of addressing relationships and the social and environmental contributors to health outcomes, such as the built environment, economic stability, education, access to food, healthcare, and other factors and available resources that affect overall health and wellness [5, 6]. The alignment between PC goals and OT philosophy reflects a natural and mutually supportive fit with the shared interest among team members of preventing negative health outcomes, optimizing independence, and improving wellness and quality of life for as many individuals and communities as possible.

OT Practice in PC

The PC setting is fast-paced and broad. The OTP is likely to encounter many different patient needs across the lifespan and across a wide breadth of presenting conditions. It is important to consider the limitations of the PC setting and the function of the OTP within this setting. Consider approaching PC OT as a triage role. If the patient's occupational deficits could be best addressed in one or a few sessions, this reduces the need for the patient to go to a separate clinic and prevents the risk of the patient being unable to follow through with a referral to access those services. However, PC is not the setting within which to conduct extensive treatment plans or to address significant occupational deficits. This would diminish the OTP's availability to best serve the patient population and the interprofessional PC team with more brief interventions for more patients. If, after an initial OT screening or OT evaluation, it is determined that the patient's needs would be better addressed through outpatient OT or by referring to a different profession, the OTP can make that suggestion and help with that referral process to an offsite provider. PC OT is a practice of brevity and breadth; offsite referrals will be necessary for more involved cases or conditions.

Example: The PCP referred Emily to the OTP for a fall risk assessment. Emily is a 56 year old woman who lives alone, reports difficulty sleeping, has high health literacy, high baseline health, and high motivation to implement OT strategies. The OTP provided sleep hygiene education during the same session as the initial evaluation, including environmental modification education. The OTP and Emily set up four, once weekly follow- up appointments. Emily also reports knee pain, and the OTP consulted with the PCP to suggest that a PT referral may also be beneficial.

Referral: Any condition or diagnosis that impairs function or involvement in daily activities may prompt an appropriate referral to the PC OTP. Educating providers is an important part of receiving appropriate referrals. OT referrals may reach the OTP via the Electronic Health Record (EHR) or by the PCP directly introducing the patient to the OTP. A direct introduction is called a "*warm handoff*" or a "*hallway handoff*" and is one of the benefits of being located in the same clinic [7]. There are times the warm handoff process interrupts an ongoing OT session, allowing the OTP to determine, based on the issues of the current patient and the new patient, if the OTP will address the new patient's issues immediately, wait a few minutes until the current session is done or have the patient return for a separate visit. No matter which of these approaches is chosen, the relationship has already been established due to the warm handoff from the PCP to the OTP. That significantly increases the likelihood that the patient will return if not seen immediately.

> **Example**: Dr. Ling's patient Elaine expressed interest in support with smoking cessation. Dr. Ling excused herself and knocked on the door of the exam room where the OTP was in session with another patient to make a request that the OTP meet with Elaine. The OTP excused herself from her session, to go with Dr. Ling to meet Elaine. The OTP provided a brief overview on OT intervention for smoking cessation, and Elaine expressed interest in working with the OTP. Elaine made an OT evaluation appointment with the front desk for another day, and the OTP returned to her session that had been temporarily interrupted by the warm hand-off referral.

Evaluation: Consider the specific populations and conditions most frequently seen at your PC site and tailor your evaluation tools to assess for occupational deficits that are related to those conditions and populations. Be mindful of the time required for assessment tools and use brief assessments when possible. Clinicians may treat patients within their own offices, or in shared treatment rooms, in which case the PC OTP may need to have portable access to assessment and intervention tools. Document OT evaluation in the EHR as soon as possible, to ensure that communication flow with other providers involved in the patient's care is current, as face-to-face communication with providers may not be possible given the potential space and time constraints.

> **Example**: An OTP integrated into an internal medicine PC clinic is working with Garret, a 79 year old man who lives with his wife in a one-story home and is interested in information on falls prevention and home safety. The OTP

Common Interventions

Activity Modification	Environmental Modification	Self-Management Routines
Diet and Hydration	Functional/ Cognitive Assessments	Sleep Hygiene
DME/Adaptive Equipment	Patient Education	Stress & Pain Management
Energy Conservation	Posture and Positioning	Stretches & Strengthening

Fig. 2.1 Common interventions of OTs in PC
Note: Fig. 2.1 reproduced with permission from Smith, K. & Day, M. (2018). Primary care OT: clinical and administrative templates. Pacific University doctoral thesis.

Intervention: In addition to focusing on brief evaluation processes, seek to optimize impactful interventions that require less time investment and maximize the patient's ability to utilize strategies on their own. There are many clinical services that an OTP may choose to offer to the PC team and ultimately the patient. OTPs in PC can address conditions including acute musculoskeletal injuries, developmental delays, and mental health needs [8, 9]. See Fig. 2.1 for an overview of common interventions that are often appropriately delivered in a PC OT context. See the **Conditions Addressed by Occupational Therapy in Primary Car**e section for condition-specific intervention strategies for PC OT practice.

Example: The OTP met with Carol, a 23 year old coffee barista developing initial symptoms of carpal tunnel syndrome. The OTP worked with Carol for four sessions in total, and at the end of the OT plan, Carol was able to independently demonstrate job-specific activity modifications and ergonomics and reduce her overall experience of carpal tunnel syndrome symptoms.

Communication: Consistent communication with the interprofessional team is essential in PC, as the PCP will be generating referrals to all available providers, including the PC OTP, and the PCP is ultimately responsible for directing the patient's plan of care. PCPs often work closely with a medical assistant (MA), who supports the PCP in patient communications, referral flows, patient rooming, and documentation. As mentioned above, there may be other professions who will also be working together in PC, and the PC OTP must understand the roles and scopes of practice of the various professionals located at the specific PC clinic where they are working. This serves to ensure patient needs are met by the most appropriate provider available.

Example: The OTP walked past a MA typing in the EHR. The MA asked the OTP if OT would be beneficial for a patient experiencing stress and anxiety. The MA explained that the PCP was hoping to connect the patient to the PC psychologist, but that the psychologist was out at meetings today. The OTP briefly explained the OT role in stress management including self-management routines, pacing, and energy conservation. The MA suggested that OT may be an excellent fit for the patient's needs, as the patient's stress is related to their challenges with managing their chronic lupus independently while feeling successful at work. The MA communicated to the PCP and the patient was able to initiate services with the OTP that day.

Summary

The holistic and contextual OT philosophy and the evolving PC approach share many common goals and interests. When delivering OT services in PC, be mindful of the overall preventative and population-health perspective, as well as the importance of addressing patient needs in the context of their communities. The importance of interprofessional collaboration and communication cannot be overstated as this is critical to ensure the needs of patients are expeditiously and effectively addressed, while at the same time ensuring the providers are all working at the top of their license. All OTPs are prepared through their training to practice as PC OTPs if they choose to do so, and this book will support OTPs in tailoring their services to the needs identified at their specific PC site.

References

1. Office of Disease Prevention and Health Promotion. Healthy people 2020. Access to primary care. 2020. https://www.healthypeople.gov/2020/topics-objectives/topic/social-determinants-health/interventions-resources/access-to-primary.
2. Patient-Centered Primary Care Collaborative. Investing in primary care: a state-level analysis. 2019. https://www.pcpcc.org/sites/default/files/resources/pcmh_evidence_report_2019.pdf.
3. Bodenheimer TS, Smith MD. Primary care: proposed solutions to the physician shortage without training more physicians. Health Aff. 2013;32(11):1881–6. https://doi.org/10.1377/hlthaff.2013.0234.
4. Trembath F, Dahl-Popolizio S, Vanwinkle M, Milligan L. Retrospective analysis: most common diagnoses seen in a primary care clinic and corresponding occupational therapy interventions. Open J Occup Ther. 2019;7(2):1539. https://doi.org/10.15453/2168-6408.1539.
5. American Occupational Therapy Association. Occupational therapy in the promotion of health and well-being. Am J Occup Ther. 2020;74(3):1–14. https://doi.org/10.5014/ajot.2020.743003.
6. American Occupational Therapy Association. Role of occupational therapy in primary care. Am J Occup Ther. 2020;74(Supplement 3):7413410040p1–7413410040p16. https://doi.org/10.5014/ajot.2020.74S3001.
7. Smith K, Day M, Muir S, Dahl-Popolizio S. Developing tailored program proposals for occupational therapy in primary care. Open J Occup Ther. 2020;8(1):1–13. https://doi.org/10.15453/2168-6408.1630.
8. Dahl-Popolizio S, Rogers O, Muir SL, Carroll J, Manson L. Interprofessional primary care: the value of occupational therapy. Open J Occup Ther. 2017;5(3):1363. https://doi.org/10.15453/2168-6408.1363.
9. Dahl-Popolizio S, Manson L, Muir S, Rogers O. Enhancing the value of integrated primary care: the role of occupational therapy. Fam Syst Health. 2016;34(3):270–80. https://doi.org/10.1037/fsh0000208.
10. Mitchell P, Wynia M, Golden R, McNellis B, Okun S, Webb CE, Rohrback V, Von kohorn, I. Core principles and values of effective team-based health care. Washington, DC: Institute of Medicine; 2012. www.iom.edu/tbc

Chapter 3
Administrative and Operational Considerations

Katie Jordan and Ashley Halle

Strategic Plan: Needs Assessment of Site, Population, and Stakeholders

Whether you are already engaged in PC or PC-related services or looking to get started, it's important to first consider the strategic priorities of your plan. Because of the breadth and depth of people, populations, and stakeholders in PC, it is vital to reflect on your strategic priorities for engaging in PC settings. Below is a list of considerations when reflecting on your strategic plan.

- Business plan or proof of concept plan

    - There are numerous tools available to support developing a business plan that will prompt and guide you through the process. While a formal business plan may be needed for contracting, negotiating for space, or acquiring a business loan, a proof of concept plan can sometimes be a more logical and accessible place to start. Generally, a proof of concept plan involves research to determine the viability of your ideas, testing those ideas by talking with stakeholders, and then involving stakeholders in the development of your plan. One way to approach your plan is by using a SWOT (Strengths, Weaknesses, Opportunities, and Threats) analysis to discover the needs of your site(s), population(s), and stakeholder(s). A SWOT analysis template can be found online.

K. Jordan (✉)
University of Southern California, University Clinical Services, Los Angeles, CA, USA
e-mail: mkjordan@usc.edu

A. Halle
University of Southern California, University Clinical Services, Los Angeles, CA, USA

University of Southern California, Chan Division of Occupational Science and Occupational Therapy, Los Angeles, CA, USA
e-mail: halle@chan.usc.edu

© Springer Nature Switzerland AG 2023
S. Dahl-Popolizio et al. (eds.), *Primary Care Occupational Therapy*,
https://doi.org/10.1007/978-3-031-20882-9_3

- SWOT analysis online resources:

  MindTools.com SWOT Analysis https://www.mindtools.com/pages/article/newTMC_05.htm
  LivePlan.com What is a SWOT Analysis and How to Do It Right: With Examples https://www.liveplan.com/blog/what-is-a-swot-analysis-and-how-to-do-it-right-with-examples/

- Vision and mission
  - A vision document contains current goals but also inspires a path forward toward your ideal future state. A vision document can be exhaustive or short and to the point, depending on the current stage of development you are in for your PC practice. It should set achievable aspirational targets and must be a reflexive document that you continue to refine over time.
  - A mission statement explains your purpose, explaining what you are currently doing and why.
  - The vision and mission of your practice may be combined into one document, but it's important that you clearly define each and that you continue to modify the document(s) when making strategic decisions as circumstances or priorities change.

- Learn your stakeholders, what matters to them and why
  - PC is a broad practice area, and there are many stakeholders whose interests must be considered. Below is Table 3.1: *Stakeholder Interests*, which includes

Table 3.1 Stakeholder interests

Stakeholder	Considerations
Consumers of the service (patients)	Experience, access (to providers, space, and support), cost, quality/outcome
Families/caregivers/ significant others	Caregiver support and resources, access, experience
Referring providers (DO, MD, PA, NP, optometry, etc.)	Internal and external providers that refer (or do not refer) to OT, perceived barriers and supports, workflow and clinical pathways, space
Health system and/or facility ownership/leadership	Integration into a health system vs. standalone practice, leadership expectations and vision, risk tolerance, culture
Payers	Payer policy, payer mix, access to payers (billing, coding office support), documentation requirements
Students and volunteers	Experience, educational goals/requirements, strengths and skills
Researchers	Current and potential collaborations, opportunity for synergies, how research will be used
Professional and support staff	Clinical and operational workflow, culture of the team(s), perceived needs/supports
OTPs	Current or previous attempts to connect OT services, desired future state, employment options and benefits, advancing OT practice

initial stakeholders but depending on your setting, there may be others. After listing all invested stakeholders, the next step is to engage them. Your site might already have an advisory group of some kind or you might need to reach out to individuals to begin building relationships to help you understand what is important to each stakeholder and why, especially regarding PC access, services, workflow, and operations.

Resources

- General business plan free online resources:

  – U.S. Small Business Association website https://www.sba.gov/business-guide/plan-your-business/write-your-business-plan
  – SCORE is another organization that offers information regarding writing business plans:
  – https://www.score.org/business-plans-startup-assistance-resources

- Specific OT in PC business plan development resource:

  – Developing Tailored Program Proposals for Occupational Therapy in Primary Care [1]. https://scholarworks.wmich.edu/ojot/vol8/iss1/11/

- Vision statements:

  – TopNonProfits.com 30 Example Vision Statements https://topnonprofits.com/examples/vision-statements/
  – ProjectManager.com A Guide to Writing the Perfect Vision Statement https://www.projectmanager.com/blog/guide-writing-perfect-vision-statement-examples

- Mission statements:

  – https://www.missionstatements.com/

Understand Your Environment

The physical, policy, temporal, and cultural environments in which your target PC practice is located adds important context for planning. Below are some key areas for reflection. Building expertise in these areas can take time. Practitioners should use resources, if available at your clinical site, such as legal counsel, compliance officers, and billing and coding experts for support and guidance. While professionals in these offices may not be familiar with OT's role in PC, they can serve as subject matter experts and can advise you on questions related to regulatory, compliance, and reimbursement issues.

- Regulatory

  Understanding regulatory constraints and supports is an important step in building a sustainable practice. Answering questions about the regulatory context of your target PC environment can help you construct the most sustainable model for your practice while also helping you avoid barriers (see Table 3.2).

Table 3.2 Regulatory considerations

Key questions	Key considerations
How is your space licensed and/or accredited?	Space where healthcare services are delivered is generally regulated by local, state, and/or national rules. A PC space may be licensed as a specific type of space that creates parameters around how services are delivered there. Additionally, PC sites may hold a special accreditation that designates the level of service that they provide
Who are the stakeholders that have knowledge regarding licensure and/or accreditation of your target PC practice?	Depending on the breadth and depth of your clinical site, the administration or leadership would typically know what licensure and which accreditations are active at your site. If there is a legal or compliance office, they would also be able to provide more information on this question
What impact might space licensure or accreditation have on your practice plan?	Licensure and/or accreditation set rules and parameters for service development, delivery, access, and outcomes. Understanding how these rules impact your strategic plan is important for building a successful and sustainable practice. For example, you planned to conduct a therapeutic group in the waiting room in the evenings but your site is restricted from providing clinical services outside of licensed patient room areas. Understanding these constraints and supports is important for building your program and your credibility with your site and referring providers
Are there carve-out spaces that are not licensed or are licensed differently to consider in your planning?	Understanding how space is allocated and for what purpose may take some time, but it's an important first step for sustainable program development
How are services furnished for different types of providers or in different service lines?	Depending on how a space is licensed and/or accredited healthcare professionals may fall into different categories. For example, in some spaces, an OTP may be considered part of the facility and not able to bill for professional services. In another scenario, the OTP may be able to bill fee-for-service the same way a physician would bill in many PC settings
Are certain services required and/or required in specific spaces?	Licensure and/or accreditation may protect access to certain services by supporting their availability. PC sites that are designated as a Federally Qualified Healthcare Center (FQHC), for example, often have access to population health funds that could potentially support program development led by an OTP
Are any services prohibited under existing licensure and/or accreditation?	Licensure and/or accreditation may protect consumers by limiting access to certain services by restricting their availability

Table 3.3 Reimbursement considerations

Key questions	Key considerations
How are services in your target setting funded? What are the current and prospective funding sources that you need to consider?	If your site is currently billing fee-for-service, consider which CPT® codes will be useful to describe your planned services. AOTA offers members a quick reference document for the codes most commonly used by OTPs (see the 2022 CPT® Codes for Occupational Therapy, at AOTA.org). There are other mechanisms by which your services as an OTP may be covered. Access your experts within your professional associations and at your site to discuss the ways in which services are developed and delivered to explore how OT might support or expand programs and services
What is the payer mix for the population(s) you are targeting?	If you are billing using fee-for-service, it's important to understand the payers that need to authorize and reimburse for OT services at your site. Each payer has their own policy and while there are some consistencies, it's important to appreciate the variability as there may be opportunities to innovate
Is there a contracting office that you need to meet with to discuss your plans?	There are often steps needed to establish a workflow plan for reimbursement. For example, OT may need to be added as a service to the site payer contracts, authorization may be required per those contracts before initiating OT services, and there may be limits (diagnosis, number of sessions, type of intervention) on the type of services that OT can be reimbursed for by that payer
What payment models are feasible in your setting? (fee-for-service, alternative payment models, grant funding, etc.)	Explore the possibilities and be open to trying new ideas. Reimbursement in health care is a moving target, which creates opportunities for innovation
What if reimbursement is denied?	Ensure you are notified if reimbursement is denied as you typically have the opportunity to appeal this decision. If denied, the responsible party (often the patient) may be billed for the total service or the practice may simply write off the billed charges without informing the billing provider. This can lead to consumer dissatisfaction and/or a large and often unnecessary loss of revenue

Reimbursement

Establishing and maintaining a sustainable practice requires attention and resources toward current and future reimbursement mechanisms. A successful practitioner must establish how the service will be funded in current and future states of the practice [2] (see Table 3.3).

Compliance

It is critical that you are aware of the rules and regulations that might impact the development, clinical offerings, and viability of your PC service line (see Table 3.4). In addition to ethical practice and high provider integrity, a strong compliance liaison or office can support and protect all stakeholders in complex healthcare settings.

Table 3.4 Compliance considerations

Key questions
Does your site have a compliance expert or office that can provide guidance on regulatory, reimbursement, and legal questions?
Is there a risk officer or office that can support risk and liability issues and concerns?
Are there existing policies and procedures regarding who or what office has oversight of policy?
Are there employment and/or labor laws to consider at your site? A healthcare attorney can be helpful when determining the best structure for your status at your site (independent contractor, consultant, employee, etc...)
Is there a general counsel office or a consulting attorney with healthcare expertise where you can direct questions? • Potential Stark issues • Anti-kick-back violations • Conflict of interest and/or commitment • Privacy of protected health information (HIPAA concerns)

PC Populations

As mentioned in the section on stakeholders, understanding the details of your facility is essential to establishing OT services. PC can occur in many different locations and serve patients with a variety of different needs. In a 2018 study, the 10 most common clinician-reported reasons for visits in global PC were upper respiratory tract infection, hypertension, routine health maintenance, arthritis, diabetes, depression or anxiety, pneumonia, acute otitis media, back pain, and dermatitis [3]. While this global picture of the needs frequently addressed in PC is helpful to understand the variety of PC issues, it is critical to remember that PC clinics can look very different from each other. Oftentimes, PC is connected to Family Medicine, where the provider works with patients across the lifespan and across all healthcare-related needs. However, this does not capture all of PC. Some PC settings may be more focused on a specific age group, such as pediatrics or geriatrics. Others may be focused on addressing a certain diagnosis or concern, such as diabetes or homelessness. It is essential to understand the needs of your clinic, the population they serve, and their individual clinic priorities [4].

Regulatory Considerations

Health care is a highly regulated industry. There are regulatory support and constraints from local, state, federal, and private agencies to consider. Below is a list of some of the regulatory bodies that might influence the design and sustainability of your PC practice (see Table 3.5).

Note: The names of the organizations have been provided as well as the link to current resources. If the links provided become inactive, you can find the resources by searching the name of the organization.

Table 3.5 Regulatory considerations

Regulatory body	Key considerations
Centers for Medicare and Medicaid Services (CMMS) Regulatory guidance: https://www.cms.gov/Regulations-and-Guidance/Regulations-and-Guidance Manuals: https://www.cms.gov/Regulations-and-Guidance/Guidance/Manuals/index	CMMS is a federal agency that is part of the U.S. Department of Health and Human Services (DHHS). They have oversight of the Medicare and Medicaid programs and have a powerful influence over healthcare policy as more than 50% of health care is funded by this agency [2]
Federally Qualified Health Centers (FQHC) CMS guidance: https://www.cms.gov/Center/Provider-Type/Federally-Qualified-Health-Centers-FQHC-Center Health Resources and Services Administration: https://www.hrsa.gov/opa/eligibility-and-registration/health-centers/fqhc/index.html HRSA fact sheet: https://bphc.hrsa.gov/sites/default/files/bphc/about/healthcenterfactsheet.pdf	FQHCs are community-based healthcare centers that provide primary and preventive care services to under-served populations regardless of their ability to pay for care. FQHCs must meet strict regulatory standards, have an established sliding scale for payment, and be governed by a board that includes consumers. FQHCs are generally paid using a prospective payment system (PPS) that is based on their costs for medically necessary PC and qualified preventive care services
State Department of Health and Human Services National Conference of State Legislatures (NCSL): https://www.ncsl.org/	State health departments regulate offices to support health care, mental health, public health, social services, and other health-related services. In addition to regulatory oversight, state health departments often convene task forces and workgroups to create guidelines and enforce best practices in health and social service areas
Agency for Healthcare Research and Quality (AHRQ) is part of DHHS and defines the qualities of a Patient Centered Medical Home (PCMH): https://pcmh.ahrq.gov/page/defining-pcmh PCMH supports: https://pcmh.ahrq.gov/page/pcmh-foundations	A PCMH is a model for the organization of preventive and PC. A PCMH must achieve five main functions: comprehensive care, patient-centered care, coordinated care, accessible services, high quality and safety standards
National Committee for Quality Assurance (NCQA) payment methodology, grant funding, etc.) https://www.ncqa.org/	The NCQA collects data that measures the quality of performance for healthcare sites and providers. NCQA provides health plan accreditation based on quality indicators and PCMH certification based on meeting standard criteria and quality outcomes
The Joint Commission (TJC): https://www.jointcommission.org/ The Joint Commission Resources: https://www.jcinc.com	TJC is an accrediting body that provides standards for quality, performance, and environment. They accredit and/or certify healthcare organizations and programs including PC settings. To comply with Medicare's condition of participation, hospitals and other healthcare organizations may use an accrediting agency, like TJC, to meet the mandatory CMS evaluation

Setting Configurations

Using language from the Six Levels of Collaboration/Integration from the SAMHSA-HRSA Center for Integrated Health Solutions (CIHS) [5], below are examples of space configurations for PC settings. They are presented in order from most transformed/integrated practice to lowest, starting with Integrated, then Co-Located, and then Coordinated Off-Site.

1. **Integrated:** Providers work together in the same space, within the same facility, where some or all of the office/practice space is shared.
2. **Co-located:** Providers work in the same facility, but not necessarily the same offices. Space is shared by team members. Teams may be in the same room or within the same building.
3. **Coordinated Off-site:** This is a referral model where providers work in separate facilities and refer off-site. They may even have separate organizational and health record systems, and communication is minimal.

Pros and Cons (see Tables 3.6 and 3.7).

Table 3.6 Pros and cons of shared space configurations

Pros	Cons
Easier to communicate with team members	Personal space may be limited
Able to consult and problem-solve difficult cases with team members	Lack of privacy
Team cohesion and bonding	Volume of noise
Patients don't need to go to multiple locations	
Patients see providers working as a team which can improve patient confidence in their care	

Table 3.7 Pros and cons of separated space configurations

Pros	Cons
May have more space	Can be challenging to communicate with team
Space could be more tailored for OT use	Team can feel disconnected
More privacy	Volume of noise
	Patients need to go to multiple locations
	Increased likelihood patients will not be seen. As patients are sent out, the likelihood of them falling through the cracks in the system increases

Synchronous vs. Asynchronous Collaboration

Synchronous collaboration means that services from more than one team member are provided simultaneously, while asynchronous services are provided one team member at a time. Synchronous collaboration and sharing of space offers benefits to team members such as the ability to problem-solve in real time. However, if space is limited or schedules do not permit, this is not always feasible. Asynchronous collaboration and space utilization allows the same space to be used by multiple team members, but means that communication between providers does not happen in real time.

Reimbursement Models

- **Fee-for-service**: fee-for-service billing can include billing existing Current Procedural Terminology (CPT®) codes, as well as private pay rates for OT evaluation and services. Table 3.8: CPT® *Codes for OT* lists CPT® codes that are often billed by OTPs, but there are additional codes that can be used for other services provided in PC (e.g., wheelchair management, wound care, orthotic fabrication, and training). A comprehensive book of all CPT® codes may already be owned by the practice or can be purchased annually from the American Medical Association. In addition, AOTA generates an annual list of frequently used CPT® codes for OTPs that is accessible to members at AOTA.org

Table 3.8 CPT® codes for OT

CPT® codes often used by OTPs	Code number	Narrative description
Evaluation/ re-evaluation codes	**Untimed codes**	Level of complexity dictates code used
Occupational therapy evaluation, low complexity	97165	Requires low complexity clinical decisions based on a problem-focused assessment
Occupational therapy evaluation, moderate complexity	97166	Requires moderate analytic complexity required to make decisions, client may present with comorbidities that affect function
Occupational therapy evaluation, high complexity	97167	Requires high analytic complexity required to make decisions, multiple options to consider
Occupational therapy re-evaluation	97168	Re-evaluation requires assessment of changes in patient functional or medical status with revised plan of care

(continued)

Table 3.8 (continued)

CPT® codes often used by OTPs	Code number	Narrative description
Intervention codes	**Timed codes—15 min increments**	Most of intervention codes are timed
Self-care/home management training (ADLs)	97535	Self-care/home management training (e.g., activities of daily living [ADLs] and IADLs). May include safety training and education in use of adaptive devices
Therapeutic activities	97530	Therapeutic activities (i.e., functional activities used to improve functional/occupational performance)
Community/work reintegration training	97537	Community/work reintegration training (e.g., shopping, managing money, transportation, non-work and work-related activities and/or work environment/modification evaluation, work task analysis, use of assistive technology device/adaptive equipment)
Therapeutic procedure; therapeutic exercise	97110	Therapeutic procedure or exercise to develop strength and endurance, range of motion, and flexibility
Therapeutic procedure; group	97150 (untimed code)	Therapeutic procedure(s) group (2 or more) with constant attendance by the practitioner
Therapeutic interventions; cognitive function	97129	Therapeutic interventions that focus on cognitive function (e.g., attention, memory, problem solving, and other cognitive function skills). May include development of compensatory strategies to improve functional performance
Orthotic and prosthetic management and training	97760 (initial encounter orthotics) 97761 (initial encounter prosthetics) 97763 (subsequent encounters both orthotics/prosthetics)	Orthotics/prosthetics—includes assessment, fitting, training/management of orthotics/prosthetics for the upper/lower extremities, and trunk

- Be thoughtful in choosing your codes. To demonstrate your distinct skill set as an OTP, especially when using a code that other professions also utilize. Your documentation must clearly articulate the skilled OT perspective of your intervention. Your documentation must support why that code aligns with the diagnosis you are addressing and the treatment you provided. We've provided this guide to support choosing the most appropriate code for the activity they are doing. The documentation must support the code. Examples:

  If you use "therapeutic exercise," you should document how the exercise you are doing facilitates function and supports the functional goal in your intervention plan.

If you are using "therapeutic activity," your documentation must explain how the activity facilitates or supports improvement in functional performance as related to your goals set in your intervention plan.

**Note: Brief narrative descriptions reflect the 2020 Current Procedural Terminology (CPT®) [6] code definitions and are provided here for ease of reference; however, these descriptions should not be considered the legal definitions. We recommend referencing the actual code descriptions in the CPT® manual to ensure accuracy of code choice.

- **Bundled Payments for Care Improvement (BPCI) Initiative**
  - The Bundled Payments for Care Improvement (BPCI) initiative comprises four broadly defined models of care, which link payments for the multiple services that beneficiaries receive during an episode of care. Under the initiative, organizations enter into payment arrangements that include financial and performance accountability for episodes of care. These models may lead to higher quality and more coordinated care at a lower cost to Medicare. Information on BPCI is accessible at the CMS.gov website. OTPs can be powerful collaborators to achieve BPCI quality outcome indicators, which is an important point to convey to the practice.

- **Federally Qualified Health Centers (FQHCs)**
  - FQHCs are generally paid based on their costs using a prospective payment system (PPS). OT services may be accounted for in their encounter rates. In addition, group medical visits may include different providers, like OTPs, in an encounter. In addition, FQHCs may have access to population health and wellness funding that could cover the cost of programming developed or led by an OTP.

- **Grant Funding**
  - Although not sustainable, grant funding can be very helpful to initiate OT involvement in a PC setting and demonstrate our distinct value on the PC team. Grant funding may be useful to demonstrate the feasibility of an idea or expand an existing service to provide more comprehensive health promotion in PC.

- **Telehealth** (Chap. 4)
  - Telehealth services may be provided and funded in varying ways depending on the type of setting, payer, type of provider, client preference and ability, and technology available. Before initiating telehealth services, it is important to understand patient consent, state licensure laws, site policy and procedure, and payer restrictions and supports for telehealth services. Table 3.9: *Telehealth services* lists some telehealth services that OTPs may provide and resources for each.

Table 3.9 Telehealth services

Telehealth service	Description	Code(s)	Resources
E-visits	Established patient initiated communication or inquiry	98970, 98971, 98972, G2061, G2062, G2063	AOTA update: CMS expands therapy E-visit services during COVID-19 outbreak[a] CMS: Medicare telemedicine health care provider fact sheet[b]
Telephone assessment and management (no video)	New or established patient	98966 98967 98968	CMS: Medicare and Medicaid programs; policy and regulatory revisions in response to the COVID-19 Public Health Emergency[c]
Virtual check-ins	Contact with an established patient. May be telephone, audio/video, text, email	G2012, G2010	CMS: Medicare Telemedicine Health Care Provider Fact Sheet[d]
Telehealth visits	Evaluation and intervention billed using CPT® codes, but eligible code set for telehealth may be restricted	CPT® codes	CMS: List of Telehealth Services[e] AOTA: Billing Telehealth Services under Medicare[f] Occupational Therapy and Telehealth: State Statutes, Regulations, and Regulatory Board Statements[g]

[a] https://www.aota.org/Practice/Manage/telehealth/Nonphysician-Evisits.aspx
[b] https://www.cms.gov/newsroom/fact-sheets/medicare-telemedicine-health-care-provider-fact-sheet
[c] https://www.cms.gov/files/document/covid-final-ifc.pdf
[d] https://www.cms.gov/newsroom/fact-sheets/medicare-telemedicine-health-care-provider-fact-sheet
[e] https://www.cms.gov/Medicare/Medicare-General-Information/Telehealth/Telehealth-Codes
[f] https://www.aota.org/Advocacy-Policy/Federal-Reg-Affairs/News/2020/Billing-Telehealth-Services-Medicare.aspx
[g] https://www.aota.org/~/media/Corporate/Files/Advocacy/State/telehealth/Telehealth-State-Statutes-Regulations-Regulatory-Board-Statements.pdf
Note: As of this writing, telehealth rules, regulations, best practices, and reimbursement policies are updating regularly due to the COVID-19 pandemic of 2020. Be sure to check with your local OT association, AOTA, and your practice managers to ensure that your use of telehealth is compliant with current regulations and best practices

Managing Barriers

Below are some examples of common potential barriers to OT in PC, as well as strategies for overcoming these barriers. A recommendation to apply to all barriers is to network and develop a wide range of contacts to help you problem-solve. Reach out to interprofessional team members, staff, community members, and acquaintances outside of your organization to help you problem-solve barriers.

1. Resources and support—limited resources (funding, time, space, energy, enthusiasm) can result in challenges in moving your services and ideas forward. Recommend focusing on addressing issues that are easiest to change and that are supported by the practice/team members. If the team is unreceptive, it will impede your success.

    Examples:

    - Focus on fostering relationships with providers, staff, and administrators who are interested in transforming practice, rather than those who are not.
    - If a PCP is receptive, start offering OT services for patients who need lifestyle modification guidance (HTN, diabetes, obesity, etc.). Once you can show results, you can approach the more resistant team members and gradually expand the services you offer.

2. Technology—Use of telehealth and digital monitoring can be a challenge, especially when systems don't "speak" to each other, or even if providers have different note formats. If possible, design or redesign systems with IT department to maximize collaboration and communication.

3. Culture—OT isn't part of the "primary team" and is considered an "ancillary" rather than professional service.

    - Advocacy is essential to address this barrier. It is critical to demonstrate your distinct value. See examples in "Resources and Support" above.

Considerations for Success

1. **Return on Investment (ROI):** In the context of fee-for-service models, Alternative Payment Models (APMs), and other health care initiatives, a business argument may be effective. Return on Investment (ROI) is a way to measure profitability and benefit resulting from an investment. In this case, an organization's "investment" in OT produces desired outcomes ("returns"), thus demonstrating the value of the profession in PC. For example, by augmenting the physician—patient interaction, OTPs can help facilities or entities meet quality standards, improve patient satisfaction, achieve quality reporting metrics, or enhance referrals to other service lines [7]. Below are some ways to consider demonstrating a ROI.

    - **Consultative service with referral tracking and conversion monitoring:** One way to approach ROI could be by demonstrating that consultations in PC result in an increase in referrals to OT services, as well as increased likelihood that referred patients schedule and complete their OT evaluation. The OTP can track the number of referrals referred and the number completed, thus demonstrating the financial and experiential benefit of patient access to OT services.

- **Consumer experience:** Demonstrating enhanced consumer experience and increased patient satisfaction through measurable surveys (e.g., Likert scale questions) can demonstrate patient satisfaction with the addition of OT to the practice. Satisfied patients are less likely to leave their health system and spend their healthcare dollars at another facility.
- **Provider experience:** Burnout is extremely prevalent among PCPs, which can increase turnover. OT on PC teams can help off-set this burden and support PCPs by addressing issues related to behavioral health, lifestyle, and other issues that do not require the medical and diagnostic skill set of the PCP. This will allow the PCP more time to attend to diagnostic and prescribing needs of the patients. This can improve provider satisfaction and decrease turnover which reduces the expense associated with recruiting, hiring, and training new providers.
- **Meeting required metrics and quality reporting:** Including OT in PC may help clinics and other team members meet certain criteria required of them, such as patient outcomes and annual screenings. OT services may positively impact individual or site/group quality reporting outcomes.

2. **Measuring your impact**: To demonstrate proof of concept, efficacy of individual service, and impact on the clinic, providers, consumers, and larger population, it's imperative that the OTP systematically collect, analyze, and disseminate data. Table 3.10: *Measuring your impact* includes types of data the OTP may collect and use to support OT service and communicate to stakeholders.

Table 3.10 Measuring your impact

Type of data	How to use it
Clinical outcomes	Demonstrate efficacy for services
Quality outcomes	Participate in quality reporting, support measurement of quality in clinic
Process outcomes	Examine workflow and develop flexible responses to improve efficiency, access, and experience of stakeholders
Consumer experience	Patient satisfaction and engagement data is useful in understanding the experience of consumers and care-givers and supporting their access and needs in your system
Provider experience	Address referring provider feedback and adapt practice to support your team members and larger clinic or system goals
Population health	Population health data can support service line development and expand OT's role and contribution in PC

Communicate and Disseminate Your Work

Growing OT's roles in PC requires a community of providers sharing their experiences, clinical expertise, research results, and advocacy efforts with all stakeholders [4]. If you are involved in providing, developing, or supporting OT's role in any PC setting, it's critical that you publish and present your work to educate others and build a community of practice that can provide more capacity to expand OT's distinct role in this emerging practice area.

References

1. Smith K, Day M, Muir S, Dahl-Popolizio S. Developing tailored program proposals for occupational therapy in primary care. Open J Occup Ther. 2020;8(1):1–13. https://doi.org/10.15453/2168-6408.1630.
2. Jordan K, Sandhu K. The occupational therapy manager. 6th ed. North Bethesda: AOTA Press; 2019.
3. Finley CR, Chan DS, Garrison S, Korownyk C, Kolber MR, Campbell S, Eurich DT, Lindblad AJ, Vandermeer B, Allan GM. What are the most common conditions in primary care? Systematic review. Can Fam Physician. 2018;64(11):832–40.
4. Jordan K. Occupational therapy in primary care: positioned and prepared to be a vital part of the team. Am J Occup Ther. 2019;73(5):1–6. https://doi.org/10.5014/ajot.2019.735002.
5. Substance Abuse and Mental Health Services Administration. Center for Excellence of Integrated Health Solutions [CIHS'] Standard Framework for Levels of Integrated Healthcare. 2022. https://www.thenationalcouncil.org/wp-content/uploads/2020/01/CIHS_Framework_Final_charts.pdf?daf=375ateTbd56
6. American Medical Association. CPT 2020 Professional Edition. Washington, DC: American Medical Association; 2020.
7. Halle AD, Mroz TM, Fogelberg DJ, Leland NE. Occupational therapy and primary care: updates and trends. Am J Occup Ther. 2018;72(3):1–6. https://doi.org/10.5014/ajot.2018.723001.

Chapter 4
Telehealth

Katie Smith and Sue Dahl-Popolizio

What is Telehealth?

- The AOTA position paper on Telehealth in Occupational Therapy defines telehealth as "The application of evaluative, consultative, preventative, and therapeutic services delivered through information and communication technology" [1].

Why Use Telehealth?

- Providing on-location services

  - OT is most true to its origins when it is practiced within the native context of the patient. Telehealth transcends traditional environmental boundaries by enabling the OTP to interact with and observe the patient in their home environment, while still remaining available to the PC team in the office.
  - Telehealth allows the OTP to address issues in the patient's home without being physically in the patient's home. This is an important option for PC therapists as patients who are not home-bound do not qualify for a home visit and patients who prefer to be seen remotely have that option available.

K. Smith (✉)
Revolutionary Alignment, LLC, Detroit, MI, USA
www.RevolutionaryAlignment.com

S. Dahl-Popolizio
Arizona State University, Phoenix, AZ, USA

AT Still University, Mesa, AZ, USA
e-mail: sdahlpopolizio@atsu.edu; sue.dahlpopolizio@asu.edu

© Springer Nature Switzerland AG 2023   31
S. Dahl-Popolizio et al. (eds.), *Primary Care Occupational Therapy*,
https://doi.org/10.1007/978-3-031-20882-9_4

- Supporting the goals of The Triple Aim [2] and the fourth goal in the Quadruple Aim:

  - (1) Improving the individual experience of care

    Telehealth improves access to OT services, prevents delays in care caused by personnel shortages, travel, and other barriers, facilitates communication and care coordination [3], and can be a compassionate and clinically relevant choice for patients with limited mobility, time, or energy.
    Patients receiving telehealth care report high levels of satisfaction with their care [3].

  - (2) Improving the health of populations

    Telehealth is effective in programs designed for patients with mobility impairments, aging in place, chronic disease management, home exercises, adaptive equipment, home modifications, and quality of life improvement [3], all of which are applicable to PC OT.

  - (3) Reducing the per capita costs of care for populations

    Many studies indicate the clinical efficacy of interventions delivered via telehealth [3]. By retaining a high level of clinical efficacy while also reducing transition time between patients, as well as office space, lobby accommodations, and other facility costs, telehealth may serve to reduce PC office overhead costs without sacrificing care.

  - (4) Reducing provider burn-out and increasing job satisfaction by

    Allowing the OTP to see more patients by eliminating commute time and the room change time.
    The ability of the OTP to offer reduced wait times between visits and increase access to care.
    Offering another service delivery platform that OTP, patients, and caregivers found satisfactory.

- Considering transmissible infections

  - With in-person OT services, the patient and the therapist are in the same room together, with a closed door for privacy and without guaranteed access to ventilation. This increases the exposure for the therapist and the potentially immuno-compromised patient to droplet-transmissible infection, including COVID-19. Telehealth eliminates this risk entirely.
  - As more services are delivered via telehealth during the COVID-19 pandemic, more research was possible to be conducted on how telehealth can most effectively be utilized moving forward [4].

How to Use Telehealth?

- Telehealth Decision Guide [5]

    - AOTA publication to help practitioners determine when and how to use telehealth for clients and considerations for use at each step.
    - Review the AOTA position paper on telehealth [1].
    - Does my state allow telehealth OT?

        AOTA's state by state chart of telehealth laws [6].
        AOTA's list of state actions affecting OT's use of telehealth in light of the COVID-19 pandemic.

    - Will I get reimbursed for telehealth?

        Rules for telehealth reimbursement vary by payer, and while most insurances are currently reimbursing for OTPs to use telehealth, the rules regarding acceptable codes can vary, and rules may change as emergency orders due to COVID-19 expire.
        State regulations regarding which professions can use telehealth and how it can be used vary as well, so be sure to check with your state organization and your licensing board regarding this. AOTA's list of commercial payer coverage of telehealth [7].

- A variety of populations and conditions have been effectively treated via telehealth including: [8]:

    - Pediatrics
    - Geriatrics
    - Developmental delays
    - Cognitive issues
    - Mental/behavioral health
    - Hand/upper extremity issues/injuries
    - Neurological issues
    - Orthopedic issues
    - Swallowing issues

- A variety of interventions have been effectively provided via telehealth [8]:

    - Evaluations
    - Visual motor integration
    - Functional fine motor skill retraining
    - Therapeutic exercises
    - Activities of daily living and instrumental activities of daily living
    - Caregiver education/coaching
    - Behavioral health interventions
    - Cognitive retraining/interventions
    - Feeding/swallowing treatments

- Safety and ethical considerations
  - AOTA Advisory on Telehealth Ethics [9].
  - All patients need to be informed of: the risks and benefits of using telehealth, their rights as patients and responsibilities (including the right to refuse treatment), and organizational policies for the retention and storage of audio and video recordings and electronic health records [8].

    Risks include:
    Possible technological connection issues and a plan to address any issues should be established before the visit (e.g., if secure video connection is unstable, provide a call-in phone number).
    Security and confidentiality issues, depending on the telehealth platform and electronic health record system used (such as HIPAA compliance) and the possibility that someone in proximity could overhear the session.
    Any potential injury as a result of lack of physical contact with the therapist during the telehealth session.

  - Consider obtaining emergency contact information and current location address for the patient, in case emergency support services need to be deployed to patient's location during telehealth session.
  - Continue to adhere to licensing regulations, code of ethics, and scope of practice while using telehealth, including close attention to supervision regulations when working with students or COTAs [10].
  - Telehealth may allow a therapist to treat patients across state lines if indicated by your practice location or if your patients travel out of state and require your services. If this need arises, the OTP should check to see if their state is a member of the OT Interstate Professional Licensing Compact [11]. Check with AOTA and with your home state licensing board to determine steps required to treat patients across state lines.

References

1. American Occupational Therapy Association. Telehealth in occupational therapy. Am J Occup Ther. 2018;72(Supplement_2):7212410059p1–7212410059p18. https://doi.org/10.5014/ajot.2018.72S219.
2. Institution for Healthcare Improvement. IHI Triple Aim Initiative. 2020. http://www.ihi.org/Engage/Initiatives/TripleAim/Pages/default.aspx
3. Cason J. Health policy perspectives—telehealth and occupational therapy: integral to the triple aim of health care reform. Am J Occup Ther. 2015;69:6902090010p1. https://doi.org/10.5014/ajot.2015.692003.
4. Totten AM, McDonagh MS, Wagner JH. The evidence base for telehealth: reassurance in the face of rapid expansion during the COVID-19 pandemic. Rockville: Agency for Healthcare Research and Quality (US); 2020.
5. American Occupational Therapy Association. Occupational therapy telehealth decision guide. 2020. https://www.aota.org

6. American Occupational Therapy Association. Occupational therapy and telehealth: state statutes, regulations and regulatory board statements. 2022. https://www.aota.org
7. American Occupational Therapy Association. Commercial payer telehealth coverage. 2021. https://www.aota.org
8. Dahl-Popolizio S, Carpenter H, Coronado M, Popolizio NJ, Swanson C. Telehealth for the provision of occupational therapy: reflections on experiences during the covid-19 pandemic. Int J Telerehabil. 2020;2(2):1–16. https://doi.org/10.5195/ijt.2021.6382.
9. Estes J. The American Occupational Therapy Association advisory opinion for the Ethics Commission Telehealth. 2017. http://www.aota.org
10. American Occupational Therapy Association. Guidelines for supervision, roles, and responsibilities during the delivery of occupational therapy services. Am J Occup Ther. 2014;68(Suppl. 3):S16–22. https://doi.org/10.5014/ajot.2014.686S03.
11. Pudeler M. State legislative forecast: COVID-19 and state budgets, telehealth, and the interstate licensure compact. North Bethesda: American Occupational Therapy Association; 2020. https://www.aota.org

Chapter 5
Conducting Research

Mansha Mirza, Sue Dahl-Popolizio, and Katie Smith

Why Do We Need Research on OT in PC?

- U.S. healthcare delivery is transitioning from fee-for-service reimbursement to value-based payment models [1]. As a result of this transition:

  - Evidence supporting the use of interventions provided for the specific diagnoses treated is increasingly required.
  - Providers are reimbursed for improved patient outcomes rather than for the amount of services they deliver [2] (i.e., reimbursed for patient improvement rather than type and number of codes billed).
  - Clinical accountability to patients is critical.

- With value-based models and with the remaining fee-for-service models:

  - Credible evidence is needed to inform clinical decisions.
  - Third-party payers are tying funding to empirically supported treatments [3].

- Therefore, it is imperative to strengthen the evidence base for OT services in PC.

  - The American OT Association (AOTA) strongly promotes clinical accountability through evidence-based practice. One example of AOTA's many efforts in this regard is the publication of evidence-based practice guidelines [4].

M. Mirza (✉)
University of Illinois Chicago, Chicago, IL, USA
e-mail: mmirza2@uic.edu

S. Dahl-Popolizio
Arizona State University, Phoenix, AZ, USA

AT Still University, Mesa, AZ, USA
e-mail: sue.dahlpopolizio@asu.edu; sdahlpopolizio@atsu.edu

K. Smith
Revolutionary Alignment, LLC, Detroit, MI, USA
www.RevolutionaryAlignment.com

© Springer Nature Switzerland AG 2023   37
S. Dahl-Popolizio et al. (eds.), *Primary Care Occupational Therapy*,
https://doi.org/10.1007/978-3-031-20882-9_5

These guidelines present a summary of promising interventions in a variety of practice areas, which are grounded in a synthesis of the best available evidence.

- This information is intended to help clinicians better respond to their patients' needs as well as communicate the benefits of OT services to external audiences [4]:

    Physicians
    Nurses
    Medical assistants
    Office staff
    Other providers (social workers, physical therapists, chiropractors, psychologists, etc.)
    Administrators in the practice
    Public Health Professionals
    Community stakeholders who have an interest in the PC practice and can influence referrals to the practice and the providers (faith leaders, community leaders, policy makers, etc.)

- Clinical research is needed to help inform a robust set of practice guidelines and justify the presence of OT in PC contexts [5].
- Research has been described as "a prologue and epilogue" [6] to clinical practice.

    - As prologue, OTPs in PC can use available evidence to inform and justify their choice of interventions;
    - As epilogue, practitioners can assess the effectiveness of selected interventions and adapt them as needed to improve patient outcomes.

- Gathering clinically relevant evidence related to PC OT services serves the profession by:

    - identifying and implementing interventions that are most likely to benefit patients,
    - advocating for competitively compensated OT positions within PC practices, and
    - establishing our professional autonomy and credibility within interdisciplinary PC teams.

What Is the Current Status of Research on OT in PC?

- The National Institute for Disability, Independent Living, and Rehabilitation Research identifies four stages of intervention research [7].

    - Exploration and discovery
    - Intervention development

- – Intervention efficacy
- – Scale-up evaluation

- These stages are intended to facilitate scientific development of interventions by clarifying where research activities and related evidence fall and where evidence is lacking.
- ***Stage 1 Exploration and discovery***: intended to lay the foundation for future intervention development [7].

  - – May include describing existing clinical models for implementing OT in PC settings as well as identifying barriers to and facilitators for integration of OT services in PC.
  - – Examples:

    A group of Canadian researchers conducted a series of studies to document examples of OT services in PC after a provincial push for inclusion of OT in PC settings.

    - Donnelly and colleagues (2016) [8]:

      - – **Format:** online survey with 52 practitioners who identified as working in PC settings.
      - – **Purpose:** to identify existing OT roles and scope of practice within PC.
      - – **Findings:** OT services (adaptive, preventive, and health promotion training) were provided to individual PC patients primarily in the clinic, then via home care and community-based services. Group-based and community-level interventions were less frequently reported. Integrated practice was hindered by a limited understanding of OT among other PCPs and communication challenges.
    - Donnelly and colleagues (2013) [9]:

      - – **Format:** case studies involving semi-structured interviews at four family health clinics in Ontario, Canada, which employed OTPs as part of the interprofessional team.
      - – **Purpose:** to explore barriers and facilitators for OT integration in PC services.
      - – **Findings:** strategies that could facilitate integration of OTPs in PC teams include

        co-location of services
        OT access to EHRs
        interprofessional team meetings and teaching rounds
        training residents and educating other professionals on the role of OT to increase referrals
        collaborating with physicians who can champion the importance of OT
        coordinating OT services within pre-existing programs such as chronic disease self-management [9]

Similar foundational studies have also been conducted in the United States, where integration of OT services in PC is still in the early stages.

- Trembath and colleagues (2019) [10].

  - **Format:** retrospective analysis of ICD-10 codes used by a PCP.
  - **Purpose:** to determine whether the most common conditions seen in PC could benefit from existing OT interventions.
  - **Findings:** of the 15 most common conditions seen in PC, 100% could be benefit from OT treatment of the condition directly, or the treatment of issues underlying the condition, or common comorbidities that occur with the condition [10].

- Dahl-Popolizio and colleagues (2017) [11].

  - **Format:** cross-sectional survey-based study involving descriptive group comparisons.
  - **Purpose:** to determine receptiveness of both OTPs and PCPs to the inclusion of OTPs on the PC team.
  - **Findings:** Overall, both PCPs and OTPs were supportive of including OTs on the interprofessional PC team. Any concerns expressed were primarily related to clarification of OT's role on the team and reimbursement [11].

- Winship and colleagues (2019) [12].

  - **Format:** qualitative study including semistructured interviews with clinic patients and staff as well as review of staff meeting transcripts.
  - **Purpose:** to investigate opportunities for OTPs in a PC team within a complex care clinic.
  - **Findings:** clinic staff struggled to meet patients' medical needs due to resource limitations, concurrent mental health issues, and cognitive behavioral problems. Patients' unmet needs extended beyond disease management and also included community mobility, ADLs, and IADLs. OTPs can play a dual role in PC providing direct services to meet patient needs and consulting with other providers on use of adaptive technologies and modified educational materials to meet needs of patients with a wide range of sensory and cognitive abilities [12].

- Koverman and colleagues (2017) [13].

  - **Format:** a descriptive study on the steps taken before and lessons learned after the implementation of an 8-week pilot OT program in a geriatric PC clinic housed in a large academic medical center.
  - **Purpose:** to outline structures and processes that could support OT integration in PC.

  – **Findings:** strategies that facilitated successful implementation of the program included:

  > reviewing PC practices within the medical center
  > conducting a survey with PC clinicians and office managers to gather their perspectives on OT
  > marketing OT services to referral sources such as physicians, nurse practitioners, and physician assistants
  > Data were recorded on: average number of patients seen per day, most common diagnoses seen, most frequent interventions offered (ADL training and fall prevention). Data were used to seek approval for the program to be made permanent [13].

The studies described above provide a foundation for introducing OT services in PC by:

(1) describing the landscape of PC services,
(2) assessing needs of PC patients, and
(3) identifying successful models of practice.

These studies tell us what OT services *could* be provided in PC settings. However, they do not tell us what targeted OT interventions *should* be provided, i.e., interventions with proven effectiveness for PC patients. Studies that focus on intervention development represent a step forward in this direction.

- ***Stage II Intervention development*** [7]: focuses on developing OT interventions for PC patients, testing how feasible they are in PC clinics, determining how acceptable they are for patients, and evaluating their potential to improve outcomes.

  – Examples:

  Pyatak and colleagues (2019) [14].

  - **Format:** Pilot randomized controlled trial (RCT) focusing on an eight session OTP-led diabetes management program based on Lifestyle Redesign®.
  - **Purpose:** to examine the implementation feasibility and preliminary clinical outcomes of the intervention at a safety-net PC clinic.
  - **Findings:** The intervention was found to be acceptable to patients and other staff. Pre- and post-intervention comparisons of patient data indicated promising improvements in control of HbA1c levels, diabetes self-management behaviors (e.g., medication adherence, diet changes, and foot care), overall health including mental health, physical function, and pain [14].

Mirza and colleagues (2020) [15].

- **Format:** Feasibility study that used an RCT design to compare two OTP-delivered interventions—(1) a manualized intervention informed by the person-environment-occupation (PEO) framework that comprised six treatment sessions (three in person and three by phone); sessions combined lifestyle modification and chronic disease self-management with environmental modifications and physical activity; (2) a chronic disease care coordination intervention that involved eight weekly phone sessions focusing on counseling patients about diet, symptom management, medication management, community resources, and referral management.
- **Purpose:** to compare the feasibility, acceptability, and preliminary efficacy of the two interventions for PC patients 50 years and over with heart disease, arthritis, and uncontrolled diabetes.
- **Findings:** Both interventions were associated with improved scores on patient perception of chronic illness care, with biggest improvement seen in self-reported physical and mental health. The authors found that the PEO-informed intervention was feasible to deliver in the context of a busy PC clinic. Patients were very satisfied with the intervention, and PCPs supported its integration in the clinic [15].

- The two studies described above exemplify how we, as a field, are beginning to develop interventions that are specifically designed to address the clinical context and healthcare needs of PC patients. While these interventions show promise, further efficacy testing is needed before they are considered evidence-based and can be widely adopted in PC settings.

- *Stage III Intervention Efficacy*: experimental testing of promising interventions under strictly controlled conditions [7].

  - Testing conditions might include specific criteria for patients who qualify for the intervention and a strict schedule and protocol for delivering the intervention.
  - Some researchers further divide this stage into "pure efficacy testing" and "real-world efficacy testing" [16].

    Pure efficacy testing: the intervention is provided in research settings, such as a research laboratory, and by research-based providers.
    Real-world efficacy testing: the intervention is provided in community settings, such as a PC clinic, and by community-based clinicians who do not have a research affiliation or training [16].

  - Efficacy studies can also involve measuring the strength of the relationships between an intervention and outcomes [7].
  - It may also be possible to isolate patient factors (such as age, comorbidities) and environmental factors (such as family income, access to social support) that influence intervention effects.

Example:

- Are older patients with diabetes less or more likely to benefit from PC OT services compared with younger patients? Are geriatric PC patients with strong social support more likely to benefit from OT services than those without it?

– At the time of writing, there were no examples of OT research studies that focused on testing the efficacy of PC interventions, indicating a gap in scientific development of the evidence base. The few studies that do exist are non-U.S. based.

Examples:

- Richardson and colleagues (2010) [17].

  – **Format:** RCT comparing standard rehabilitation care with a PC intervention involving collaborative goal-setting between patients and rehabilitation providers (OT and PT), individual treatment as needed, and a 6-week group workshop that combined information on chronic disease self-management with information on rehabilitation care, exercise principles, and assistive devices.
  – **Purpose:** to examine the effects of OT and physical therapy (PT) services for adults with chronic illness at an interprofessional PC center in Ontario, Canada.
  – **Findings:** Compared with those who received standard rehabilitation care in the community, those who received the PC intervention were more satisfied with services and had significantly fewer planned hospital days. However, contrary to the authors' expectations, the PC intervention did not significantly improve patients' self-reported health status nor did it significantly reduce their emergency room visits [17].

- Richardson and colleagues (2012) [18].

  – **Format:** Quasi-experimental design used to compare PC patients with chronic illnesses who received a multi-component rehabilitation intervention (including OT) with age and sex-matched controls who received usual care.
  – **Purpose:** to determine if PC patients with chronic conditions who received the multi-component rehabilitation intervention (function-based individual assessment and action planning, group-based self-management workshops delivered over 5 weeks, and an online personal record system) exhibited less functional decline than similar patients in another clinic who received usual care.
  – **Findings:** Statistically significant differences were noted between the intervention and control groups in physical functioning and

physical performance Outcomes related to healthcare utilization, self-efficacy for chronic disease management, and self-rated health were not significantly different [18].

- Garvey and colleagues (2015) [19].
    - **Format:** Pragmatic feasibility RCT comparing a waitlist control group to PC patients receiving an OTP-led self-management support program. The 6-week intervention involved individual goal- setting and weekly group sessions addressing topics such as fatigue management, healthy eating, physical activity and mental health, medication management, and healthcare communication.
    - **Purpose:** to test the effectiveness of the OTP-led self-management support program for older adults with multiple chronic conditions in Dublin, Ireland.
    - **Findings:** The intervention was found to be effective in improving patients' participation in various activities, their perceived satisfaction with activity performance, their achievement of self-determined goals,, their self-efficacy, ADL independence, and quality of life [19].

- The above studies establish the efficacy of OT interventions in improving patient outcomes in PC. However, these interventions would need to be adapted and reassessed for feasibility within the U.S. healthcare context before replication in PC settings in the United States.

- ***Stage IV Scale-up evaluation:*** Tests whether an intervention that performs well during efficacy testing is effective in improving outcomes in a real-world setting [7].

    - Includes the following:

        Implementing a promising intervention without the strict controls applied during the intervention efficacy stage.
        Identifying factors that help or hinder successful replication of the intervention in different settings [7].
        May include adapting OT interventions for PC that have established efficacy in other clinical settings, such as out-patient or community rehabilitation.

    - Examples:

        Multiple systematic reviews [20–22] have found that OT interventions, such as training in daily living skills, home safety assessments, and referral for assistive devices, are effective in improving and maintaining functional independence and participation in daily life activities among those aging with and without chronic illnesses. Occupation-focused health promotion interventions have also demonstrated gains in quality adjusted life years among healthy older adults [23].

The Well Elderly study [24] and its predecessors [25, 26].

- **Format:** A series of RCTs to evaluate the effectiveness of a 9-month program, later labelled Lifestyle Redesign, focused on embedding health promotion strategies into the daily lives of community-dwelling older adults.
- **Purpose:** to determine the short- and long-term effects of a preventive lifestyle-based OT intervention.
- **Findings:** Short-term and long-term beneficial effects on participants' health, function, and quality of life [25, 26]. A 6-month version of the program implemented with ethnically diverse older adults also demonstrated beneficial effects on a variety of outcomes including pain, vitality, social functioning, mental health, and life satisfaction [24].
- Although an important precursor for OT interventions focusing on health promotion and primary prevention, the Lifestyle Redesign program was not implemented in PC settings. Therefore, its efficacy for PC patients is uncertain.

- OTP in PC can draw upon established programs, such as Lifestyle Redesign [24–26], to inform their own practice. At the same time, they need to use clinical judgment to adapt these programs, so they are suitable for their specific patient population and feasible for their organization's capacity and demands.

What Role Can Clinicians Play in Expanding the Evidence Base on OT in PC?

- For many clinicians, the prospect of engaging in research can be intimidating. This section demystifies the research process by describing:
  - Basic types of research design
  - Suggesting which designs are most appropriate for PC clinic research
  - Resources needed to conduct different research studies
  - How clinicians can contribute to research

- Types of research design
  - *Randomized control trials* (RCTs):

    Considered the most sophisticated research design within most healthcare disciplines. If conducted well, evidence generated by such studies is considered to be highly reliable and credible [27].
    The Well Elderly study by Clark et al. [24] and the Canadian PC study by Richardson et al. [17] described previously are examples of RCTs.

RCTs are complicated to execute and entail strict conditions such as

- control or comparison group whose participants do not receive the studied intervention
- random assignment of participants to the control/comparison and intervention groups
- measurement of consistent outcomes before and after for each group and comparing outcomes between groups using advanced statistical procedures [27]

RCTs are unfeasible in typical clinic situations for several reasons

- they are time consuming and resource-intensive to plan and implement, and strong research knowledge and experience is usually required.
- the clinic or organization might be ethically opposed to the idea of withholding interventions from the control group, a necessary condition for an RCT.
- studies using an RCT design often offer financial or gift incentives to encourage patient participation in study procedures, which is unsustainable and unrealistic in real-world clinical settings as patients typically do not receive payment of any type to receive healthcare services; typically the patient is required to pay something such as a copay or deductible

- *Quasi experimental studies:*

  Although not considered as rigorous as RCTs, they can be used to answer similar research questions and conduct similar analyses as an RCT [28]. There are many different types of quasi-experimental study designs.

  - For example, it would be possible to compare aggregate outcomes between groups; however, groups are naturally occurring and not generated for the purpose of the study.
  - This feature makes quasi-experimental studies more amenable for OTPs working in PC, though collaboration with an experienced researcher might still be warranted.
  - For example, the second study conducted by Richardson and colleagues and described in the previous section [18], used a quasi-experimental design to compare outcomes for patients at two different family practice clinics. The study intervention, which involved OT services, was implemented in one clinic only. Patients at the second clinic, where OT services had not been introduced yet, served as a naturally occurring control group.

  Quasi-experimental study design also serves as a model for scaling up OT services across multiple clinics within a large healthcare system. Services could be introduced in one clinic with other clinics serving as control sites. Statistical analyses could be used to compare outcomes for patients between clinics. If OT services are found to be beneficial, a strong case could be made for expanding services to other sites.

– *Single-subject design* [29] (SSDs):

Might be better suited to full-time clinicians who are already integrated in a PC practice.
Typically involves one patient at a time who is closely observed for specific outcomes (e.g., number of falls, time spent in active leisure activities).

- While there are different types of single subject designs, typically, the patient is monitored on these outcomes during a baseline period (i.e., when the intervention has not begun yet), whilst receiving the intervention, and for a specific time period after the intervention is completed [29].
- Single subject designs often appeal to clinicians as they represent only a slight departure from regular clinical practice. These study designs are relatively easy to incorporate into clinical routines and focus on generating evidence for immediate practical use rather than creating new knowledge and testing unknown interventions.
- External validity (how applicable study findings are to different patients and settings) is limited with a single subject study but can be enhanced by replicating the study with multiple patients across different clinical sites [29].
- SSDs are considered a critical foundation on which more sophisticated research studies can be built [30]. These are considered a rigorous methodological approach especially when research on a topic, such as PC, is in its nascent stages and we are still in the initial phases of developing appropriate interventions [30].

– *Observational Study* [31].

Data are collected and analyzed as they naturally exist [31].

- In PC this could involve tracking diagnoses of patients and services provided at each clinic.
- The study by Trembath and colleagues (2019) [10] described previously is an example of an observational study where OT researchers analyzed existing clinical data to identify common diagnoses seen in a PC practice. Studies such as this help to reduce some of the uncertainty regarding the role of OT in PC and what practice can look like in PC settings.

Data from multiple practices can be pooled for a larger sample size. Electronic health records (EHRs) can also be harnessed for patient data.

- Example:
  - Ingram and colleagues (2017) [32].

    Format: observational study analyzing EHR data including contact with clinic-based community health workers (CHWs) and chronic disease indicators such as HbA1c (glycated hemoglobin), body mass index (BMI), blood pressure, and blood lipid profile.
    Purpose: to evaluate the effect of Community Health Worker (CHW) integration on chronic disease-related health indicators at two federally qualified health centers delivering PC.
    Findings: Some improvement in chronic condition indicators noted between groups [32].

  - A similar study design could be used to evaluate the effects of OT integration in PC clinics.
- Clinicians may also consider research as an entry point into PC practice.
  - For example, a clinician can plan a small-scale experimental intervention and offer it under the auspices of an evaluation study at a PC practice. They can then present the evaluation results to the PC practice to support permanent integration of the OTP on the team.
- Regardless of the research design selected, clinician researchers must be aware of, and adhere to, ethical guidelines for conducting research with human participants.
  - The U.S. federal government requires that all research studies involving humans must be overseen by a board of experts [33]. Most academic institutions and some large healthcare organizations have an in-house board of experts, also known as an institutional review board (IRB) [33].
  - As many community-based health centers and stand-alone clinics do not have access to an IRB, clinicians working in such settings can establish partnerships with academic OT programs. They can then submit their research protocol to be reviewed, approved, and overseen by the IRB at their academic partner's institution. This will ensure that their research study is conducted in accordance with ethical guidelines and that their research results can be published and disseminated.

Challenges for Future Research on OT Services in PC

- The integration of OT services in PC settings is still in a nascent stage. As a result, many aspects of PC are unfamiliar to OTPs, both clinicians and researchers. This section summarizes some challenges that can be anticipated when planning OT research in PC.

– One critical challenge is developing standardized empirically supported interventions. Intervention development and testing entails strict controls and thorough documentation of procedures and outcomes [34]. Intervention developers
must document their procedures in manuals, including guidelines and strategies for each patient contact. To ensure that the intervention is delivered consistently in a standardized manner, interventionists must be trained in the
process [34].

However, these procedures leave little room for flexibility and improvisa-
tion in response to the unique needs and circumstances of each patient [35].
Therefore, it is important to develop intervention manuals that allow for indi-
vidualization and flexibility whilst recommending a consistent overarching
protocol.

Recent examples in the field recommend a stepwise process of intervention
development. This involves incremental revisions in the intervention protocol
after observing its viability and utility in small-scale pilot and feasibility studies [36, 37]. This allows the researcher to identify aspects of the intervention
that are too rigid for the administering clinician to be able to respond to emerging patient needs without disrupting the study protocol [35].

– Another challenge for research on OT in PC is aligning traditional OT outcomes with outcomes important to the PC clinic. For some health centers,
tracking specific outcomes is required for third-party reimbursement, quality
monitoring, and obtaining/maintaining a desired provider status such as
patient centered medical home (PCMH) level.

For example, a set of core measures for PC have been developed by the
Core Quality Measure Collaborative [38] This collaborative approach
unites multiple stakeholders including health insurance administrators,
Centers for Medicare and Medicaid Services (CMS) leaders, representa-
tives from the National Quality Forum (NQF), national physician organizations, employers and consumers.

Examples of PC outcomes identified by this Collaborative include percentage of adult patients with controlled blood pressure, percentage of adult
patients with controlled HbA1c levels, rates of preventive cancer screening, and depression remission [38].

None of the above outcomes are overtly occupation-focused. Yet if we
demonstrate that OT services contribute to these outcomes, we can make a
strong case for including OT in PC clinics. To address this challenge,
OTPs can

• offer interventions related to health promotion or medication management, which are more likely to be aligned with the above clinical
outcomes.

• select proximal outcomes related to occupational aspects of everyday
life and health management and distal outcomes related to vitals or
laboratory indicators.

- reframe PC outcomes in the context of occupation (e.g., health management is an occupation and preventive screenings are essential tasks within this occupation, medication adherence is an ADL).
- use generic PC assessments (e.g., The Duke Health Profile, the PROMIS-29), these assessments often have global domains, e.g., physical, mental, social, general, perceived health, self-esteem, anxiety, depression, pain, and disability which can be used to demonstrate treatment effectiveness in domains within the OT scope of practice,

  – Patients in PC settings who are not receiving external rehabilitation care are likely to be higher functioning. It is difficult to demonstrate improvement in an ambulatory patient population that is already functioning at the high end of most OT assessments [15]. This phenomenon is called *ceiling effects*[39]. Following strategies can be used to measure change in high functioning patients seen in PC:

- OTPs can use more general assessments already used and understood by other PC team members such as those mentioned above (The Duke, the PROMIS-29).
- OTPs can document and measure our role in improving occupational engagement and performance related to chronic disease self-management. For example, when medication adherence is viewed as an ADL, a patient with uncontrolled diabetes is not independent with medication management if they are simply able to take their medication. If they are taking it 50% of the time, and their HbA1c level is 9 or above, they clearly require assistance. If the OTP documents the intervention provided, and medication adherence increases to 100% with an HbA1c level of 6.5, those are outcomes that support the OTP's role in the PC team.
- OT researchers must be open to the idea of *no change* or *lack of decline* or *slower rate of decline* as a positive outcome of OT interventions in PC, as there is a growing body of research supporting this approach [40].
- This line of thinking is better aligned with the main premise of PC which is to prevent secondary complications and specialist referrals.

  – Example:
  – Siemonsma and colleagues (2018) [41]:

    Format: Two types of intervention were compared, usual physical therapy (PT) and functional task exercise (FTE) PT. A control group of older adults not receiving any PT services was also included in the comparison.
    Purpose: to examine the effectiveness of PT for improving ADL performance in community dwelling older adults with complex health problems.

Findings: The researchers found that ADL performance deteriorated slightly for both PT and FTE groups. However, the control group, which did not receive any PT, deteriorated significantly more. Researchers concluded that although PT intervention did not *improve* daily functioning, it reduced further deterioration which occurs with aging and chronic disease [41].

- OT researchers and practitioners in PC can focus on outcomes such as maintenance of HbA1c levels for longer time periods or fewer hospitalizations and office visits compared with similar age peers who have similar chronic conditions. This will allow us to demonstrate the effectiveness of OT in PC while underscoring its distinct role and value.

- In summary, there is a need to expand the evidence base to support integration of OT services in PC. Clinicians working in PC or related practice settings can play an important role in this endeavor. The PC setting offers many non-traditional opportunities to measure the effectiveness of OT interventions in this setting. This chapter offers suggestions and ideas for research projects that clinicians can realistically participate in or initiate. We hope the information presented in this chapter allows readers to envision themselves at the forefront of evidence-based OT practice in PC.

References

1. Truong K. CMS launches new value-based payment models for primary care in 2020. 2020. https://medcitynews.com/2019/04/cms-launches-new-value-based-payment-models-for-primary-care/?rf=1.
2. Putera I. Redefining health: implication for value-based healthcare reform. Cureus. 2017;9(3):e1067. https://doi.org/10.7759/cureus.1067.
3. McCauley JL. Guidelines and value-based decision making: an evolving role for payers. N C Med J. 2015;76(4):243–6.
4. Lieberman D, Scheer J. AOTA's evidence-based literature review project: an overview. Am J Occup Ther. 2002;56(3):344–9. https://doi.org/10.5014/ajot.56.3.344.
5. Killian C, Fisher G, Muir S. Primary care: a new context for the scholarship of practice model. Occup Ther Health Care. 2015;29(4):383–96. https://doi.org/10.3109/07380577.2015.1050713.
6. Kenneth J. Ottenbacher; research: its importance to clinical practice in occupational therapy. Am J Occup Ther. 1987;41(4):213–5. https://doi.org/10.5014/ajot.41.4.213.
7. Administration for Community Living. NIDILRR frameworks. 2019. https://acl.gov/aging-and-disability-in-america/nidilrr-frameworks.
8. Donnelly CA, Leclair LL, Wener PF, Hand CL, Letts LJ. OT in primary care: results from a national survey. Can J Occup Ther. 2016;83(3):135–42. https://doi.org/10.1177/0008417416637186.
9. Donnelly C, Brenchley C, Crawford C, Letts L. The integration of OT into primary care: a multiple case study design. BMC Fam Pract. 2013;14:60. https://doi.org/10.1186/1471-2296-14-60.

10. Trembath F, Dahl-Popolizio S, Vanwinkle M, Milligan L. Retrospective analysis: most common diagnoses seen in a primary care clinic and corresponding occupational therapy interventions. Open J Occup Ther. 2019;7(2):6.

11. Dahl-Popolizio S, Muir S, Davis K, Wade S, Voysey R. Occupational therapy in primary care: determining receptiveness of occupational therapists and primary care providers. Open J Occup Ther. 2017;5(3):1–12. https://doi.org/10.15453/2168-6408.1372.

12. Winship JM, Ivey CK, Etz RS. Opportunities for occupational therapy on a primary care team. Am J Occup Ther. 2019;73(5):7305185010. https://doi.org/10.5014/ajot.2019.030841.

13. Koverman B, Lydia R, Stoykov M. Occupational therapy in primary care: structures and processes that support integration. Open J Occup Ther. 2017;5(3):12.

14. Pyatak E, King M, Vigen CLP, Salazar E, Diaz J, Schepens Niemiec SL, Shukla J. Addressing diabetes in primary care: hybrid effectiveness-implementation study of lifestyle redesign® occupational therapy. Am J Occup Ther. 2019;73(5):7305185020. https://doi.org/10.5014/ajot.2019.037317.

15. Mirza M, Gecht-Silver M, Keating E, Krischer A, Kim H, Kottorp A. Feasibility and preliminary efficacy of an occupational therapy intervention in a primary care clinic. Am J Occup Ther. 2020;74(5):7405205030p1–7405205030p13. https://doi.org/10.5014/ajot.2020.039842.

16. United States Department of Health and Human Services. NIH stage model for behavioral intervention development. https://www.nia.nih.gov/research/dbsr/nih-stage-model-behavioral-intervention-development.

17. Richardson J, Letts L, Chan D, Stratford P, Hand C, Price D, Law M. Rehabilitation in primary care setting for persons with chronic illness—a randomized controlled trial. Prim Health Care Res Dev. 2010;11:382–95. https://doi.org/10.1017/S1463423610000113.

18. Richardson J, Letts L, Chan D, Officer A, Wojkowski S, Oliver D, Kinzie S. Monitoring physical functioning as the sixth vital sign: evaluating patient and practice engagement in chronic illness care in a primary care setting—a quasi-experimental design. BMC Fam Pract. 2012;13:29. https://doi.org/10.1186/1471-2296-13-29.

19. Garvey J, Connolly D, Boland F, Smith SM. OPTIMAL, an occupational therapy led self-management support programme for people with multimorbidity in primary care: a randomized controlled trial. BMC Fam Pract. 2015;16:59. https://doi.org/10.1186/s12875-015-0267-0.

20. Orellano E, Colon WI, Arbesman M. Effect of occupation- and activity-based interventions on instrumental activities of daily living performance among community-dwelling older adults: a systematic review. Am J Occup Ther. 2012a;66(3):292–300. https://doi.org/10.5014/ajot.2012.003053.

21. Orellano E, Colon WI, Arbesman M. Systematic review of occupation- and activity-based health management and maintenance interventions for community-dwelling older adults. Am J Occup Ther. 2012b;66(3):277–83. https://doi.org/10.5014/ajot.2012.00332.

22. Steultjens EM, Dekker J, Bouter LM, Jellema S, Bakker EB, van den Ende CH. Occupational therapy for community dwelling elderly people: a systematic review. Age Ageing. 2004;33(5):453–60. https://doi.org/10.1093/ageing/afh174.

23. Zingmark M, Nilsson I, Fisher AG, Lindholm L. Occupation-focused health promotion for well older people: a cost-effectiveness analysis. Br J Occup Ther. 2015;79(3):153–62. https://doi.org/10.1177/0308022615609623.

24. Clark F, Jackson J, Carlson M, Chou CP, Cherry BJ, Jordan-Marsh M, Azen SP. Effectiveness of a lifestyle intervention in promoting the well-being of independently living older people: results of the well elderly 2 randomised controlled trial. J Epidemiol Community Health. 2012;66(9):782–90. https://doi.org/10.1136/jech.2009.099754.

25. Clark F, Azen SP, Zemke R, Jackson J, Carlson M, Mandel D, Hay J, Josephson K, Cherry B, Hessel C, Palmer J, Lipson L. Occupational therapy for independent-living older adults: a randomized controlled trial. JAMA. 1997;278(16):1321–6.

26. Clark F, Azen SP, Carlson M, Mandel D, LaBree L, Hay J, et al. Embedding health-promoting changes into the daily lives of independent-living older adults: long-term follow-up of OT intervention. J Gerontol B Psychol Sci Soc Sci. 2001;56(1):60–3.

27. Kabisch M, Ruckes C, Seibert-Grafe M, Blettner M. Randomized controlled trials: part 17 of a series on evaluation of scientific publications. Deutsches Arzteblatt Int. 2011;108(39):663–8. https://doi.org/10.3238/arztebl.2011.0663.
28. Schaw CF. Quasi-experimental designs. In: Breakwell GM, Smith JA, Wright DB, editors. Research methods in psychology. 4th ed. Thousand Oaks: Sage; 2012. p. 75–92.
29. Engel RJ, Schutt RK. Single-subject design. In: Fundamentals of social work research. Thousand Oaks: Sage; 2009. p. 139–75.
30. Kottorp A, Fisher AG. Evidence-based occupational therapy 2.0: developing evidence for occupation. Jpn Occup Ther Res. 2015;34:349–54.
31. Portney LG, Watkins MP. Observational designs. In: Portney LG, Watkins MP, editors. Foundations of clinical research. Upper Saddle River: Prentice Hall Health; 2009. p. 277–99.
32. Ingram M, Doubleday K, Bell ML, Lohr A, Murrieta L, Velasco M, Carvajal SC. Community health worker impact on chronic disease outcomes within primary care examined using electronic health records. Am J Public Health. 2017;107(10):1668–74. https://doi.org/10.2105/AJPH.2017.303934.
33. DePoy E, Gitlin LN. Protecting the boundaries. In: Introduction to research: understanding and applying multiple strategies. 4th ed. St. Louis: Mosby; 2011. p. 148–59.
34. Nezu AM, Nezu CM. Ensuring treatment integrity. New York: Oxford University Press; 2008.
35. Ng MY, Weisz JR. Annual research review: building a science of personalized intervention for youth mental health. J Child Psychol Psychiatry. 2016;57(3):216–36. https://doi.org/10.1111/jcpp.12470.
36. Blanche EI, Fogelberg D, Diaz J, Carlson M, Clark F. Manualization of OT interventions: illustrations from the pressure ulcer prevention research program. Am J Occup Ther. 2011;65(6):711–9. https://doi.org/10.5014/ajot.2011.001172.
37. Pyatak EA, Carandang K, Davis S. Developing a manualized occupational therapy diabetes management intervention: resilient, empowered, active living with diabetes. OTJR. 2015;35(3):187–94. https://doi.org/10.1177/1539449215584310.
38. Centers for Medicare and Medicaid Services. Core measures. 2017. https://www.cms.gov/Medicare/Quality-Initiatives-Patient-Assessment-Instruments/QualityMeasures/Core-Measures.
39. Salkind NJ. Encyclopedia of research design. Thousand Oaks: Sage Publications, Inc.; 2010. https://doi.org/10.4135/9781412961288.
40. Apóstolo J, Cooke R, Bobrowicz-Campos E, Santana S, Marcucci M, Cano A, Holland C. Effectiveness of interventions to prevent pre-frailty and frailty progression in older adults: a systematic review. JBI Database Syst Rev Implement Rep. 2018;16(1):140–232. https://doi.org/10.11124/JBISRIR-2017-003382.
41. Siemonsma PC, Blom JW, Hofstetter H, van Hespen ATH, Gussekloo J, Drewes Y, van Meeteren NLU. The effectiveness of functional task exercise and physical therapy as prevention of functional decline in community dwelling older people with complex health problems. BMC Geriatr. 2018;18:164.

Chapter 6
Trauma-Informed Approaches

John V. Rider and Katie Smith

Introduction

Decades of work in the field of trauma have generated multiple definitions of trauma and explanations for its impact on everyday functioning. While there is no universal definition of trauma, the following concept was generated based on existing definitions and an expert panel by the Substance Abuse and Mental Health Services Administration (SAMHSA) [1]: "Individual trauma results from an event, series of events, or set of circumstances that is experienced by an individual as physically or emotionally harmful or life threatening and that has lasting adverse effects on the individual's functioning and mental, physical, social, emotional, or spiritual well-being" [1]. Examples of trauma include but are not limited to experiencing or observing physical, sexual, or emotional abuse, exposure to violence, discrimination, neglect, natural disasters, bullying, terrorism, a motor vehicle accident, food insecurity, life-threatening incidences, poverty, and having a family member with a mental health or substance use disorder.

To further understand the evolving nature of trauma, SAMHSA has developed the "Three Es" of trauma: *events, experiences,* and *effect* [1]. For example, when a person is exposed to a traumatic *event*, how they *experience* it greatly influences the lasting adverse *effects* of carrying the weight of that trauma. *Events* and circumstances may be a single or repeated occurrence of trauma. It is important to be aware that the individual's *experience* of these events or circumstances determines if it is a traumatic event. For example, a particular event may be experienced as traumatic for one individual and not for another. Trauma is therefore related to how an

J. V. Rider (✉)
School of Occupational Therapy, Touro University Nevada, Henderson, NV, USA
e-mail: jrider@touro.edu

K. Smith
Revolutionary Alignment, LLC, Detroit, MI, USA
www.RevolutionaryAlignment.com

© Springer Nature Switzerland AG 2023
S. Dahl-Popolizio et al. (eds.), *Primary Care Occupational Therapy*,
https://doi.org/10.1007/978-3-031-20882-9_6

individual labels or assigns meaning to the event and how it physically and psychologically disrupts them. A range of personal factors, including cultural beliefs, availability of social supports, or the individual's developmental stage, informs the experience of an event [1]. The long-lasting adverse *effects* of the event are a critical component of trauma and may occur immediately or emerge at a future time. Often, individuals may not recognize the connection between the traumatic events and the adverse effects impacting their everyday life. Examples of adverse effects that OTPs may address include the inability to cope with normal everyday stresses, inability to trust and benefit from relationships or social connection, inability to manage executive functioning, inability to regulate behavior or control the expression of emotions appropriately, etc. [1]. Moreover, traumatic effects, which can range from a constant state of arousal to numbing or avoidance, eventually wear a person down, physically, mentally, and emotionally [1].

Trauma contributes to mental health and functional difficulties among all ages. Exposure to trauma early in life increases a person's lifelong potential for serious health problems and engaging in health risk behaviors [2–4]. For people with mental and substance abuse disorders, trauma is an almost universal experience [1]. Awareness of trauma's impact is growing among PC providers, including OTPs working in PC, and providers realize the value of trauma-informed approaches to care. Although trauma still holds a significant stigma in the United States, trauma survivors have begun to powerfully and systematically share their paths to recovery, igniting the development of trauma-informed approaches.

The Need for Trauma-Informed Approaches in PC

It is important to recognize that individuals who have experienced trauma do not only seek services in behavioral or mental healthcare settings. Responses to traumatic experiences can manifest in behaviors at any level of care throughout the healthcare system, including PC. Because trauma does not respect age, gender, socioeconomic status, race, ethnicity, geography, or sexual orientation, *OTPs working in PC will inevitably work with a client that has experienced trauma*. Traumatic experiences have been shown to have an impact on health and an individual's responsiveness to health interventions, further demonstrating a need for OTPs to understand and address trauma using trauma-informed care and evidence-based practice [5–7].

Experiencing trauma at any point in life, but especially during childhood, significantly increases the risk of serious chronic health problems. Evidence indicates that trauma increases the risk of chronic lung, heart, and liver disease, as well as depression, sexually transmitted diseases, and tobacco, alcohol, and illicit drug abuse [5–7]. Furthermore, adverse childhood experiences (ACEs) are prevalent among individuals living in the United States. Two-thirds of adults report experiencing at least one ACE, and one in five reports experiencing three or more [8]. Individuals with multiple ACEs are more likely to engage in health-risk behaviors, more likely to be obese, and have higher rates of heart disease, stroke, liver disease, lung cancer, chronic obstructive pulmonary disease, and autoimmune disorders than the general population, further illustrating the downstream consequences of trauma in childhood [9]. As PC aims to address a large majority of personal healthcare needs, recognizing the significant role that trauma plays in physical and psychological health is imperative to providing evidence-based, holistic, and person-centered care.

Evidence-based interventions for trauma responses have been developed; however, they have been integrated most heavily within the behavioral and mental healthcare system. Despite the progress of trauma-informed care within this setting, based on the voice of trauma survivors, interventions within only one aspect of the healthcare continuum are not enough [1]. Beyond clinical interventions, an approach informed by trauma is needed across healthcare settings, especially in PC. *A trauma-informed approach is distinct from trauma-specific interventions, which are designed specifically to address the consequences of trauma and facilitate healing.* Adopting a trauma-informed approach is not accomplished by implementing a single technique or "one-and-done" items on a checklist. While utilizing a trauma-informed approach includes trauma-specific interventions and assessments, it also requires constant attention, caring awareness, sensitivity, and often a cultural change at the organizational level to incorporate fundamental trauma principles throughout the PC practice.

A Trauma-Informed Approach

A trauma-informed approach assumes that an individual is more likely than not to have a history of trauma. Additionally, it recognizes the presence of trauma symptoms and acknowledges the role trauma may play in an individual's life. Using a trauma-informed approach, OTPs can strive to deliver what is commonly referred to as "trauma-informed care" within PC settings. While multiple definitions exist [10] identified the following themes within trauma-informed care literature: (1) an awareness of how symptoms and behaviors are related to traumatic experiences, (2) an emphasis on safety, (3) an opportunity for individuals to develop or regain a sense of control over their lives, and (4) an emphasis on strengths rather than on deficiencies. Using these themes, Hopper et al. [10] developed the following definition of trauma-informed care:

"Trauma-Informed Care is a strengths-based framework that is grounded in an understanding of and responsiveness to the impact of trauma, that emphasizes physical, psychological, and emotional safety for both providers and survivors, and that creates opportunities for survivors to rebuild a sense of control and empowerment."

Importantly, trauma-informed care emphasizes physical, psychological, and emotional safety for *providers* and *survivors*, indicating consideration for OTPs themselves, colleagues, and clients. OTPs can advocate for an inclusive work environment that considers trauma experienced by providers and staff, in addition to clientele, when developing policies and procedures.

SAMHSA has identified the following principles as the foundation of a trauma-informed approach. Notably, a trauma-informed approach is not simply following a prescribed set of practices or procedures; rather, it is adhering to key principles throughout an organization. These principles are meant to be generalizable and applied across settings, including PC. OT practice in PC should aim to reflect these principles in all aspects of care delivery.

Six Key Principles Fundamental to a Trauma-Informed Approach (SAMHSA)

1. Safety
2. Trustworthiness and Transparency
3. Peer Support
4. Collaboration and Mutuality
5. Empowerment, Voice, and Choice
6. Cultural, Historical, and Gender Issues

Clients must feel *safe* when they enter the PC offices and during their interactions with the staff and healthcare providers. OTPs can work to ensure the physical setting is safe and all interpersonal interactions promote a sense of safety. *Transparency* throughout the organizational operations fosters *trust* with clients and employees. *Peer support* refers to the use of individuals with lived experiences of trauma, sometimes referred to as "trauma survivors." OTPs can help identify ways to utilize peer support with clients to promote recovery and healing within PC settings. A trauma-informed organization recognizes that all organization members have a role to play. Because healing happens in relationships and the meaningful sharing of power and decision-making, *collaboration* and *mutuality* emphasize leveling power differences between all levels of staff and clients. When developing a more trauma-informed PC organization, OTPs can advocate for equal voices from staff, providers, and clients. The organization should recognize that trauma may be a unifying aspect in administrators' lives, those who provide services, staff, and clients, and seek to foster empowerment for all parties. OTPs should support clients in shared decision-making, *empowering* them with a *voice* and a *choice* in a treatment plan to heal and move forward. It is imperative that the organization works to combat cultural stereotypes and biases and recognizes *cultural*, *historical*, and *gender issues* that have plagued health care. Trauma-informed approaches should offer access to gender-responsive services, leverage the healing value of traditional cultural connections, incorporate policies, protocols, processes, and documentation responsive to racial, ethnic, and cultural needs, and openly address historical trauma [1]. OTPs should seek to be involved in policy and protocol development. Agner (2020) has advocated for a shift from simply being culturally competent to practicing cultural humility. Cultural humility entails being flexible, aware of bias, and having a lifelong learning-oriented approach to working with diversity [11].

Furthermore, cultural humility recognizes the role of power in healthcare interactions and supports a trauma-informed approach [11]. While OTPs traditionally have applied principles of cultural competence and humility within their individual practice, a trauma-informed approach requires the application of these concepts at an organizational level and opens doors for OTPs to contribute to trauma-informed organizational and systemic changes.

In addition to the six key principles, SAMHSA (2018) [12] has also stated that a trauma-informed program, organization, or system:

1. Realizes the widespread effect of trauma and understands potential paths for recovery
2. Recognizes the signs and symptoms of trauma in clients, families, staff, and others involved with the system
3. Responds by fully integrating knowledge about trauma into policies, procedures, and practices
4. Seeks to actively resist re-traumatization

While SAMHSA's key principles were developed to guide change at the program, organization, and system's level, it is important to recognize that these principles can and should also be applied to the individual level of healthcare providers and provide guidance for OTPs in their everyday practice.

One of the key aspects of a trauma-informed approach is that it seeks to resist re-traumatization. Re-traumatization occurs when a person re-experiences previous trauma, either consciously or unconsciously. Causes of re-traumatization include stressors similar to the original trauma's environment or circumstances, such as sounds, smells, lighting, imagery, objects, memories, or even a new relationship that mimics a previously traumatic one. OTPs in trauma-informed environments need to recognize how organizational practices may trigger painful memories and re-traumatize clients. For example, an OTP utilizing a trauma-informed approach would identify that forcing someone to recount a traumatic experience when they are not ready, using a form of restraints on an individual who had been sexually abused or placing a child who had been neglected or abandoned in a secluded room may be re-traumatizing and interfere with healing and recovery. A trauma-informed approach seeks to avoid re-traumatization, requiring additional considerations regarding the physical and socio-emotional environment, physical contact, and language used during evaluation and treatment.

SAMHSA (2014) [1] has outlined 10 domains for implementing a trauma-informed approach. While developing a trauma-informed approach requires systematic change at multiple levels of the PC organization, OTPs can serve as agents of change and initiate a shift toward trauma-informed care. Trauma-informed care does not have to be a burden to adopt, and OTPs can help stakeholders recognize that understanding the role of trauma and how a trauma-informed approach may help them meet their goals and objectives. As SAMHSA has indicated, the following domains are not simply boxes to check off; rather, they are domains of organizational change found in trauma-informed care literature.

Ten Implementation Domains for a Trauma-Informed Approach [1]

1. Governance and Leadership—The leadership and governance must support and invest in implementing and sustaining a trauma-informed approach.
2. Policy—Written policies and protocols establishing a trauma-informed approach should be an essential part of the organizational mission.
3. Physical Environment—The physical environment should promote a sense of physical and psychological safety and collaboration between staff and individuals being served.
4. Engagement and Involvement—People in recovery, trauma survivors, people receiving services, and family members receiving services should have significant involvement, a voice, and meaningful choice at all levels and areas of organizational functioning.
5. Cross-Sector Collaboration—Collaboration across sectors built on a shared understanding of trauma and principles of a trauma-informed approach is necessary.
6. Screening, Assessment, Treatment Services—Practitioners should be trained in and use evidence-based screening tools, evaluations, and culturally appropriate interventions that reflect principles of a trauma-informed approach.
7. Training and Workforce Development—On-going training on trauma and peer support throughout the organization are essential.
8. Progress Monitoring and Quality Assurance—On-going assessment, tracking, and monitoring of trauma-informed principles and effective use of evidence-based trauma-specific screening, assessments, and treatment should be implemented.
9. Financing—Financing structures should be designed to support a trauma-informed approach through training and resources for all staff.
10. Evaluation—Measures for the evaluation of service and program implementation and effectiveness should reflect an understanding of trauma and appropriate trauma-oriented research instruments.

OTPs can use their diverse training in biopsychosocial models of practice to provide recommendations for any of the above domains to further develop a trauma-informed approach in their PC practice. OTPs are well-suited to be trauma-informed care "champions" and lead the charge in PC. Doing so may open new roles and emerging responsibilities in administration and leadership in PC. These advanced positions will allow OTPs to make systematic changes and demonstrate our holistic understanding of treating the whole person while considering and attempting to understand past traumatic events and how they may influence current behaviors and coping mechanisms.

Integrating Trauma-Informed Approaches in PC

Involve the Client in the Evaluation and Treatment Process

- Client voice.
  - Aligned with OT's client-centered model, trauma-informed care approaches also advocate for the client having a voice in their own treatment planning and an active role in the decision-making process. While this can be difficult in the PC setting due to time constraints, OTPs working in a trauma-informed care approach should actively engage clients in their care and utilize their feedback as the driving force in their care plan.
  - Fette and colleagues (2019) [13] stressed that OTPs need to recognize that trauma can manifest in different ways among clients, including flat affect, defensiveness, and aggressiveness and that the client is likely trying to communicate with you through this behavior. Trauma may also present as anxiety, lack of eye contact, or hesitancy to participate in the OT encounter.

- Peer-support.
  - Peer specialists are individuals with lived trauma experience who undergo special training to be a part of the care team. Based on their similar experiences and shared understanding, they may be able to build trust with the clients more effectively and support increased engagement in treatment.
  - Peer engagement and peer support, in general, can be a powerful tool to help overcome the isolation common among individuals who have experienced trauma [14].

- Policies and procedures.
  - A PC team can also explore how it can use empowerment, voice, and choice when developing policies and procedures to provide trauma-informed services (e.g., explaining a potentially invasive procedure to a client step-by-step). OTPs can play a prominent role in developing practice materials and provider explanations that follow evidence-based guidelines and standards of care for clients with low health literacy.
  - OTPs can ensure that client education is trauma-informed and considers the potentially re-traumatizing effects of invasive or traumatic tests, procedures, or even treatments. Clients should be empowered to share their experiences, if they wish, and to direct their care.

Screen for Trauma

There are two main approaches to screening for trauma
- Upfront and universal screening.

    - Universal screening includes screening every client for trauma history as early as possible.
    - This can reduce the risk of bias.
    - While this approach may allow providers a better understanding of a client's potential trauma history, aggregate data, risk of chronic disease, and lead to targeted interventions, it may also take away the client's choice of sharing sensitive information [14].
    - Upfront screening may also lead to re-traumatization or hinder progress if appropriate interventions or referrals are not promptly initiated.

- Selective screening.

    - Selective screening for trauma may allow a trust to develop between the client and the provider before asking about any trauma history.
    - This approach may decrease the chances of re-traumatization and allow for more timely interventions and referrals.
    - Clients can be asked to share a cumulative ACE or trauma screening score after completing a questionnaire rather than identifying a specific traumatic experience, which would allow the client to decide if they want to discuss any trauma and how much detail they wish to provide [14].

- Upfront or universal screening may be more effective in PC settings, whereas selective screening may be more appropriate in behavioral health settings [14].

    - Screening frequency should be minimized to prevent continual re-traumatization, and all healthcare professionals administering the screening should be competent in trauma screening and trauma-informed approaches.
    - When screening for trauma, providers need to be prepared to offer appropriate care options, referral resources, and follow-up with trauma-related needs.

Become Trained in Trauma-Informed Approaches and Trauma-Specific Treatment Approaches

- While all PC staff should be trained in trauma-informed approaches, all clinicians evaluating and treating should also be trained in trauma-specific *treatment* approaches.

    - The National Council for Wellbeing provides training on trauma-informed care as well as "Mental Health First Aid." Mental Health First Aid [15] is a skills-based training course provided by the National Council for Mental

Wellbeing. It teaches participants about mental health and substance-use issues and how to assist someone experiencing a mental health or substance use-related crisis.

- This type of training may be beneficial in a PC setting as it prepares all staff with strategies to help someone in crisis and non-crisis situations using a trauma-informed approach. Multiple online trainings exist at the individual and organizational level for trauma-informed care.

- Additional treatment options within the scope of OT include, but are not limited to:

  - Motivational Interviewing, Mindfulness training, formal Peer Support Programs, Eye Movement Desensitization and Reprocessing (EMDR), Prolonged Exposure Therapy, Seeking Safety©, Risking Connection®, Trauma-Focused Cognitive Behavioral Therapy (TF–CBT), and Trauma-Focused Acceptance and Commitment Therapy (TFACT). OTPs in PC can pursue advanced training in these treatment techniques with trauma-specific approaches.

Effects of Trauma on Health

- OTPs need to recognize the effects of trauma on health, including coping styles and behaviors, and the need to respectfully and collaboratively discuss negative or maladaptive coping behaviors [16].
- Multiple studies have demonstrated a link between childhood trauma and lifelong health problems, such as chronic lung and heart diseases; liver disease, viral hepatitis, and liver cancer; autoimmune diseases; sexually transmitted infections; and depression and other mental health conditions [2–4].
- Children who have experienced trauma often develop coping mechanisms that may evolve into health risk behaviors, such as eating unhealthy food or overeating or tobacco, drug, or alcohol abuse. These coping mechanisms can contribute to anxiety, depression, social isolation, or chronic diseases and can be addressed by OT.
- Prolonged trauma can decrease the volume of areas in the brain responsible for cognitive function such as short-term memory, emotional regulation, and executive functioning [17].
- Trauma treatment should be tailored to each client's specific needs; however, information pertaining to population characteristics may help guide treatment. For example, it is essential to practice cultural competence and humility when working with people from diverse cultural groups, as cultural background influences how individuals respond to trauma [1].
- Members of historically marginalized populations appear to have a disproportionately higher prevalence of trauma and adverse childhood experiences and may experience a more significant impact on health compared to the general population [4, 18, 19].

PC Team Self-Awareness

Knowing One's Limits
- Raja and colleagues (2015) also highlighted the importance of knowing your own history and reactions, caring for yourself, and practicing "trauma steward-ship," which encompasses caring for clients without taking on their trauma your-self [16].
- OT interventions in PC that focus on improving function, well-being, and health can support individuals with past trauma and intensive needs [13]. However, OTPs in PC must recognize the limits of their personal knowledge and skills and be prepared to refer when needed to colleagues with advanced trauma-specific skills [13].

Whole-Person Perspective
- Deepening the embodiment of a trauma-informed approach can serve as an opportunity to get to know oneself and one's PC colleagues as healthcare provid-ers and people. The PC team is a cohesive unit of distinct human beings, and each provider brings their individual experiences and the impact of those experi-ences. The whole-person approach of OT recognizes the importance and value of seeing the self and others as whole, complete beings, inclusive of trauma history. OTPs should consider coordinating in-service sessions with local resource groups to deepen team exposure and collective integration of trauma-informed care concepts, for example, https://traumainformedoregon.org

Utilize Referral Sources and Partner with Trauma-Informed Organizations

- Interdisciplinary team.
  - Because individuals who experience trauma may have complex medical, behavioral health, and social service needs, they may be receiving care from multiple providers or need support in obtaining proper care from numerous providers.

    If PC practices or OTPs are screening for trauma, they need to be prepared to address trauma-related needs effectively and provide appropriate and timely referrals to trauma-informed practitioners across the interdisciplinary team.
- Community resources.
  - OTPs can partner with organizations within their community to develop improved services and a trauma-informed referral network. There are many

local and national resources on trauma-informed care for providers and clients. OTPs in PC should be familiar with and prepared to connect clients with these resources.

The National Council for Mental Wellbeing launched a 3-year initiative in 2017, "Trauma-Informed Primary Care: Fostering Resilience and Recovery," and is piloting a change package that will offer PC practices field-informed methods, tools, and resources to advance understanding and address the impact of trauma specifically in PC. While the results are not available at the time of writing this chapter, this project aims to make recommendations for standardized screening and assessment tools, evidence-based clinical interventions, implementation process, relevant and replicable outcome measures, and potential critical policy changes. OTPs working in PC can utilize this resource and review the results and recommendations with the entire PC team.

Here are some additional resources:

- A large trauma-informed care implementation resource center

  - https://www.traumainformedcare.chcs.org/

- Resources specifically relevant for children and families

  - https://www.nctsn.org/trauma-informed-care
  - https://www.parentcenterhub.org/trauma-informed-care/
  - https://www.fredla.org/resources-on-trauma-informed-care/

- Resources on ACES

  - https://www.acesaware.org/ace-fundamentals/principles-of-trauma-informed-care/

- Resources specifically relevant to PC

  - https://www.thenationalcouncil.org/consulting-areas-of-expertise/trauma-informed-primary-care/

Consider Language Choices Carefully

- Definitions of terms

  - Differing opinions

    While there is no universally accepted definition of trauma, this chapter has provided a concept of trauma developed by a key policymaker, SAMHSA.

    Menschner and Maul (2016) highlighted that some experts have encouraged open-ended definitions, believing that the idea of trauma is too broad and, if defined, may exclude individuals whose experiences do not fit within the definition but need trauma-informed services [14].

Other experts suggest that the lack of standardized terminology is actually a barrier to developing trauma-informed cross-sector collaboration and advancing the field [14].

– Awareness of impact

The language used in health care, and in this case, PC, *will* influence both the practice of providers and the experiences of clients.

Intentionally seek to use language that *reduces stigma* and *accommodates low health literacy*.

Educate clients on how traumatic experiences may contribute to their overall health and their adherence to treatment recommendations. Clients may be more likely to trust their OTPs and PCPs and follow the treatment plan if they explain how traumatic experiences contribute to their overall health instead of focusing solely on the experience of trauma itself [14].

Ask "What happened to you?" rather than "What's wrong with you?"

In a trauma-informed approach, OTPs should ask permission from the client for everything.

Create a Safe Environment

- If an individual who has experienced trauma feels physically, socially, or emotionally unsafe in the PC setting, they may experience re-traumatization. Creating a safe environment is an important step in providing trauma-informed PC. OTPs can contribute to the creation of a safe physical and social–emotional environment by providing training to the PC team and practicing some of the following recommendations [14].

  – Keep parking lots, common areas, bathrooms, entrances, and exits safe, accessible, and well lit.
  – Keep noise levels in waiting rooms to a minimum.
  – Use welcoming language on all signage.
  – Make sure clients have clear access to the door in the exam rooms and can easily exit if desired.
  – Ensure that people are not allowed to smoke, loiter, or congregate outside entrances and exits.
  – Monitor who is coming in and out of the building for safety.
  – Acknowledge that there may be aspects of the PC physical environment that you cannot change to support wellbeing.

To Create a Safe Social–Emotional Environment
- Welcome clients and ensure that they feel safe, respected, and supported.
- Ensure staff maintain healthy interpersonal boundaries and can manage conflict appropriately.
- Keep consistent schedules and procedures.
- Offer sufficient notice and preparation when changes are necessary.
- Maintain communication that is consistent, open, respectful, compassionate, and culturally responsive.
- Be aware of how an individual's culture affects how they may perceive trauma, safety, and privacy.

Protect privacy during physical examinations and in the medical record by asking for consent throughout the process. Ask for permission to touch a client, explain why it is necessary, and remain at eye level with the client whenever possible.

Conclusion

OTPs can utilize trauma-informed approaches in PC across the life span. With our advanced knowledge of the downstream consequences of trauma and the significant impact on health behavior, a comprehensive understanding of trauma and how to respond appropriately in PC is critical. As practitioners who adhere to client-centered and holistic care, we have a responsibility to understand the significant nature and widespread effects of trauma that are likely influencing many aspects of occupational performance and engagement among the clients we serve.

References

1. Substance Abuse and Mental Health Services Administration. Trauma-informed care in behavioral health services. Rockville: Substance Abuse and Mental Health Services Administration; 2014.
2. Felitti VJ, Anda RF, Nordenberg D, Williamson DF, Spitz AM, Edwards V, et al. Relationship of childhood abuse and household dysfunction to many of the leading causes of death in adults. The adverse childhood experiences (ACE) study. Am J Prev Med. 1998;14(4):245–58. https://doi.org/10.1016/s0749-3797(98)00017-8.
3. Shonkoff JP, Garner AS, Committee on Psychosocial Aspects of Child and Family Health, Committee on Early Childhood, Adoption, and Dependent Care, & Section on Developmental and Behavioral Pediatrics. The lifelong effects of early childhood adversity and toxic stress. Pediatrics. 2012;129(1):e232–46. https://doi.org/10.1542/peds.2011-2663.
4. Public Health Management Corporation. Findings from the Philadelphia Urban ACE Survey. 2013. http://www.rwjf.org/content/dam/farm/reports/reports/2013/rwjf407836.
5. Bonomi AE, Anderson ML, Rivara FP, Thompson RS. Health outcomes in women with physical and sexual intimate partner violence exposure. J Womens Health. 2007;16(7):987–97. https://doi.org/10.1089/jwh.2006.0239.

6. Campbell R, Greeson MR, Bybee D, Raja S. The co-occurrence of childhood sexual abuse, adult sexual assault, intimate partner violence, and sexual harassment: a mediational model of posttraumatic stress disorder and physical health outcomes. J Consult Clin Psychol. 2008;76(2):194–207. https://doi.org/10.1037/0022-006X.76.2.194.
7. Dutton MA, Green BL, Kaltman SI, Roesch DM, Zeffiro TA, Krause ED. Intimate partner violence, PTSD, and adverse health outcomes. J Interpers Violence. 2006;21(7):955–68. https://doi.org/10.1177/0886260506289178.
8. Pardee M, Kuzma E, Dahlem C, Boucher N, Darling-Fisher C. Current state of screening high-ACE youth and emerging adults in primary care. J Am Assoc Nurse Pract. 2017;29(12):716–24. https://doi.org/10.1002/2327-6924.12531.
9. Oral R, Ramirez M, Coohey C, Nakada S, Walz A, Kuntz A, Benoit J, Peek-Asa C. Adverse childhood experiences and trauma informed care: the future of health care. Pediatr Res. 2016;79(1–2):227–33. https://doi.org/10.1038/pr.2015.197.
10. Hopper EK, Bassuk EL, Olivet J. Shelter from the storm: trauma-informed care in homelessness services settings. Open Health Serv Policy J. 2010;3(2):80–100. https://doi.org/10.2174/1874924001003020080.
11. Agner J. Moving from cultural competence to cultural humility in occupational therapy: a paradigm shift. Am J Occup Ther. 2020;74(4):7404347010p1–7. https://doi.org/10.5014/ajot.2020.038067.
12. Substance Abuse and Mental Health Services Administration. Trauma-informed approach and trauma-specific interventions. 2018. https://www.samhsa.gov/nctic/trauma-interventions.
13. Fette C, Lambdin-Pattavina C, Weaver L. Understanding and applying trauma-informed approaches across occupational therapy settings. 2019. https://www.aota.org/~/media/Corporate/Files/Publications/CE-Articles/CE-Article-May-2019-Trauma.pdf.
14. Menschner C, Maul A. Key ingredients for successful trauma-informed care implementation. North Bethesda: SAMHSA; 2016. https://www.samhsa.gov/sites/default/files/programs_campaigns/childrens_mental_health/atc-whitepaper-040616.pdf
15. Hadlaczky G, Hökby S, Mkrtchian A, Carli V, Wasserman D. Mental health first aid is an effective public health intervention for improving knowledge, attitudes, and behaviour: a meta-analysis. Int Rev Psychiatry. 2014;26(4):467–75. https://doi.org/10.3109/09540261.2014.924910.
16. Raja S, Hasnain M, Hoersch M, Gove-Yin S, Rajagopalan C. Trauma-informed care in medicine: current knowledge and future research directions. Fam Community Health. 2015;38(3):216–26. https://doi.org/10.1097/FCH.0000000000000071.
17. Child Welfare Information Gateway. Understanding the effects of maltreatment on brain development. 2015. https://www.childwelfare.gov/pubPDFs/brain_development.pdf.
18. Andersen JP, Blosnich J. Disparities in adverse childhood experiences among sexual minority and heterosexual adults: results from a multi-state probability-based sample. PLoS One. 2013;8(1):e54691. https://doi.org/10.1371/journal.pone.0054691.
19. Schüssler-Fiorenza Rose SM, Xie D, Stineman M. Adverse childhood experiences and disability in U.S. adults. PM R. 2014;6(8):670–80. https://doi.org/10.1016/j.pmrj.2014.01.013.

Chapter 7
Transitions Across the Lifespan

Jeanne Ross Eichler and Karen M. Keptner

Introduction

Transitional periods of life can be both expected or unexpected, can occur throughout the lifespan, and can bring about changes in the way that an individual engages in their daily life [1, 2]. These changes can disrupt habits, routines, and rituals necessary to engage in important and necessary occupations. The context in which an individual engages can either support or hinder an individual's adaptation through that transition. Occupational therapists, with expert knowledge of transition can

- Promote healthy transitions through education and targeted support;
- Assist individuals in the establishment of healthy habits, routines, and rituals;
- Help individuals in restoring necessary and desired occupations;
- Modify the environment for successful engagement in occupations;
- Help the client learn how to compensate for performance skills deficits that prevent participation and engagement in important and necessary occupations.

Occupational therapy practitioners have the skills to intervene with and advocate for individuals in the process of transition so that individuals can thrive during and after important life transitions [3]. Transitions occur in large and small ways across the lifespan. In the primary care setting, paying attention to multiple aspects of transitions that are part of the lived experience for every patient may assist the

J. R. Eichler (✉)
OTonCampus, Edgewater, MD, USA

K. M. Keptner
School of Health Sciences, Cleveland State University, Cleveland, OH, USA
e-mail: k.keptner@csuohio.edu

© Springer Nature Switzerland AG 2023
S. Dahl-Popolizio et al. (eds.), *Primary Care Occupational Therapy*,
https://doi.org/10.1007/978-3-031-20882-9_7

occupational therapist as they zero in on the best and most proactive care. This short guide offers basic areas of OT opportunity for care/attention related to points of significant transition.

Developmental transitions are typical and predictable points in development that might contribute to overall health and well-being [1]. Considering overall development may result in the normalization of a concern in behavior or physical development in some cases, while in others may provide points of comparison that drive specific interventions or suggestions.

In some cases, there are **major life transitions** that involve dramatic changes in lifestyle. These transitions may include:

- Transition from home to school during early years
- Transition to adulthood
- Transition to college/career
- Transition to an age of significance (30, 40, 50, ...)
- Transitions in relationships (single to married, married to single, loss or gain of family, friends, or others close in network)
- Transitions between jobs or out of jobs (like retirement)
- Transitions in roles (becoming a parent, caregiving for a parent)
- Transitions of environment (moving, increased independence, decreased independence)
- Transitions within the healthcare system (pediatrician to internist, specialist for a health concern/change)

Paying attention to patient factors such as overall developmental stages vs. age is an important component that individualizes needs or important screens. Remember that the primary care setting may be the only place where the patient will encounter an occupational therapist. Use this time wisely and productively, as the occupational therapy lens is unique compared with other professions in PC and community settings. Consider formulating questions in the patient history or initial interview with the patient during an appointment to screen for needs related to transitions across the lifespan.

In cases involving adults, you need to carefully respect their privacy and autonomy by ensuring that you have the patient's permission to discuss their circumstances with anyone else accompanying that patient, including a caregiver. Document this permission in the chart. If the patient comes up in the caregiver's appointment, no specific information can be shared without explicit written authorization from the patient. Instead, discuss the caregiver's needs and how their health may be optimally addressed.

Multiple contexts are addressed in this section, though the list is not comprehensive. This guide intends to facilitate the thought process of the occupational therapist in primary care, prompting them to consider multiple opportunities to facilitate health and wellness in their primary care patients across the lifespan.

Transition From Home to School During Early Years

When a child has been predominantly in the home setting with the primary caregiver influence being the parent, the transition from home to school can be challenging for both the child and the parent [1]. Navigating this time provides multiple opportunities for development in the young child. Level of parent involvement may positively or negatively impact this natural growth and development process. The OTP should screen for developmental concerns for age, coach parents/caregivers and recognize adverse childhood experiences (ACEs) where applicable if the child is suspected of having experienced significant trauma (Table 7.1).

Transition to Adulthood

The transition to adulthood is most often a highly anticipated milestone for both parent/caregiver and child. This transition may occur as early as age 16 in some cases and in others may persist into traditional adult years [4]. It is becoming more common that young adults return home between major transition points, such as college/career, depending on their context. The OT role may include discussion of life skills, current areas of occupational performance (COPM), and mental health status. It may also be important to address this transition with parents/caregivers from their standpoint, making the experience of this milestone a good part of the health inventory for the annual physical exam (Table 7.2).

Table 7.1 Considerations in transitions from home to school

Stakeholders	Formal/informal assessments	Actions/plan
Child	• Developmental screens • Ages and stages (AS-Q) • Observation • ACES (where applicable)	Observe the child's behavior in the office
Parent/caregiver	• Skill checklists for parents/caregivers • Interview • Screen for depression PHQ9 • Screen for anxiety GAQ • Stress (Perceived Stress Scale)	• Discuss transition plan • Interview about experiences with smaller transitions • Acknowledge that transition involves parent as well, provide tools
Teacher/educator	• Developmental screens (refer more comprehensive issues to OP setting or school OT	Handouts about transitions (courtesy of PC practice)

Table 7.2 Considerations in transition to adulthood

Stakeholders	Formal/informal assessments	Actions/plan
Adolescent/ young adult	• Formal or informal inventory of life skills (multiple available online for free.) • COPM • Mental health screens • Screen for depression PHQ9 • Screen for Anxiety GAQ7 • Stress (Perceived Stress Scale) • Global Assessment of Functioning (GAF)	• Discuss future plans • Create planning checklists • Refer to specialists who can facilitate process as needed
Parent/ caregiver	• For caregivers of adolescents/young adults who have a disability that may impact independence, consider using a screen completed by the caregiver to determine the young adult's needs • Screen for depression PHQ9 • Screen for Anxiety GAQ7 • Stress (Perceived Stress Scale) • Global Assessment of Functioning (GAF)	• Discuss readiness for their own transition • Recommend resources for parents/caregivers

Table 7.3 Considerations in transition to higher education or the work place

Stakeholders	Formal/informal assessments	Actions/plan
Adolescent/ young adult	• Formal or informal inventory of life skills (multiple available online for free.) • COPM • Mental health screens • Screen for depression PHQ9 • Screen for Anxiety GAQ7 • Stress (Perceived Stress Scale) • Consider executive function inventory as appropriate • Global Assessment of Functioning (GAF)	• Discuss future plans • Create planning checklists • Refer to specialists who can facilitate process as needed • Talk them through multiple aspects of adulthood
Parent/ caregiver	• For caregivers of adolescents/young adults who have a disability that may impact independence, consider using a screen completed by the caregiver to determine the young adult's needs	• Discuss readiness for their own transition • Recommend resources for parents/caregivers • Online support networks are plentiful and available

Transition to College/Career

Similar to transition to adulthood, transition to a definitive location such as college/technical school or a workplace may warrant attention from the OTP in the primary care setting. Using a screen or inventory assessment such as the BRIEF may be possible in the PC setting. For those who need additional support, referral to occupational therapy in the university setting (a growing emerging area of OT practice) may assist young adults as they make this transition from an academic and personal development standpoint (Table 7.3).

Transition to an Age of Significance (30, 40, 50, …..)

Most people envision milestone ages in their lives based on what is typical in their culture. Milestone ages are often points where your patient will take a personal inventory and compare their lived experience to the "norm" [5]. Their reaction may result in no change or could lead to a crisis or somewhere in between the two. Recognizing milestone ages and asking about the lived experience provides an opportunity for the OTP to anticipate potential areas of wellness that might warrant attention (Table 7.4).

Table 7.4 Considerations in transitions to an age of significance

Stakeholders	Formal/informal assessments	Actions/plan
Patient	• Observation • Screen for mental health changes • COPM if needed • Screen for risk of common ailments per age (repetitive stress injuries, diabetes risk factors, depression) • ACES (prevention) • Relationships/support systems discussion/inventory • Wellness wheel • Screen for depression PHQ9 • Screen for Anxiety GAQ7 • Stress (Perceived Stress Scale) • Global Assessment of Functioning (GAF)	• Target common health issues that emerge at different points in lifespan as well as recognizing new skills/maturing areas per developmental theory • Milestone ages may trigger feelings of depression or regret when life has not progressed as originally envisioned/cultural milestones have not been achieved. Ask the questions
Significant others	• Observe nature of relationship/assess health of relationship through observation and dialogue • Screen for mental health issues	• Provide ways that significant others may be of support where applicable • If facilitating "late" milestones (i.e., adult child with autism leaving home or joining the workforce), follow plan for major life transitions • Do not forget that milestone ages may impact significant others independent of your patient

Transitions in Relationships (Single to Married, Married to Single, Loss or Gain of Family, Friends, or Others Close in Network)

People experience changes in relationships throughout their lifespan. Some of these changes result in very little impact and others may completely disrupt habits and routines [2]. Asking about relationships in the initial patient history/screen gives the OTP an opportunity to identify potential health and wellness risks before they occur, or if they are already present, may alert the team to address the underlying issues (Table 7.5).

Transitions Between Jobs or Out of Jobs (Like Retirement)

Employment (or lack of employment) is a significant source of stress for many adults, especially when others are dependent on them (Miller 2010). It may impact health care on a basic level because of disruption in insurance coverage. There may be opportunities for mitigating risk areas that are especially impacted by stress levels when traditional preventative healthcare use may lapse. Additionally, even with consistent healthcare coverage, changes in employment status impacts habits and routines, identity, and mental health (Table 7.6). OTP knowledge of referral sources that will accept multiple forms of payment or may be free of charge may be advantageous.

Table 7.5 Considerations in transitions in relationships

Stakeholders	Formal/informal assessments	Actions/plan
Patient	• Overall health and mobility • COPM • Screen for depression PHQ9 • Screen for Anxiety GAQ7 • Stress (Perceived Stress Scale) • Global Assessment of Functioning (GAF) • Sleep quality • ACES (per age group)	• Discuss how the patient navigated prior big transitions to predict areas that may need addressing during relationship transition • Collaborate with physician to consider increasing frequency of visits to track patient health and needs under increased stress • Create goals/project health/wellness needs • Identify additional supports/describe types of people to look for as supports
Significant others	Inventory of supports/needs in collaboration with caregiver or independently if brought up in individual appointment	Identify additional supports
Facilitators (therapists/coaches)	TBD based on needs of patient	• Referral to OP OT, life coaches, counselors • Consider encouraging co-treatment of OTP and counselor

Table 7.6 Considerations in transitions between jobs or in retirement

Stakeholders	Formal/informal assessments	Actions/plan
Patient	• Screen for depression PHQ9 • Screen for Anxiety GAQ7 • Stress (Perceived Stress Scale) • Global Assessment of Functioning (GAF) • COPM to identify opportunities to be addressed	Ask about individual identity tied to job • Discuss feelings about transition • Remember that retirement may result in the paradox of freedom and cause great disruption regardless of patient narrative • Key is to keep patient moving forward • Consider referral to OP MH OT, coach, or counselor
Significant others	With permission from patient or when patient is present: Identify observed changes in overall behavior in patient, i.e., lack of routine during day, appearance of boredom, withdrawal from friends/family/activities of interest	TBD based on patient wishes

Table 7.7 Transitions in roles

Stakeholders	Formal/informal assessments	Actions/plan
Patient (who is caring for another person)	• COPM • Assessment of body mechanics and overall function or restriction • Overall physical readiness to assume role • Psychosocial factors/readiness • Screen for depression PHQ9 • Screen for Anxiety GAQ7 • Stress (Perceived Stress Scale) • Global Assessment of Functioning (GAF)	• Review body mechanics • Discuss importance of sleep • Plan positive mental health routines, identify outlets of interest • Identify respite sources • Recognize "stopping points" where need outweighs personal capacity
Other supports	If possible, assess patient body mechanics with caregiving for actual family member	Identify other supports available Create plan for caregiver support

Transitions in Roles (Becoming a Parent, Caregiving for a Parent, Caregiving for an Adult Child)

Parents normally expect to care for the needs of their children based on a typical developmental sequence. At times, when caregiving is initiated (new parenthood) or when caregiving occurs out of sequence (care for a previously independent child/adult, care for an adult child with a disability, care for a parent/caregiver in a reverse of roles), this can create an opportunity for the OTP to examine the situation and offer a holistic overview of potential needs to preserve health and wellness presents itself (Table 7.7).

Transitions in Environment (Moving, Increased Independence, Decreased Independence)

Transitions at the most basic level are disruptions in a person's daily life. When an established environment changes in any way (such as a new arrangement of belongings or inhabitants) or the location completely changes (such as a move between locations, transition to a more/less restrictive environment) regardless of the patient's viewpoint of the change, moves are ranked highly on the Global Assessment of Functioning (GAF) scale [5]. Asking about significant transitions, including a move or change in living context, presents an opportunity for the occupational therapist to recognize and collaborate with the patient and other team members on needs resulting from this very physical transition (Table 7.8).

Transitions in the Healthcare System (Pediatrician to Internist, Specialist for a Health Concern/Change)

Transitioning to a new provider in primary care signals a change in the social context of a client and is important to their overall health and wellbeing. If a client changes location, has a new medical need, or loses a provider, they will need to seek out a new provider.

Considerations for choosing a new provider (Table 7.9):

Table 7.8 Transitions in environment

Stakeholders	Formal/informal assessments	Actions/plan
Patient	• Screen for depression • Observation • COPM • ADL/IADL assessment/inventory (where needed.) • Screen for depression PHQ9 • Screen for Anxiety GAQ7 • Stress (Perceived Stress Scale) • Global Assessment of Functioning (GAF)	• Discuss typical response to change during other major transitions • *Transition to more restrictive environment (ALF/SNF/Hospice):* Facilitate discussion for end of life wishes • *Transition to less restrictive environment (adult transitioning out of parent home):* Facilitate discussion of additional supports that may be needed • Provide information about what to expect/look for
Significant other/ other caregivers	Discussion (where authorized by patient.)	• When patient has provided a release to discuss case with a significant other: • Determine need for OT follow- up for patient • Identify/anticipate additional referrals needed

Table 7.9 Important considerations for occupational therapists who must help clients navigate a medical care transition

Theme	OT assessment/observations	Intervention ideas
Accessibility and inclusion	• Ask about payment sources for medical care • Assess client's ability to arrange for transportation to new location • Assess physical location of building where provider is located for accessibility features needed by client • If needed, is telehealth an option for services? • Does the provider understand the client's cultural context?	• Explore transportation options • Problem-solve perceived accessibility issues • Navigate physical barriers • Role play problem solving cultural issues • Help client advocate for accessibility and inclusion needs
Self-determination/self-advocacy	• Locus of control informal questionnaire (multiple examples available online) • ARC self-determination scale (adolescents with disabilities)—free http://www.ou.edu/education/centers-and-partnerships/zarrow/self-determination-assessment-tools/arc-self-determination-scale • AIR self-determination assessments (student, parent, educator/therapist) free http://www.ou.edu/education/centers-and-partnerships/zarrow/self-determination-assessment-tools/air-self-determination-assessment	• Questioning strategies to help client recognize and understand their needs • Role-play self-advocacy skills • Help client write down or voice memo questions for the provider's office • Discuss needs and how to advocate for/make a plan for attaining those needs
Relative mastery/competence	Relative Mastery Scale	• Role-play client–provider interactions • Help client generate a list of important questions to consider asking their new provider
Satisfaction	Numeric rating scale (0–10) COPM	• Dialogue with patient to set healthcare goals and envision an optimal relationship with their provider/practice • List what is important to them and discuss it

This new provider must have **the skills or specialty** that meet the needs of the client within the **health payment structure** in which they are enrolled. The provider must also be in a location that is **accessible** to the client (via private transportation or public bus system). Even if a provider is located within an accessible location, the physical office might present barriers that are not conducive to the client's needs (e.g., signage is not clear). If it is determined that the provider's office is accessible, it might not be inclusive, due to cultural differences or unconscious bias that is only observed in communication with staff and the provider themselves.

Considerations for establishing rapport with a new provider:

Meeting a new provider involves a number of **social skills** (on both the part of the provider and the client) that will influence whether or not the client is **satisfied** with the new provider and to assess whether there is client–provider fit. The client must feel that they can **determine** and **advocate** for their needs.

Occupational therapists can work with individual clients to address perceived barriers when transitioning to a new provider. They may also have a role in educating providers in how to make their offices more accessible and inclusive.

Summary

Transitional periods of life can be both expected or unexpected, can occur throughout the lifespan, and can bring about changes in the way that an individual engages in their daily life. These changes can disrupt habits, routines, and rituals necessary to engage in important and necessary occupations. The context in which an individual engages can either support or hinder an individual's adaptation through that transition. Occupational therapists, with expert knowledge of transition, can

- Promote healthy transitions through education and targeted support;
- Assist individuals in the establishment of healthy habits, routines, and rituals;
- Help individuals in restoring necessary and desired occupations;
- Modify the environment for successful engagement in occupations; and
- Help the client learn how to compensate for performance skills deficits that prevent participation and engagement in important and necessary occupations.

Occupational therapy practitioners have the skills to intervene with and advocate for individuals in the process of transition so that individuals can thrive during and after important life transitions.

References

1. Orentlicher M, Schefkind S, Gibson R, editors. Transitions across the lifespan: an occupational therapy approach. North Bethesda: AOTA Press; 2015.
2. Schlossberg NK, Waters EB, Goodman J. Counseling adults in transition. 2nd ed. New York: Springer; 1995.
3. American Occupational Therapy Association. Occupational therapy practice framework: domain and process. Am J Occup Ther. 2020;74(Supplement 2):7412410010. https://doi.org/10.5014/ajot.2020.74S2001.
4. Arnett JJ. Emerging adulthood: a theory of development from the late teens through the twenties. Am Psychol. 2000;55(5):469–80. https://doi.org/10.1037/0003-066x.55.5.469.
5. Miller TM, editor. Handbook of stressful transitions across the lifespan. New York: Springer; 2010.

Part II
Conditions Addressed by Occupational Therapy in Primary Care

Chapter 8
Addiction and Substance Use Recovery

Nicole Villegas

Introduction

Substance use, behavioral engagement and addictions observably impact occupational performance. As an OTP, you have the foundational tools to assess the impact of unhealthy substance use and/or behavioral engagement on daily life and support clients to make changes for their wellness. These changes can improve performance and satisfaction in roles, habits, and routines, within the recovery process. "Recovery is a process of change through which people improve their health and wellness, live self-directed lives, and strive to reach their full potential" [1].

- **Substance Use and Addiction:** The Diagnostic and Statistical Manual of Mental Disorders (DSM-5) provides classification and diagnostic guidance for substance-related and addictive disorders for the following 10 classes of drugs *(repetitive use of substance(s) despite negative consequences in daily life, due to physiological and/or behavioral dependence)* [2]:

  - Alcohol
  - Caffeine
  - Cannabis
  - Hallucinogens
  - Inhalants
  - Opioids
  - Sedatives, hypnotics, and anxiolytics
  - Stimulants (amphetamine-type substances, cocaine, and other stimulants)
  - Tobacco
  - Other (or unknown) substances

N. Villegas (✉)
Boston University, Boston, MA, USA
e-mail: nlvilleg@bu.edu

© Springer Nature Switzerland AG 2023
S. Dahl-Popolizio et al. (eds.), *Primary Care Occupational Therapy*,
https://doi.org/10.1007/978-3-031-20882-9_8

- **Behavioral Engagement and Addiction:** Growing evidence highlights areas of potential behavioral addiction *(repetitive engagement in behavior(s) despite negative consequences in daily life, due to physiological and/or behavioral dependence)* [2–5].

  - Gambling disorder (classified in the DSM-5)
  - Kleptomania (classified in the DSM-5)
  - Technology use (computer game, internet, social networks)
  - Working
  - Pornography
  - Exercise
  - Food
  - Other repetitive behaviors with negative consequences

- **The Mechanisms of Addiction:** The human brain is wired for a reward system, evolutionarily supporting basic needs such as eating, procreating, and social interaction. Drugs and some repetitive behaviors activate the brain's reward system and elicit feedback in the form of pleasure, euphoria, and increased energy, and/or analgesic, anesthetic, or "numbed out" effects; these experiences can be described as a "high." The physiological understanding of this process continues to evolve within neuroscience; up-to-date research can provide details on current understandings [6]. The effects of these drugs and behaviors can have a negative impact on engagement in meaningful occupations. People may engage in them despite negative consequences, leading to neglect of adaptive daily life activities and the preoccupation of engagement with the substance or behavior. This complex interaction between brain chemistry, genetics, psychosocial experience, trauma history, environment and occupational engagement can lead to addiction. Like other chronic and persistent health conditions, people in recovery can explore various treatment options, experience relapse, and live in remission.

- **Prevention:**

  - Diagnosable substance use disorders and mental disorders are likely to appear on the clients' diagnosis list, but this requires the substance use or engagement in behavior is at a level that meets the DSM-5 criteria or is otherwise determined by the PCP to fit the diagnosis codes. Clients with symptoms or behaviors that do not qualify for a formal diagnosis may benefit from preventative OT services to decrease substance use or decrease the behavioral engagement that is negatively impacting their daily lives.

    Through a prevention lens, providers may consider the areas of behavior change within the continuum of *nonuse* and addiction. As demonstrated by Fig. 8.1: *Continuum of Nonuse and Addiction*, all designations of use and engagement are connected to each other and based on occupational engagement within the recovery process. The highlighted area between

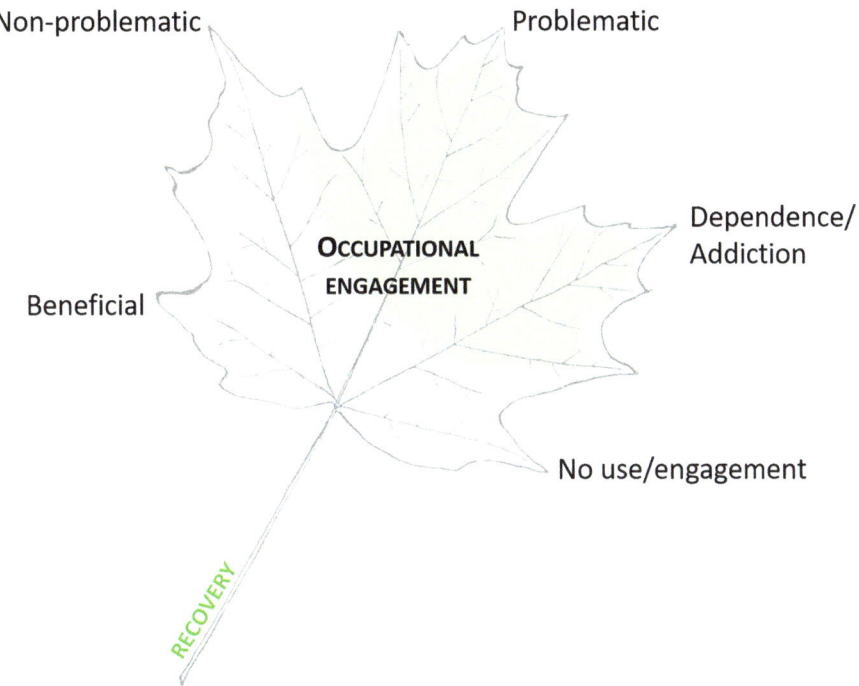

Fig. 8.1 Continuum of nonuse and addiction

Nonproblematic and *Dependence/Addiction* designates areas of prevention where brief intervention and treatment is most likely to result in
behavior change. Intervention at this level can decrease risk of related
chronic comorbidities. Prevention efforts and treatment approaches for
addiction are generally as successful as those for other chronic diseases [7].

Role of the PCP

- The PCP can be the first provider to identify a potential substance use issue. A
  widely used approach to early intervention is called Screening, Brief Intervention,
  and Referral to Treatment (SBIRT) [8]. Screening assesses severity of use, brief
  intervention includes conversation-based intervention for motivation toward
  behavior change, and referrals are made to appropriate specialty care. PCPs will
  also manage any prescribed medications or outside referrals and will collaborate
  with the other team members to ensure client needs are met.

- **Screening:** PC services may have established protocols for screening for substance use disorder. If not, advocate for universal screening to decrease stigma of substance use, addiction and recovery; it can increase likelihood that clients will explore this area with their PCP even if it was not their main reason for seeking care in a given visit.
- **Brief Intervention:** Client-centered discussion of screening scores; education on clinical criteria for substance-use disorders and impacts on health; motivational interviewing to elicit behavior change; and goal setting.
- **Referral to Treatment:** The client may be directed immediately to a higher level of care if their need is a safety concern or an emergency. Clients may also be referred to any of the following resources.

   Medication Assisted Treatment (MAT): The PCP may manage MAT to address biological mechanisms of addiction by relieving withdrawal symptoms and interrupting cravings. The ability of the PCP to prescribe certain medications may depend on the practice setting's governing body and certification (e.g., SAMHSA-certified Opioid Treatment Programs) [6].

   In-house OT, other behavioral health providers, social workers, addictions specialists, or peer mentors/support specialists.

   Services outside of the setting, including community-based services that range from outpatient care to in-patient treatment. Friends, family, or community members of the client may also be referred to community-based support.

Common Comorbidities

- People living in recovery of substance use disorders and/or behavioral addictions are likely to have multiple comorbidities. They are at risk for polysubstance use and living in environments that support continued substance use. The complex relationship of substance use or behavioral engagement despite negative consequences may lead to negative physical, social, and occupational impacts.
- Comorbidities of substance use include [9, 10]:

   - Diabetes (Chap. 19)
   - Hypertension (Chap. 26)
   - Chronic Obstructive Pulmonary Disorder (COPD) (Chap. 13)
   - Liver disease
   - Osteoporosis
   - Certain types of cancer
   - Mental disorders (co-occurring disorder)
   - Often occurring alongside and resulting from trauma (Chap. 6)
   - Related to subsequent physical injury, sleep disturbances and insomnia, poor pain management (Chaps. 27, 34).

- Comorbidities of behavioral engagement and addiction may also include:
  - Mental disorders
  - Subsequent injuries, such as repetitive strain injury (RSI) (Chap. 35)
  - Vision impairments (Chap. 36)
  - Self-neglect
  - May not present physical cues of relapse or overuse like substance use

Role of the OTP

OTPs are distinctly skilled to address behavior change to prevent compounding negative impacts on daily life and enhance occupational engagement in meaningful roles and activities. In PC, they do this in brief interactions and in collaboration with the PCP.

Occupational Impact

- The consequences of substance use and behavioral engagement have the potential to impact all areas of occupation, with varying degrees.
- Addiction as occupation: the activities of obtaining, using, and experiencing substances are occupations that the person engages in [11].

  - Within the continuum of nonuse and addiction, a person may utilize various resources to fill their needs to obtain a substance or maintain a behavior. These resources may impact financial management, home maintenance, ability to care for others, or meet their basic ADL needs.
  - Areas of occupation that enhance quality of life may be neglected, such as engagement in school, work, or leisure.
  - Most often, friends, family, or community will experience relationship changes with the client; this occupational impact may ultimately support recovery or continued use.

OT Areas of Emphasis

- **Distinct OTP skills include:** activity analysis, occupation-based interventions, and integrating understanding of client factors and systems on daily life activity. The OTP can provide valuable consultation to the clinical team about the impacts of the substance or behavior on areas of occupation, especially as they relate to other health maintenance and management outcomes. The OTP can help the client to:

- understand the relationships between the substance use or other behavior choices with all other aspects of their life, including the beneficial and detrimental impacts of these choices.
- develop systems within their relationships, communities, and occupations that are supportive of recovery.
- strengthen skills in self-regulation, advocacy, and utilizing support for recovery.

- **Therapeutic Use of Self:**

  - **Self-reflection**: Structural violence, trauma, and stigma are few of the barriers impacting engagement in medical care, especially care for substance and behavioral addictions. As an OTP in PC, you have the valuable opportunity to provide a therapeutic interaction and relationship with clients to facilitate healing and promote continued engagement in health care. Before meeting with clients, it is helpful to reflect on your own implicit and explicit biases that may get in the way of compassionate, trauma-informed care. Post-session reflection can aid in continued professional development.

    The following questions provide structure for self-preparation:

H	How can I bring genuine positive regard, **Hope**, and praise into the session?
U	How can I make sure that we (client and therapist) have shared **Understanding** of our meeting?
L	How can I remember to **Listen** more than I talk?
A	How can I pay careful **Attention** to my client?

- **Client Autonomy and Self-Identification:**

  - Your client is the expert of their experience. When listening to their descriptions and explanations, take note of the words they use to self-identify. Ensure that you have a shared understanding of their meaning and use their chosen words.

    Example: "I notice that you describe yourself as 'an addict.' Please describe what being 'an addict' means to you....Is it okay with you if I use the word 'addict' too?"

Evaluation

- Commonly used alcohol and drug screening tools in the United States

  - Pre-screen questions asked by PCP

    How many times in the past year have you used an illegal drug or used a prescription medication for nonmedical reasons?
    How many times in the past year have you had four or more drinks in a day?

- AUDIT, or Alcohol Use Disorders Test

    10-item questionnaire
    Free, available online (https://nida.nih.gov/sites/default/files/audit.pdf)

- DAST/DAST-10, or Drug Abuse Screening Test, 10 items

    10-item questionnaire
    Free, available online (https://cde.drugabuse.gov/instrument/e9053390-ee9c-9140-e040-bb89ad433d69)

• Screening tools emphasizing impact on daily life and stages of change

- CAGE Questionnaire for Alcohol Misuse (Criticism, Annoyed, Guilty, Eye-opener)

    4-item questionnaire
    Free, available online (https://www.hopkinsmedicine.org/johns_hopkins_healthcare/downloads/all_plans/CAGE%20Substance%20Screening%20Tool.pdf)

- RAFFT Screening Tool (Relax, Alone, Friends, Family, Trouble)

    5-item provider administered questionnaire
    Free, available online (https://www.porticonetwork.ca/web/knowledgex-archive/amh-specialists/screening-for-cd-in-youth/screening-sud/rafft)

- Readiness to Change Questionnaire for Alcohol Misuse

    12-item questionnaire
    Free, available online from the National Drug and Alcohol Research Centre (https://ndarc.med.unsw.edu.au/sites/default/files/ndarc/resources/TR.019.pdf)

• Comorbid Screening

- GAD-7—General Anxiety Disorder 7

    7-item questionnaire
    Free, available online (https://adaa.org/sites/default/files/GAD-7_Anxiety-updated_0.pdf)

- PHQ-9—Patient Health Questionnaire 9 (Depression Screen)

    9-item questionnaire
    Free, available online (https://www.apa.org/depression-guideline/patient-health-questionnaire.pdf) or access *PHQ-9* in "Appendix"

- Example session outline

Ask permission	Ask the client's permission to discuss the PCPs assessment and the agreed upon plan to speak with you
Complete screens	With permission from the client, proceed with a full screen or follow- up questions to completed screens
Assess occupational impact Listen for areas of change talk	Explore occupational impact: • Ask *how do you spend your time? What roles are important to you?* • Inquire about activities, roles, habits, and routines impacted by substance use and/or behavioral engagement Explore use/engagement directly: • Ask *"What are the good things about your [substance use/ behavioral engagement]? What are the not so good things about it?"* Focus on occupational performance • Ask *"Have you previously thought about cutting back or quitting?" "If you cut back or quit, how would [engagement in occupation] change?"*
Provide feedback Elicit change talk	Provide trauma-informed feedback on results of screen, assessments, and clinical analysis of conversation. Assess for shared understanding Elicit change talk through motivational interviewing techniques. • Describe *"based on your answers on the screens and your descriptions of your daily life, it sounds like…[occupational impact]."*
Provide education and guidance on occupational performance	When the client expresses readiness to hearing education and suggestions, provide guidance on next steps to promote change toward recovery
Identify immediate next step Identify goal(s)	Ask *"If you were to make a change today, what would be your first step?"*
Closing	Collaboratively summarize session, reinforce client strengths, instill hope for change, and arrange follow-up • Ask *"What are the main takeaways of our conversation today?"* Share your summary • Review next steps for both client and therapist

Intervention Strategies

Suggested client interaction strategies and intervention tools with examples:

- **Make It Concrete** *(realistic, detailed, observable).*

    - Write down relevant facts of discussion (client or therapist, depending on client factors).
    - Focus on one activity or area of occupation to address.
    - Use visuals to orient and guide the conversation.

        Printout of the 8 Dimensions of Wellness.

    – Identify immediate next steps for progress.

> On the way home today, I will buy two beers and a flavored seltzer instead of three beers.
> Today, I will start using the alarm we set and enjoy my last caffeinated beverage between 4:00 p.m. and 5:00 p.m.

    – Set up tools for adherence to plan based on client factors.

> Phone alarms, reminder note in wallet,

    – Identify and/or set up social supports.
    – Set a clear plan for the next encounter (call, in-office appointment) to support follow through.

- **Addiction and Trauma Education.**

    – Provide education in a trauma-informed model to normalize experience and continue to establish trust and rapport.

> "What we know about trauma/addiction is _____ because/ to ____."

    - Example: What we know about trauma is that trauma survivors often started using substances to either prevent feeling greater pain, to feel something at all, or because it was forced onto them.

> "For people who experience trauma/addiction it can be difficult/supportive to_____"

    - Example: For people who experience addiction, it can be supportive to have someone in our life who is living in remission and can share their experience.

- **Stages of Change and Motivational Interviewing.**

    – Stages of Change: Prochaska and Diclemente's Six Stages of Change (https://tnchildren.org/wp-content/uploads/2014/11/Stages-of-Change.pdf).   See 'Appendix' for *Stages of Change* instructional handout for OTPs.
    – Motivational Interviewing: (https://www.ihs.gov/california/tasks/sites/default/assets/File/BP2015-4_TeachingSBIRTFacultyGuideSession3Part2.pdf).

> See 'Appendix' for *Motivational Interviewing* assessment tool.

- **Explore Coping Skills and Meaningful Activity.**

    – Engaging in substance use or other repetitive unhealthy behavior often serves as a primary coping skill. How will clients manage occupational performance changes, stress, or other triggers without their substance or behavior? How will they grieve the loss of the substance or behavior? [12]. This is an opportunity to enhance current supportive occupational engagement, re-introduce meaningful occupations from the past, or introduce new skills, activities, or occupations.

- Cognitive Behavioral Therapy (CBT) provides an approach to guiding clients in identifying antecedents and consequences to behaviors; it can help clients identify and utilize alternate coping tools to address antecedents before substance use or behavioral engagement. OTP education about the approach may be beneficial for skilled inclusion of CBT-based skill building during brief treatment [13].
- For many people who have experienced trauma and/or who use substances or behaviors to cope, it may be difficult to notice and identify a large range of emotions. For instance, a person may only identify *anger* and *happiness* as their emotions. A skilled OTP can cue for further identification of emotions to assist the client in exploring areas for change, as it relates to their roles and occupations. This is done through mutual trust and positive reinforcement of exploration. Visual aids may be beneficial to demonstrate an array of emotions.

- **Interoception and Self-reflection** [14, 15]

  - Interoception, or one's sense of the internal state of the body, may be impaired for this population due to trauma or repetitive, unhealthy engagement in substance or behavior. Interoceptive awareness can be practiced and utilized as additional information to aid in decision making.
  - Enhanced interoceptive awareness can help clients have more immediate information about their body's experience and needs. This information can inform health decisions, including use of substances or behaviors to self soothe.
  - For instance, a client may learn that engaging in a phone call with their primary support person helps them feel a sense of calm in their body (e.g., decreased heart rate, relaxed shoulders) and they may choose to call the support person to gain those effects.
  - It is important that OTPs utilizing this approach are skilled in understanding sensory systems and trauma-informed care. Strengths and impairments in clients' metacognition and executive function must be considered when providing interventions in interception skill building.

Other Considerations and Resources

Documentation and Billing

- Refer to the *Administrative and Operational Considerations* chapter for more information regarding reimbursable codes (Chap. 3).
- Codes for preventative counseling, smoking cessation counseling, AUDIT/ DAST, health risk assessment test, health behavior assessment and intervention may be billed. SBIRT provided by an OTP may be reimbursed through Medicare/ Medicaid incident to billing. See state-specific guidelines.

- OTPs may bill for frequently used treatment codes, such as therapeutic activity, as they relate to management of chronic disease diagnoses.
- Direct care services provided by OTPs may be paid out-of-pocket or using health savings account (HSA) or flexible savings account (FSA) funds. See direct access states, licensing board, and state-specific guidelines.

Suggested Referrals

- Appropriate referrals may include:
    - Behavioral health, social work, peer groups, treatment centers, outpatient programs, and community-based support groups and resources
- Build your toolbox
    - Establish relationships with community-based organizations for treatment outside of PC. This will help make the transition for clients as easy as possible, increasing likelihood that they will follow through with instructions.
    - Gather information about digital therapeutics: phone and computer applications for reminders, coaching, and peer-support communities for recovery.

Additional Resources

- Substance Abuse and Mental Health Services Administration
    - https://www.samhsa.gov
    - 1-800-662-HELP (4357)
- Practice resources
    - SBIRT:

        https://www.thenationalcouncil.org/program/center-of-excellence/
        https://www.masbirt.org/besst

    - Core Addictions Practice—Participant's Resource Guide, available from:

        https://collaborativetoolbox.ca/

- Trauma-informed practices.
    - https://traumainformedoregon.org/
- Find therapists, treatment centers.
    - https://findtreatment.gov/
    - https://www.psychologytoday.com/us/therapists

References

1. U.S. Department of Health and Human Services, Substance Abuse and Mental Health Services Administration. Recovery and recovery support. https://www.sanhsa.gov/find-help/recovery.
2. American Psychiatric Association. Diagnostic and statistical manual of mental disorders. 5th ed. Washington, DC: American Psychiatric Association; 2013. https://doi.org/10.1176/appi.books.9780890425596.
3. Alavi SS, Ferdosi M, Jannatifard F, Eslami M, Alaghemandan H, Setare M. Behavioral addiction versus substance addiction: correspondence of psychiatric and psychological views. Int J Prev Med. 2012;3(4):290–4.
4. Alimoradi Z, Lin CY, Broström A, Bülow PH, Bajalan Z, Griffiths MD, Ohayon MM, Pakpour AH. Internet addiction and sleep problems: a systematic review and meta-analysis. Sleep Med Rev. 2019;47:51–61. https://doi.org/10.1016/j.smrv.2019.06.004.
5. Journal of Behavioral Addictions. AK Journals. 2012–2020. https://akjournals.com/view/journals/2006/2006-overview.xml.
6. Volkow ND, Boyle M. Neuroscience of addiction: relevance to prevention and treatment. Am J Psychiatr. 2018;175(8):729–40. https://doi.org/10.1176/appi.ajp.2018.17101174.
7. NIDA. Principles of drug addiction treatment: a research-based guide (third edition). 2018. https://www.drugabuse.gov/publications/principles-drug-addiction-treatment-research-based-guide-third-edition.
8. Pace CA, Uebelacker LA. Addressing unhealthy substance use in primary care. Med Clin N Am. 2018;102(4):567–86. https://doi.org/10.1016/j.mcna.2018.02.004.
9. NIDA. Common comorbidities with substance use disorders. 2020. https://www.drugabuse.gov/node/pdf/1155/common-comorbidities-with-substance-use-disorders.
10. John WS, Zhu H, Mannelli P, Schwartz RP, Subramaniam GA, Wu LT. Prevalence, patterns, and correlates of multiple substance use disorders among adult primary care patients. Drug Alcohol Depend. 2018;187:79–87. https://doi.org/10.1016/J.DRUGALCDEP.2018.01.035.
11. Bonsaksen T. Addiction as occupation? Br J Occup Ther. 2015;78(3):205–6. https://doi.org/10.1177/0308022615575025.
12. Chambers RA, Wallingford SC. On mourning and recovery: integrating stages of grief and change toward a neuroscience-based model of attachment adaptation in addiction treatment. Psychodyn Psychiatry. 2017;45(4):451–74. https://doi.org/10.1521/pdps.2017.45.4.451.
13. Institute for Quality and Efficiency in Health Care (IQWiG). Cognitive behavioral therapy. Köln: IQWiG; 2016.
14. Paulus MP, Stewart JL. Interoception and drug addiction. Neuropharmacology. 2014;76(PART B):342–50. https://doi.org/10.1016/j.neuropharm.2013.07.002.
15. Price CJ, Hooven C. Interoceptive awareness skills for emotion regulation: theory and approach of mindful awareness in body-oriented therapy (MABT). Front Psychol. 2018;9:1–12. https://doi.org/10.3389/fpsyg.2018.00798.

Chapter 9
Alzheimer's Disease

Katelyn Fell and Jyothi Gupta

Introduction

Alzheimer's disease (AD) is a degenerative neurocognitive disorder typically seen in older adults, with first symptoms appearing in the mid-60s. Memory and executive functions of the brain deteriorate and impact everyday activities depending on the severity. In severe forms, the individual cannot recognize family members and the individual becomes totally dependent on a caregiver for everyday functioning. AD is characterized by abnormal clumps called amyloid plaques and tangles of neurofibrillary elements with tau protein. Neuronal connections are also compromised, and this impacts the ability of the brain to process information [1, 2].

Sub-Types

- **Early onset AD (young-onset)** is an uncommon form of AD affecting people younger than age 65 and is thought to occur in about 5–6% of individuals with AD [3].

    - Early onset AD is identified as either sporadic (not caused by genetics) or familial (likely to run in families) [3].
    - Familial type early onset AD has been linked to a genetic mutation of one of three genes (APP, PSEN 1, and PSEN 2) [3]. Genetic testing for these mutations is available.

K. Fell (✉)
University of St. Augustine for Health Sciences, St. Augustine, FL, USA
e-mail: kfell@usa.edu

J. Gupta
University of Texas Medical Branch, Galveston, TX, USA
e-mail: jygupta@utmb.edu

© Springer Nature Switzerland AG 2023
S. Dahl-Popolizio et al. (eds.), *Primary Care Occupational Therapy*,
https://doi.org/10.1007/978-3-031-20882-9_9

Mild vs. Major Neurocognitive Disorder (NCD) Due to AD

The fifth edition of the *Diagnostic and Statistical Manual of Mental Disorders* further describes NCD as *major* NCD or *mild* NCD [4].

- **Mild NCD:** Diagnostic criteria for *mild* NCD include a modest decline in cognitive function that does not interfere with the capacity for independence in everyday activities [4].
- **Major NCD:** Diagnostic criteria for *major* NCD includes significant cognitive decline which interferes with independence in everyday activities [4]. *Major* NCD is further categorized by the severity of symptoms using the terms *mild* (impacting IADL performance), *moderate* (impacting both ADL and IADL performance), and *severe* (dependence in both ADL and IADLs) [4, 5].

Disease Stages

Most commonly, AD is described as progressing through three primary stages: early, middle, and late stages. A seven-point Global Deterioration Scale (GDS) may be used for more clinically and diagnostically complex assessments [6]. The progression and clinical presentation of AD varies significantly for each individual, though usually appears in a hierarchical pattern [6]. Early stages present with more mild impairment in higher level cognitive functions and memory, resulting in decreased ability to perform IADLs or complex work, leisure, or driving tasks. Middle stages may result in further declines impacting the individual's ability to effectively complete ADLs and basic self-care tasks. Later stages result in significant impairment in both cognitive and motor functions, requiring assistance from caregivers for functional mobility and self-care, with progressive impairment in language and communication skills as well [6].

Stages [7]

- **Preclinical AD**
    - No outward symptoms visible at this stage
    - Imaging may identify the presence of amyloid-beta deposits in the brain

- **Mild Cognitive Impairment (MCI) due to AD**
    - Mild cognitive changes that do not significantly impact daily functioning

- **Mild Dementia due to AD (Early)**

  – Decreased short-term memory, complex problem-solving, word finding
  – Personality changes including being withdrawn, irritability, apathy
  – May require assistance with IADLs (financial management, household management, medication management, shopping, managing appointments)

- **Moderate Dementia due to AD (Middle)**

  – Increasingly poor judgment and confusion, greater memory loss
  – May require assistance with ADLs (dressing, bathing, toileting, grooming, feeding)

- **Severe Dementia due to AD (Late)**

  – Requires assistance with all self-care and mobility
  – Loss of communication skills
  – Difficulty swallowing

Role of PCP

There is currently no effective treatment to cure or reverse the disease course for AD. However, early recognition and diagnosis is important to intervene with appropriate referrals in the earliest stages of the disease and allow for the individual to remain in the community for as long as possible, before requiring a higher level of care or institutionalization [6]. Medical management should include identifying and treating other conditions which might further exacerbate symptoms and disability [6]. Finally, the primary focus should be to maximize function and independence, establish a safe environment, and reduce behavior disturbances through patient and family education, and also engagement of all members of the primary care team.

Common Comorbidities

- Anxiety (Chap. 11)
- Depression (Chap. 18)
- Delirium

Suggested Referrals
- Geropsychologist
- OT
- Physical therapy (PT)
- Speech language pathologist
- Support groups

Role of OTP

The role of an OTP in working with individuals with AD in PC includes using a client-centered approach which emphasizes the client's abilities rather than focusing on impairment. OTPs do this by providing actionable strategies that can be employed and modified as needed, across the lifespan.

Occupational Impact

Due to the progressive nature and impact on cognitive, motor, and behavioral functioning, AD greatly impacts occupational performance. Early stages of the disease may involve only mild cognitive impairments, resulting in declining IADL function while maintaining independence with ADLs. As the disease progresses, further decline in cognitive, motor, and behavioral functioning will result in decreased:

- ability to perform ADLs and further loss of ability with IADLs
- functional mobility
- leisure
- social participation

The primary symptoms of AD impact occupational abilities and include impaired memory and new learning. Individuals may also experience a gradual decline in other cognitive domains and exhibit behavioral symptoms [4].

- Cognitive symptoms [4]:
  - Complex attention: sustained, selective, divided, processing speed.
  - Executive function: planning, decision making, sequencing, working memory, error correction
  - Learning and memory: short-term, long-term, reasoning, comprehension, orientation
  - Language: expressive, receptive, word finding, fluency, and rhythm.
  - Perceptual motor: visual perception, visual-constructional, praxis, proprioception, balance, postural control, hand–eye coordination, bilateral integration, FMC, GMC
  - Social cognition: recognition of emotions, body language, understanding social norms
- Mood and behavioral symptoms [8]:
  - Depression (Chap. 18)
  - Apathy
  - Agitation
  - Psychotic features
  - Combativeness
  - Wandering

OT Areas of Emphasis

OTPs facilitate continued participation in meaningful occupations and address quality of life across the disease continuum for those living both in the community and in long-term care settings. As the disease progresses and memory and new learning decline, incorporating the individual's past life experiences and roles may be helpful in engaging the client and enhancing participation [9]. Establishing a daily routine may also help to reduce behavioral outbursts and enhance participation. Throughout the course of the disease process, OTPs will:

- Facilitate participation in meaningful occupations.
- Make recommendations for appropriate durable medical equipment (DME), adaptive equipment, or assistive devices as needed.
- Consider functional mobility and community mobility needs.
- Address upper extremity function/coordination.
- Provide caregiver and family education/training.
- Educate on community resources including support groups, transportation, and exercise/activity classes.

Evaluation

A comprehensive evaluation which assesses cognition, motor function, and psychosocial components of the individual is vital. Developing an occupational profile will provide information about specific client factors and contexts which may support or hinder performance. Additionally, frequent functional reassessment is necessary as the disease progresses and the needs of the individual change. With an OT on the PC team, this can be done frequently as the client is seen in the PC office for issues other than their AD. Addressing these issues in PC also facilitates communication among the PC team members.

Areas of Assessment

Due to cognitive impairment associated with AD, the cognitive and perceptual requirements of any given assessment must be considered by the OTP. Depending on the stage of the disease, some assessments may not be appropriate. When possible, we have included links to sites where you can find assessments. Many of these assessments can also be obtained through Shirley Ryan Abilities Lab website.

- Cognitive function (memory, new learning, executive functions, attention)
    - Montreal Cognitive Assessment (MoCa), Mini Mental Status Exam (MMSE), Mini-Cog, Allen Cognitive Level (ACL), Cognitive Performance Test,

Executive Function Performance Test, Cognitive Assessment of Minnesota, Routine Task Inventory-Expanded

- Fine Motor Coordination
  - 9 Hole Peg Test, Minnesota Rate of Manipulation Test, Purdue Pegboard, Jebson Hand Function Test
- Gait and Balance
  - Timed Up and Go (TUG), Berg Balance Scale, Tinetti, Activities-Specific Balance Confidence Scale, Five Times Sit to Stand Test, Functional Reach Test
- Psychosocial Components
  - Functional Behavior Profile, WHOQol-BREF, Patient Health Questionnaire (PHQ-9). See Appendix for *PHQ-9*, Beck Depression Inventory, Cornell Scale for Depression in Dementia, Geriatric Depression Scale
- ADLs Performance
  - Canadian Occupational Performance Measure (COPM), Barthel Index, Kohlman Evaluation of Living Skills (KELS), Assessment of Motor and Process Skills
  - ADL Situation Test, Katz Activities of Daily Living, Assessment of Motor and Process Skills (AMPS), Performance Assessment of Self-Care Skills
- IADL
  - Direct Assessment of Functional Abilities, Kitchen Task Assessment, Lawton Instrumental Activities of Daily Living Scale, Independent Living Scale

Other Considerations for Assessment

- Hearing and vision: additional sensory impairments may result in further functional deficits [6, 10].
- Communication abilities
- Feeding and swallowing abilities
- Home modification needs
- Social support systems
- Community resources
- End-of-life care

Intervention Strategies

Specific OT interventions will vary depending on the stage of the disease process and the individual needs of the client. OT intervention may include the following, as appropriate for the stage of the disease:

- Activity modification and use of adaptive equipment
- Cognitive skills; memory supports
- Routine management/establishment
- Functional mobility training
- Home exercise program (flexibility, functional strength training, endurance)
- Leisure exploration
- Family and caregiver education/training
- End-of-life care

Mild Stage

Mild memory impairment, word finding difficulties, or complex problem solving may be impaired at this stage. Routine ADLs such as dressing, bathing, and grooming are likely to remain intact, while more complex IADL tasks, such as managing finances, home management, driving in unfamiliar environments, or medication management, may be performed with less accuracy, efficiency, or safety due to cognitive symptoms.

These individuals may still live independently in the community and therefore benefit from training in memory strategies, establishment of routines, home safety assessments, and identification of IADL tasks, such as meal preparation, shopping, and transportation, that may require activity modification or assistance from caregivers and other support services. Use of environmental memory aids and visual cues such as calendars, signs, and notebooks may be effective compensatory strategies for improving occupational performance [5, 6].

Promoting physical activity including aerobic, balance, and resistance training may help to improve or maintain ADL performance, functional mobility, and sleep [5].

Leisure and social participation may become more difficult during this stage of AD. Providing opportunities and encouraging caregivers/others to initiate socialization may allow for continued participation and help the individual to maintain a positive self-concept despite experiencing changes in cognitive and motor function [6].

New, complex learning may be difficult at this stage. Use of errorless learning techniques has been shown to be effective in improving occupational performance [5]. Caregiver education and training on use of simple and direct instructions may improve communication between the individual and caregiver. Establishing a support network is important as the disease progresses and the individual will likely require increased assistance from caregivers. Caregiver training and education on strategies to allow the greatest levels of independence, while fostering a safe environment is a primary goal.

Moderate Stage

Individuals in the moderate stage of AD are not safe to live independently. The progression of cognitive impairment is likely to impact even routine ADL functions and individuals may require assistance or cueing from caregivers for accurate completion of daily tasks such as feeding, dressing, toileting, and bathing. There may also be changes in sleep and wake cycles including night-time wandering. Caregiver education on sleep hygiene, adequate physical activity during the day, reducing environmental stimuli, and addressing safety precautions related to wandering is beneficial [5].

Most IADLs are too complex for the individual to complete independently, though with assistance and activity modifications, participation is still possible and should be encouraged when safe to do so. Social and leisure participation is further impaired and may be limited to activities that do not require complex problem-solving, decision-making, or initiation.

Safety awareness, judgment, and the ability to self correct may be impaired. Caregiver education is necessary regarding falls prevention, recommendations for appropriate assistive devices, assistance with mobility, DME, and grab bar placement throughout the home. Use of unobtrusive safety measures (e.g., camouflaged doors or silent electronic locks) may be helpful in reducing exit attempts by the client when wandering [5]. Changes in visuospatial skills including depth perception, positioning, and figure ground also increase risk for falls and accidents at the moderate stage. Removal of clutter from the environment and making important amenities (e.g., the toilet) highly visible is beneficial [5].

Communication skills are significantly impacted at this stage, making social interactions, expression of needs, and communication with caregivers even more challenging. Caregiver education on communication strategies and problem solving to help manage problem behaviors (agitation, combativeness) is vital for both the individual and caregiver [6]. Maintaining daily routines and consistencies within the environment are important for participation in overlearned tasks [6]. Routines should consist of not just ADLs and meal times but also time for exercise and physical activity, social interaction, leisure, relaxation and rest, and caregiver respite.

Severe Stage

Every aspect of cognitive functioning is impacted at this stage of the disease. Individuals require assistance with all self care and mobility. Motor skills and voluntary movement is limited, placing the individual at risk for development of contractures and pressure injuries. Caregiver education and assessment of positioning is important both for the individual's comfort and to mitigate the effects of immobility. Feeding and swallowing may also become severely impaired. Caregiver education and training on safe positioning and feeding strategies to reduce the risk for aspiration is important [6]. Communication is severely impaired and speech may be limited to only a few words, moaning, or other vocalizations. These may be expressions of discomfort, pain, or an unmet need and should therefore be assessed. OT may be involved in end-of-life care which should focus on positioning, pain management, and quality of life.

Other Considerations and Resources

See above.

References

1. National Institute on Aging. Alzheimers disease fact sheet. 2019. https://www.nia.nih.gov/health/alzheimers-disease-fact-sheet.
2. National Institute on Aging. Causes of Alzheimer's disease: what happens to the brain in Alzheimer's disease? https://www.nia.nih.gov/health/what-happens-brain-alzheimers-disease.
3. Mayo Clinic. Young-onset Alzheimer's: when symptoms begin before age 65. 2020. mayoclinic.org. https://www.mayoclinic.org/diseases-conditions/lewy-body-dementia/diagnosis-treatment/drc-20352030.
4. American Psychiatric Association. Diagnostic and statistical manual of mental disorders. 5th ed. Washington, DC: American Psychiatric Association; 2013. https://doi.org/10.1176/appi.books.9780890425596.
5. Piersol CV, Jensen L. Occupational therapy practice guidelines for adults with Alzheimer's disease and related major neurocognitive disorders. North Bethesda: AOTA Press; 2017. https://doi.org/10.7139/2017.978-1-56900-408-1.
6. Pendleton HM, Schultz-Krohn W. Pedretti's occupational therapy: practice skills for physical dysfunction. 8th ed. Amsterdam: Elsevier; 2018.
7. Mayo Clinic. Alzheimer's stages: how the disease progresses. 2019. mayoclinic.org. https://www.mayoclinic.org/diseases-conditions/alzheimers-disease/in-depth/alzheimers-stages/art-20048448.
8. Mayo Clinic. Alzheimer's disease. 2020. mayoclinic.org. https://www.mayoclinic.org/diseases-conditions/alzheimers-disease/symptoms-causes/syc-20350447.
9. McKinney A. The value of life story work for staff, people with dementia and family members. Nurs Older People. 2017;29(5):25–9. https://doi.org/10.7748/nop.2017.e899.
10. Brenowitz WD, Kaup AR, Lin FR, Yaffe K. Multiple sensory impairment is associated with increased risk of dementia among black and white older adults. J Gerontol Ser A Biol Med Sci. 2019;74(6):890–6. https://doi.org/10.1093/gerona/gly264.

Chapter 10
Amyotrophic Lateral Sclerosis

Lara Taggart and Gillian Porter

Introduction

Amyotrophic lateral sclerosis (ALS) is an upper and lower motor neuron disease which causes neuronal death that controls voluntary muscles [1]. It can be difficult to diagnose, as there is no specific test that can provide a definitive diagnosis. Therefore, diagnosing ALS involves ruling out other diseases and a detailed history of signs/symptoms.

- Classified in two groups [2]:

  - Sporadic—most common, 90–95% of cases; no known genetic link
  - Familial—5–10%; genetic mutation is the cause

- Two types of ALS [2]:

  - Spinal ALS—most signs/symptoms observed in the limbs/trunk; paralysis or death typically within 3–5 years
  - Bulbar ALS—signs/symptoms observed in speaking, swallowing, breathing; more common in women and people over 70; paralysis or death typically within 1–2 years

- Cause of death [3]

  - Respiratory failure, pneumonia, or cardiac arrhythmias

L. Taggart (✉)
Northern Arizona University, Flagstaff, AZ, USA
e-mail: Lara.Taggart@nau.edu

G. Porter
Northern Arizona University, Flagstaff, AZ, USA

Carefree Physical Therapy, Carefree, AZ, USA
e-mail: gp288@nau.edu

© Springer Nature Switzerland AG 2023
S. Dahl-Popolizio et al. (eds.), *Primary Care Occupational Therapy*,
https://doi.org/10.1007/978-3-031-20882-9_10

- Risk factors [4]:

  - Age—typically 55–75 years old
  - Men—men slightly more likely than women to develop the disease.
  - Race/ethnicity—Caucasian and non-Hispanics; rare type of ALS (Guamanian ALS) affects residents of Guam
  - Environmental factors [5]—Smoking is the only established environmental contribution known
  - Military veterans are up to two times more likely than the general population to be diagnosed with ALS [1, 4]

Signs and Symptoms [1, 6]

Musculoskeletal
- Fasciculations in larger muscle groups, such as the arms, legs, trunk, and even the tongue
- Muscle cramps
- Spasticity (UMN) or flaccidity (LMN)
- Muscle weakness and fatigue affecting one or more limbs, neck, or diaphragm
- Slurred (dysarthria) or nasal speech
- Difficulty chewing, swallowing (dysphagia), or breathing
- Difficulty walking (tripping, stumbling, etc.)
- Wasting of hand musculature, usually thenar eminence

Nervous system
- Pseudobulbar effect—uncontrolled laughing/crying not matching a true emotional state

Respiratory system
- Breathing difficulty
- Respiratory infection and failure

Gastrointestinal
- Malnutrition
- Constipation

Cognition
- Impaired decision-making

Behavioral
- Anxiety
- Depression
- Unexplained decrease/difficulty participating in leisure activities

Disease Stages [1, 7]

There is no discreet staging; however, there is a continuum of early to late symptoms that guide interventions

- Early

  - Minimal impairment
  - This stage often occurs prior to diagnosis or is often misdiagnosed
  - Rarely seen by therapy
  - Muscles can be weak, stiff, or include twitching/fasciculations with evidence of atrophy/decreased muscle bulk
  - Symptoms/signs may be present in only one body region or have mild symptoms that affect more than one region
  - Fatigue, poor balance, slurred words, weak grip, tripping when walking

- Middle

  - Signs/symptoms becoming more apparent and widespread:

    Increased fatigue
    Increased sleeping disturbance
    Development of respiratory complications, particularly when lying flat
    Pseudobulbar effect may be present
    Weakness in swallowing may cause issues with eating, choking, and managing saliva

  - Minimum to moderate activity limitations

    Driving may be discontinued

  - Educate patient/family
  - Anticipate future needs
  - Some muscle paralysis may be evident and any muscle disuse may result in muscle contractures

- Late

  - Severe impairment

    Most voluntary muscles are paralyzed

    - Decreased ability to walk and transfer

    Severe speech difficulties or complete loss of speech
    Nutritional support often needed (PEG tube)
    Respiratory decline is severe
    Pain and muscle contractures possible

  - Dependent in all/most Activities of Daily Living (ADLs)
  - Ongoing patient/family education
  - Teaching patient-handling techniques
  - Identifying resources for support important

Role of PCP [6, 7]

The PCP will see the patient for all health issues typically seen in PC as the patient's ALS progresses. Medication interactions and the need for additional referrals and resources for family support can be managed in the PC office. For more advance cases, a referral to a neurologist may be indicated

- Diagnostic testing

    - MRI
    - CT
    - EMG
    - Spinal tap or lumbar puncture
    - US of the muscles
    - Blood test to rule out other disorders
    - Muscle biopsy
    - Genetic testing
    - Respiratory testing, such as vital capacity and pulmonary function

- Medical management/palliative care

    - Supportive systems required

        Feeding tube/nutritional support
        Respiratory support, noninvasive (BiPAP) or invasive (tracheostomy with respiratory)
        Adaptive equipment
        Assistive devices (power chair)

    - Medications approved by FDA to slow disease progression of ALS

        Rilutek
        Radicava

    - Medication approved by FDA to manage pseudobulbar effect

        Neudexta

    - Botox to address swallowing muscles
    - Psychotropic medications to manage depression and anxiety
    - Medications for pain management

- Referrals

    - Multidisciplinary ALS clinic, if available

        Neurologist specializing in ALS
        OT, PT, SLP, dietary, respiratory
        Social services

  – Local ALS association

     Loan closet for equipment
     Support group for patient and/or care partner(s)
     Literature/resources including recent research
     Transportation for medical appointments

  – Assistive Technology Act Programs (ATAPs)

Common Comorbidities

- hypertension
- depression (Chap. 18)
- anxiety (Chap. 11)
- hyperlipidaemia
- ischemic heart disease/arrhythmia
- osteoarthritis (Chap. 12)
- cancer (*primarily* prostate and breast)

Role of OTP

ALS is a condition that is devastating to both the patient and their families. As the outcome is always death, the OTP on the primary care team can help the patient and their family navigates the functional decline of the patient with strategies to prolonged ROM and strength, while simultaneously providing adaptive equipment and strategies. This section focuses on the progression of physical decline; however, with the behavioral health skill set, the OTP can also address comorbid behavioral health issues. Providing help to the patient and family with adjustment to illness, and in the transitions that occur as this disease progresses to its ultimate outcome is a critical role for the OTP in PC as well.

Occupational Impact [8]

Many aspects of function are affected and will need treatment. Maintenance of occupational performance focuses on:

- Optimizing strength and ROM using home exercise programs
- Maintaining function in ADL and Instrumental Activities of Daily Living (IADLs) through use of Assistive Devices or Adaptive Devices

  – Important to secure a power chair for mobility and possible use as bed as disease progresses [1]

- Decreasing fatigue in the neck and extremities through use of orthotics
- Managing pain and energy using joint protection and energy conservation techniques
- As function declines

  - Mobility and self-care become increasingly difficult
  - Home evaluations/in-home therapy will be important

    Continued assessment of respiration and swallowing

  - Care partner education and training:

    Optimizing safety with positioning, transfers, and maintenance of skin integrity
    Enabling communication using augmentative equipment
    Identify and obtain equipment to support mobility and positioning
    Environmental modifications for safety and to support mobility as possible

  - Optimize social participation

OT Areas of Emphasis

Physical changes as a result of weakness, spasticity, sensory problems, pain, and decreased endurance and ROM necessitate OT services to enhance mobility, upper extremity function, and overall conditioning to reduce falls and maintain participation. Assisting the patient and family with adjustment to illness and end-of-life concerns will also be addressed by the OTP in the PC setting.

Evaluation

Assessments for clients with ALS should be based on clearly defined levels of function and the individual's needs and priorities. Many assessments are available at the Shirley Ryan Ability Lab website.

- ALS Functional Rating Scale

  - Evaluates functional status and can be used to monitor change over time
  - Free, available online (https://www.sralab.org/sites/default/files/2017-07/PMandR_ALSRatingScale033111.pdf)

- ADL and IADL assessments should be included in all evaluations to determine ongoing functional ability
- Upper extremity ability

  - Purdue Pegboard, 9-hole peg test or other timed upper extremity function tests
  - Range of Motion (ROM) and Manual Muscle Testing (MMT)

- Fatigue is shown to affect physical quality of life and can be assessed with the Multidimensional Fatigue Inventory (MFI) or other screening measures (https://www.med.upenn.edu/cbti/assets/user-content/documents/Multidimensional%20Fatigue%20Inventory%20(MFI).pdf).
- As communication and swallowing decline assessment and intervention is required to ensure that nutritional needs and social participation are maintained. Because of disease progression, re-evaluation at each visit is required.
- St Louis University Mental Status (SLUMS) Examination for cognition to measure orientation, memory, attention, executive function.

Intervention Strategies [8]

OT intervention strategies are in relation to disease stage/progression

- **Early**
  - Ambulatory, no problems with ADL, mild weakness

    Normal activities, moderate exercise in unaffected muscles, active ROM, and strength exercise
    No equipment

    - Consider beginning the acquisition of a power chair given the amount of time to fit, manufacture, deliver, and train to use a chair

    Energy conservation techniques

- **Middle**
  - Ambulatory likely with impairment, moderate weakness in certain muscles, increased fatigue

    Modification in living; modest exercise; active, assisted range of motion exercises
    Assistive devices, use of hands free devices, electronic tablet

  - As atrophy progresses, patients may benefit from orthotics to avoid contractures and keep joints in functional positions. Examples:

    a short or long thumb spica can be used to maintain the ability to pinch
    A volar wrist orthosis with an MCP point flexion strap can reduce the MCP hyperextension and IP joint flexion positioning that impedes the ability to grip and pinch, and that allow contractures to develop
    For patterns and pictures of orthoses, see *Common Orthoses in Primary Care* in Appendix

  - Ambulatory likely with impairment or wheelchair confined, severe weakness in specific muscles, increased dependence due to difficulty with ADLs; marked fatigue

> Adaptations to continue active life; active, assisted, passive ROM exercise; joint pain management
> Smart technology, adaptive devices, home equipment and environmental controls

- **Late**

  - Wheelchair confined, dependent, marked leg and arm weakness

    > Passive ROM exercise, pain management, decubitus ulcer prevention
    > Smart technology, adaptive devices, home equipment, environmental controls, wheelchair

  - Bedridden (confined to power chair common), unable to perform ADLs, maximal assistance required

    > Passive ROM exercise, pain management, prevention of decubitus ulcers and venous thrombosis
    > Smart technology, adaptive devices and home equipment to assist caregiver(s), environmental controls, wheelchair

Other Considerations and Resources

- Exercise considerations throughout all stages [1, 8]

  - Oxygen saturation level—oxygen saturation level will be low because oxygen is unable to get to the alveoli (ventilation), not because oxygen cannot get to the body's tissues (oxygenation). This means O_2 Sat may not be a reliable measurement during treatment
  - Active and passive ROM, strengthening, endurance, stretching, and home breathing programs are appropriate at various stages of the disease and are effective for minimizing secondary complications
  - Attention to overexertion, potential secondary problems, muscle spasms, and careful monitoring of fatigue are important to a successful exercise program
  - Encourage enjoyable sports and leisure activities while maintaining safety
  - Discourage high-resistance exercise (not shown to be any more beneficial than moderate-resistance exercise)
  - Training on energy conservation is essential to avoid negative impact on daily activities

- Equipment considerations throughout all stages [1]

  - Adaptive equipment for ADLs

    > Reacher
    > Dycem
    > Suction toothbrush

    Invisible guard plate
    Meal lifter
    Self-feeder
    Spill-proof guards
    Utensil holder
    Headmaster cervical collar
    Mobile arm support

– Durable medical equipment

    Bathtub/shower bench
    Lift chair/seat
    Hoyer lift
    Pivot transfer device
    Hospital bed
    Grab bars
    Handheld shower equipment
    Bedside commode or raised toilet seat
    Bidet
    Stair glide

– Adaptive equipment for IADLs

    Bluetooth wireless foot mouse
    Bilateral arm support
    E-write tablet
    Tablet with text-to-speech app or eye gaze to speech

– Assistive devices for mobility

    Ankle-Foot Orthoses (AFOs)—consider prefabricated or over-the-counter options to avoid delay in manufacturing custom (this device will be short-term)
    Power chair

References

1. Wing MK, Carter V. Treatment concepts for persons with ALS. Medbridge. 2020. https://www.medbridgeeducation.com/course-player/play/27453.
2. ALS News Today. Types of ALS. https://alsnewstoday.com/forms-of-als/?cn-reloaded=1.
3. Arbesman M, Sheard K. Systematic review of the effectiveness of occupational therapy for people with amyotrophic lateral sclerosis. Am J Occup Ther. 2013;68:20–6. https://doi.org/10.5014/ajot.2014.008649.
4. National Institute of Neurological Disorders and Stroke. Amyotrophic lateral sclerosis fact sheet. 2013. https://www.ninds.nih.gov/Disorders/Patient-Caregiver-Education/Fact-Sheets/Amyotrophic-Lateral-Sclerosis-ALS-Fact-Sheet.

5. Armond C. Medscape. What causes amyotrophic lateral sclerosis. 2019. https://www.medscape.com/answers/1170097-81833/what-causes-sporadic-amyotrophic-lateral-sclerosis-als.
6. Muscular Dystrophy Association. Amyotrophic Lateral Sclerosis fact sheet. 2019. https://www.mda.org/sites/default/files/2019/03/MDA_ALS_Fact_Sheet_March_2019.pdf.
7. Muscular Dystrophy Association. Amyotrophic lateral sclerosis: assistance in stages of ALS.   https://www.mda.org/disease/amyotrophic-lateral-sclerosis/medical-management/assistance-in-stages-of-als.
8. Radomski MV, Trombly Latham CA. Occupational therapy for physical dysfunction. 7th ed. Philadelphia: Lippincott Williams & Wilkins; 2008.

Chapter 11
Anxiety

Chantelle Rice Collins and Marissa Marchioni

Introduction

Anxiety is an emotion characterized by feelings of fear and tension accompanied by physical symptoms. Anxiety is normal and can be healthy, but when anxiety becomes excessive, it impacts engagement in daily activities. Anxiety is the most common mental health diagnosis in the world. Approximately 18% of the U.S. population reports anxiety every year, and a lifetime prevalence of 33% [1–3]. The United States and other high-income nations have higher rates of anxiety when compared to lower income nations [4]. While anxiety onset typically occurs in early adolescence through young adulthood [5], onset can occur across the lifespan [6]. Women are twice as likely as men to experience anxiety [5, 7]. The prevalence of anxiety disorders varies among different racial groups, with white Americans having the highest rates of diagnosis for all anxiety disorders except post-traumatic stress disorder, which is most prevalent among African Americans [8].

Diagnostic Criteria

Anxiety disorder is characterized by excessive worry and fear, intrusive thoughts, and physical symptoms including a racing heart and muscle tension. The criteria below are taken from the Diagnostic and Statistical Manual of Mental Disorders, 5th Edition (DSM-5):

1. Excessive anxiety and worry occurring more days than not for at least 6 months, about several events or activities.

C. R. Collins (✉) · M. Marchioni
University of Southern California, Los Angeles, CA, USA
e-mail: Chantelle.Rice@med.usc.edu; Marissa.Marchioni@med.usc.edu

© Springer Nature Switzerland AG 2023
S. Dahl-Popolizio et al. (eds.), *Primary Care Occupational Therapy*,
https://doi.org/10.1007/978-3-031-20882-9_11

2. The individual finds it difficult to control the worry.
3. Three (or more) of the following six symptoms:

   (a) Restlessness or feeling keyed up or on edge
   (b) Being easily fatigued
   (c) Difficulty concentrating or the mind going blank
   (d) Irritability
   (e) Muscle tension
   (f) Sleep disturbance

4. The anxiety, worry, or physical symptoms cause clinically significant distress or impairment in functioning
5. The disturbance is not attributable to the physiological effects of a substance or another medical condition
6. The disturbance is not better explained by another mental disorder [1]

Categories of Anxiety

- **Generalized anxiety disorder (GAD)**

  GAD is characterized by excessive anxiety and worry accompanied by physical or cognitive symptoms that last for at least 6 months. The individual's worry and anxiety can focus on a variety of topics and are considered very difficult to control [1]. While one of the more common anxiety diagnoses, generalized anxiety disorder can have the most significant impact on health-related quality of life and a patient's ability to participate in roles and routines [9].

- **Panic disorder**

  Panic attacks are defined as discrete experiences of intense fear or discomfort reaching peak intensity within 10 min accompanied by the presence of four DSM-5 specified symptoms. A diagnosis of panic disorder is warranted when panic attacks are recurrent and followed by either a concern about having more panic attacks or maladaptive behavior changes related to the attacks [1]. Due to the intensity of panic attacks, people often seek medical attention for fear of having a heart attack due to chest pain and shortness of breath.

- **Phobias**

  Phobias are an overwhelming fear of something specific that results in avoidance of a specific thing or situation. When the feared situation or thing is unavoidable, an individual experiences extreme anxiety [1].

- **Social Anxiety Disorder**

  Social anxiety is defined as a significant fear of one or more social or performance situations in which there is a potential for observation or examination from others or exposure to people who are unfamiliar. When exposed to these situations a person's anxiety increases, often leading an individual to avoid these situations entirely or endure them with serious discomfort [1].

- **Separation Anxiety Disorder**

  Separation anxiety disorder (SAD) is the excessive fear of being separated from specific persons or pets that is not considered developmentally appropriate. A diagnosis of SAD is made when the fear is considered persistent and severe [1]. Typically considered a childhood anxiety disorder (prevalence 4.1%), separation anxiety disorder can be diagnosed in adults (prevalence 6.6%) [10].

- **Obsessive-Compulsive Disorder**

  Obsessions center on thoughts, urges, or mental images that cause anxiety, whereas compulsions are repetitive behaviors that a person feels an urge to carry out in response to obsessive thoughts [1].

- **Post-Traumatic Stress Disorder**

  Occurring in 5–10% of the population, post-traumatic stress disorder (PTSD) can develop after exposure to a precipitating event, such as threatened or actual death, sexual violation, or serious injury. The four diagnostic clusters include re-experiencing, avoidance, negative cognitions and mood, and arousal [1].

Diagnoses That Mimic Anxiety But Are Not Anxiety

The signs and symptoms of anxiety resemble other conditions, necessitating careful exploration of differential diagnoses in order to provide appropriate treatment. While anxiety may be the primary diagnosis or the secondary diagnosis in response to another physical or chronic condition, the presence of additional symptoms may suggest that an alternative diagnosis is possible, check with the PCP to discuss. Examples of diagnoses that mimic anxiety include:

- Cardiac issues
- Endocrine conditions
- Gastrointestinal conditions
- Inflammatory conditions
- Metabolic conditions
- Neurologic conditions
- Respiratory conditions

Symptoms of anxiety	
Intrusive thoughts	• Unwanted thoughts or mental images that are distressing or disturbing such as the expectation of death, catastrophic events, or personal failure [11]
Somatic symptoms	• Symptoms that are experienced as bodily or physical sensations such as fatigue, muscle tension, sweating, cardiac or gastrointestinal sensations [12]
Behavioral symptoms	• Increased or decreased behaviors that are secondary to anxiety such as increased health risk behavior, avoidance of anxiety-producing situations, or decreased engagement in daily activities [13]

Role of PCP

In collaborating with the PCP, it can be helpful to understand their role and priorities. While the PCP will also engage in the screening and assessment of anxiety, it is unlikely that they will have the time and training for counseling. They will order relevant labs and tests to screen for medical conditions that may be the primary cause of the anxiety or anxiety-like symptoms. They will also prescribe and adjust medications as well as refer to mental health specialists as needed. Over the lifespan of the patient, they will provide surveillance and monitoring to identify times when anxiety symptoms are relapsing or at risk for relapsing.

Common Comorbidities

Anxiety is as prevalent as depression but underdiagnosed and undertreated much to the detriment of patients [14]. Among patients who attend PC appointments, it is estimated that 10–25% have an anxiety disorder [15], and those with depression have a 25–54% likelihood of having current GAD [16]. Depression and anxiety have similar impacts on occupational engagement and given their similarities in symptomology and the significant likelihood of co-occurrence, it should be part of clinical practice to screen for depression when a patient has an anxiety diagnosis. This is especially true in the presence of symptoms such as sadness, hopelessness, anger or irritability, and loss of interest in normal activities (see Chap. 18) [17].

Similarly, individuals living with chronic physical illnesses often have comorbid anxiety diagnosis. While their primary reason for visiting PC is typically to discuss their physical conditions, practitioners should be mindful of signs and symptoms of anxiety and be prepared to screen these patients. When living with a chronic illness, fear and worry about prognosis, as well as feeling overwhelmed with disease management and recommended behavior changes are common.

Common diagnoses with comorbid anxiety [18]
- Heart disease
- Stroke
- Cancer
- Migraines [19]
- Multiple sclerosis [20]
- Parkinson's [21]
- Autism [22–24]

Factors Contributing to Anxiety

The etiology of anxiety is complex, and it is often a combination of the factors below that increase an individual's risk. In addition to utilizing standardized screening tools for anxiety, understanding how underlying factors can contribute to anxiety will support the PC OTP in effectively collecting relevant information from the client and creating effective treatment plans and interventions.

Contributing factor	Potential impact
• Family history and genetics	• Having first-degree relatives with a diagnosis of anxiety increases the likelihood of heritability [25] • Research suggests that certain genes are linked with anxiety and heritability could be as high as 30% [26]
• Brain chemistry	• Neurotransmitters such as serotonin, norepinephrine, and gamma-aminobutyric acid (GABA) are associated with anxiety [27]
• Personality	• Persons with anxiety tend to be sensitive in nature, the signs of which they can identify beginning as early as childhood
• Life events and culture	• Life events and circumstances ranging from parenting styles, to messages learned and absorbed in school and religion, to the loss of a loved one influence anxiety across the lifespan • Many cultures emphasize refraining from explicitly discussing personal emotions • Culture impacts the tendency to seek help and treatment-seeking delay [28] • Culture of origin shapes the expression of anxiety

Role of OTP

OTPs in PC settings work with interprofessional colleagues to appropriately screen, evaluate, and treat patients with anxiety. Anxiety is often first addressed in PC as either the reason for visit or a co-occurring condition. Considering the role of comorbid mental and behavioral health conditions on overall health, the OTP on the PC team is well positioned to address anxiety as it affects many acute and chronic conditions.

Occupational Impact

All aspects of a patient's life are impacted by anxiety. Substantial quality of life impairments for people with anxiety disorders across several domains of functioning including perceptions of health, social relationships, home, work, and family life [38]. A common feature of anxiety is the use of "safety behaviors" such as avoidance, escape, or other "coping" behaviors, resulting in decreased participation in an array of occupations and roles [39]. For example, decreased role functioning at work impacts components affecting productivity including decreasing work performance, attendance, and opportunities for work [40]. Similarly, impairments in social functioning and quality of life are seen among individuals with anxiety, especially with comorbid depression [41]. As with all interventions, treatment of anxiety should be client-centered and might include a variety of techniques and topics [42, 43].

OT Areas of Emphasis

The areas the OTP will focus on includes assessing the effect anxiety is having on the patient's life and providing actionable strategies that the patient can employ to achieve condition self-management. In PC, the focus of treatment is to provide brief interventions with strategies the patient can easily apply after they leave. As the visits are shorter and on an "as-needed" basis compared to traditional mental health, the focus of treatment is alleviating stress to improve daily quality of life with sustainable skills.

Evaluation

Screening

Patients may come to the OTP with anxiety as their known diagnosis and presenting concern, or the OTP may decide to screen for anxiety for reasons such as

- The patient has a condition commonly comorbid with anxiety
- PCP has expressed concern about anxiety
- Patient expresses concerns about anxiety, symptoms of anxiety, or a change in the severity of anxiety

Screening for anxiety disorders is particularly important when the patient presents with the common signs and symptoms of anxiety listed in the sections above [29]. There are multiple screening tools that can be used to support the diagnosis of anxiety and its severity. If patients in a particular PC setting are at high risk for specific types of anxiety (e.g., PTSD or OCD), the OTP should use screening tools specific to those diagnoses. Some common screening tools include:

- Generalized Anxiety Disorder 7 (GAD-7) [30]
- Generalized Anxiety Disorder Questionnaire-IV (GAD-IV) [31]
- Depression Anxiety Stress Scales (DASS-21) [32]
- Overall Anxiety Severity and Impairment Scale (OASIS) [33]

- Patient Health Questionnaire 4 (PHQ-4) [34]
- Hamilton Anxiety Rating Scale (HARS) [35]
- Primary Care PTSD Screen for *DSM-5* (PC-PTSD-5) [36]

If there is an identified diagnosis of anxiety, the team will determine the appropriate next steps with regard to referring to the appropriate providers. The PCP will determine the need for prescription medications.

Consultation

An OT consultation for anxiety is a brief encounter with the patient to determine the next steps for their health, well-being, and safety. It should also serve as an opportunity for the OTP to determine if the patient would benefit from an OT evaluation. The OTP may conduct their consultation by initiating the following:

- Gather brief information about the patient's presentation of symptoms, background, and impact on occupational performance
- Screen for safety concerns
- Offer the patient emotional support
- Establish/building rapport
- Normalize/destigmatize the patient's experience
- Assess the overall degree of impact on occupational performance and safety
- Assess the need for OT evaluation and treatment
- Assess the need for referral to psychiatry, psychology, and social work

Evaluation

During the evaluation, the OTP will conduct interviews and assessments to identify medical and therapy history, support the development of an occupational profile, and analyze occupational performance, all to develop a plan of care [37]. During an evaluation of anxiety, OTPs will specifically emphasize gathering information regarding:

- Medical history including comorbidities, prescribed medications, and therapy services utilized in the past and present (can be reviewed in the chart in advance)
- The pattern of anxiety symptoms over time, including triggers, patterns over days/weeks/months/years, and variation with occupational engagement
- Impact on occupational performance, including ADLs, IADLs, work, leisure, and social participation
- Typical daily and weekly habits and routines
- Identifying barriers to participation, e.g. excessive worry, rumination, racing heart, dizziness

- Identifying action steps to begin to overcome barriers, e.g., recognize triggers, speak with a family member, engage in healthy coping techniques
- Sources of meaning and connection, e.g., finding purpose, family, friends, spirituality
- Presence and severity of self-harm behaviors or suicidal ideation
- Patient's strengths and internal resources
- Patient's stage of change
- The patient's desired goals and objectives
- Providing brief psychoeducation regarding anxiety (see above)

Intervention Strategies

Psychoeducation

- Provision of information about symptoms, normalization of experiences, facilitation of self-management of condition, and connection to additional resources [44]

Cognitive Behavioral Therapy

- CBT is a first-line approach for anxiety disorders [45, 46]
- Includes the process of evaluating thoughts and selecting thoughts that are most adaptive, rather than allowing unsupportive and automatic thinking patterns [44]
- Additional resources at: Therapist Aid

Motivational Interviewing

- A goal-oriented communication method that supports patients in resolving ambivalence to support positive behavior changes
- Features of motivational interviewing include expressing empathy and focusing on client-centeredness, supporting change talk, developing discrepancy to resolve ambivalence, rolling with resistance, and supporting self-efficacy
- Can be used as an adjunct to CBT to increase the motivation for and commitment to intervention, particularly when intervention is challenging (e.g., during cognitive restructuring and exposure) [47]
- Additional resources at: Therapist Aid

Exposure

- Includes presenting stimuli that produce anxiety that don't present risk without engaging in anxiety "coping" behaviors
- Exposure therapy is often used as a tool adjunct with CBT and is sometimes a stand-alone treatment for social phobia, panic disorder, and OCD [48]
- Components of exposure treatment include:
  - Learning relaxation strategies
  - Developing a list of progressively challenging exposures to anxiety-provoking stimuli
  - Gradually work through exposures by staying in the situation until the anxiety subsides

Session Topics

Medication Adherence

- Medication adherence can include successfully taking medications how and when they have been prescribed and can include both medications for anxiety and other medical conditions
- Collaborative development of daily systems and processes for taking medications may be necessary to develop new habits and success with consistent use of medication [49]
- Self-stigmatization and feelings/beliefs around taking medication for a mental health concern may need to be navigated [50]

Self-Monitoring

- Part of understanding one's experience with anxiety is to become more aware of how it presents in daily life. Through tracking anxiety-related symptoms and triggers, patients can begin to recognize the interplay between their health and their participation in daily activities. Recognition of patterns can empower patients to implement behavior changes that can influence outcomes. Examples include tracking intrusive thoughts, anxiety levels at various points during the day or week, symptoms of anxiety, such as racing thoughts, heart rate, or episodes of panic.
- Self-monitoring can provide the information that a client needs to begin to successfully work with their anxiety and allow healing to occur.
- Some patients may have a difficult time recalling how they occupy their time in a typical day or week, especially patients who lack external structures such as

work or school. Tracking time use in the initial phases of treatment can support patients to set realistic expectations of how to incorporate new behaviors into their routines.

Lifestyle and Routine Modification

Lifestyle factors and behaviors do not occur in isolation and often influence one another. For example, whether someone engages in exercise will likely have an impact on their sleep patterns. Therefore, it is encouraged that an OTP address as many of the topics below as sessions and time permit when treating a patient with anxiety. Through determining the client's readiness to change specific lifestyle factors and behaviors, the OTP can assess which of the following to prioritize.

- Forming health-promoting habits and routines

  - The development of health-promoting habits and routines will serve as a foundation of self-care and anxiety management.
  - Collaborative problem-solving for scaffolding to promote self-efficacy and carry-over of identified action steps (e.g., utilize digital reminders, break a task into smaller steps, practice compassionate self-talk).

- Developing healthy eating routines

  - OTPs can address eating routines by providing education on the principles of healthy eating, helping clients engage in meal planning and preparation, and supporting clients as they adopt accountability structures.
  - Clients should be advised to avoid processed sugar and caffeine as they are known to exacerbate anxiety.
  - Eating balanced meals throughout the day and healthy blood glucose regulation can support anxiety management [51].

- Engaging in physical activity

  - Physical activity can reduce symptoms of short-term anxiety and long-term anxiety, especially moderate to vigorous exercise [39].
  - The benefits of exercise for anxiety management require consistency over the long term. Patients should meet the guidelines for at least 150 min of exercise weekly, including a combination of aerobic, anaerobic, and flexibility exercises.
  - OTPs can support patients as they initiate engagement in exercise, recognizing that this can be challenging for patients with anxiety, particularly with somatic symptoms or fears related to health. To overcome activity avoidance, the OTP should support the client in identifying activities they have safely enjoyed in the past or might enjoy currently. Through task analysis and scaffolding, the OTP can help the patient conceptualize how to incorporate exercise into their daily and weekly routines and facilitate participation.
  - (see *Walk to Run Program* in Appendix).

- Sleep hygiene
    - Sleep disturbances have a bi-directional relationship with anxiety; OTPs can support patients in decreasing environmental, cognitive, and behavioral barriers to sleep [52, 53]
    - The OTP should address sleep hygiene by supporting the client as they:

        Establish appropriate sleep/wake times
        Identify a wind-down/sleep preparatory routine
        Eliminate stimulating activities before sleep
        Modify the environment

    - Patients at risk for insomnia should be screened and referred appropriately
    - (see **Sleep Hygiene** and **Weekly Sleep Log** handouts in Appendix)
- Substance use
    - Substance use disorders are highly co-morbid with anxiety disorders, and negative affect may exacerbate substance use; Treating anxiety and substance use disorders concurrently result in improved outcomes [54]
- Time management
    - Time management skills are crucial for patients hoping to implement changes to habits and routines and is a component to problem-focused stress coping

        Provide strategies for increased time awareness
        Assess tools used for scheduling and planning
        Identify barriers to effective time use

    - (see **Schedule** handout in Appendix)
- Self-regulation and stress management
    - Sensory processing

        Some studies have found an association between self-reported anxiety and responsiveness to sensory stimuli [55]
        Sensory processing impairments in childhood may be associated with anxiety in adulthood through difficulties managing emotional distress

    - Relaxation training, mindfulness, and acceptance-based techniques

        Attending to and controlling physiological arousal through the use of techniques such as diaphragmatic breathing, progressive muscle relaxation, and visualization [44]
        (see **Mindfulness, simplified** and **Mindfulness, higher literacy level** handouts in Appendix)

- Progressive muscle relaxation

    - Progressively tense and release muscles with a slowly paced (e.g., 4–6 s), synchronized diaphragmatic breathing
    - (see ***Progressive Muscle Relaxation*** handout in Appendix)

- Diaphragmatic breathing

    - Deep breathing focused on rhythmic inhalations and exhalations resulting in movement of the abdomen and stimulation of the vagus nerve

- Visualization

    - Relaxing engagement of imagery associated with a pleasant place, incorporating imagining of aspects of the sensory environment

Increase awareness of experiences in the moment, practicing acceptance, and values-driven actions [44]

Community Integration

- Social Skills Development and Participation

    - Social skills training supports individuals with social anxiety and supports increased social engagement as well as alleviation of anxiety symptoms [56]

- Work and School Engagement

    - Developing strategies for improved role performance in the areas of work and/or educational performance is a form of problem-focused coping that support the management of anxiety
    - The worker/student role is associated with specific stressors including performance stress and fears of insufficiency, social stress such as supervisor oversight or peer conflict, and health or safety concerns related to the environment [57]

- Spiritual Participation

    - Daily spiritual experience is a protective factor against stress and mental health concerns [52]
    - OTPs can integrate spirituality into discussions about the meaning of occupations, navigate barriers to participation in spiritual activities, and support use of spiritual expression as a coping mechanism [58]

Ongoing sessions should entail collaborative goal setting to ensure that the client is implementing behavior changes that will support successful anxiety management.

Other Considerations and Resources

Discharge, Health Maintenance and Relapse Prevention, and Recovery

At the time of discharge, the OTP will re-administer any clinical assessments and outcomes, assess progress toward long-term goals, and engage the patient in planning for continued health maintenance and relapse prevention and recovery. Upon discharge, the OTP will determine the course of follow-up with the patient. One benefit of working in a PC setting is the potential for the OTP to check-in with the patient at their next PC visit to provide encouragement, accountability, and opportunities for further follow-up.

References

1. American Psychiatric Association. Diagnostic and statistical manual of mental disorders: diagnostic and statistical manual of mental disorders. 5th ed. Washington, DC: American Psychiatric Association; 2013.
2. National Institute of Mental Health. Anxiety disorders. 2018. https://www.nimh.nih.gov/health/topics/anxiety-disorders/index.shtml. Accessed 10 Mar 2019.
3. Bandelow B, Michaelis S. Epidemiology of anxiety disorders in the 21st century. Dialogues Clin Neurosci. 2015;17(3):327.
4. Ruscio AM, Hallion LS, Lim CCW, et al. Cross-sectional comparison of the epidemiology of DSM-5 generalized anxiety disorder across the globe. JAMA Psychiatry. 2017;74(5):465–75.
5. Kessler RC, Berglund P, Demler O, Jin R, Merikangas KR, Walters EE. Lifetime prevalence and age-of-onset distributions of DSM-IV disorders in the National Comorbidity Survey Replication. Arch Gen Psychiatry. 2005;2:593–602.
6. Lenze EJ, Wetherell JL. A lifespan view of anxiety disorders. Dialogues Clin Neurosci. 2011;13(4):381–99.
7. Institute for Health Metrics and Evaluation (IHME). Findings from the global burden of disease study 2017. Seattle: IHME; 2018.
8. Asnaani A, Richey JA, Dimaite R, Hinton DE, Hofmann SG. A cross-ethnic comparison of lifetime prevalence rates of anxiety disorders. J Nerv Ment Dis. 2010;198(8):551–5. https://doi.org/10.1097/NMD.0b013e3181ea169f.
9. Comer JS, Blanco C, Hasin DS, Liu SM, Grant BF, Turner JB, Olfson M. Health-related quality of life across the anxiety disorders: results from the national epidemiologic survey on alcohol and related conditions (NESARC). J Clin Psychiatry. 2011;72(1):43–50.
10. Shear K, Jin R, Meron Ruscio A, Walter E, Kessler R. Prevalence and correlates of estimated DSM-IV child and adult separation anxiety disorder in the national comorbidity survey replication. Am J Psychiatry. 2006;163(6):1066–73. https://doi.org/10.1176/ajp.2006.163.61074.
11. Romero-Sanchiz P, Nogueira-Arjona R, Godoy-Ávila A, Gavino-Lázaro A, Freeston MH. Differences in clinical intrusive thoughts between obsessive–compulsive disorder, generalized anxiety disorder, and hypochondria. Clin Psychol Psychother. 2017;24(6):O1464–73.
12. Mallorquí-Bagué N, Bulbena A, Pailhez G, Garfinkel SN, Critchley HD. Mind-body interactions in anxiety and somatic symptoms. Harv Rev Psychiatry. 2016;24(1):53–60.
13. Kirk A, Meyer JM, Whisman MA, Deacon BJ, Arch JJ. Safety behaviors, experiential avoidance, and anxiety: a path analysis approach. J Anxiety Disord. 2019;64:9–15.

14. Kroenke K, Spitzer RL, Williams JB, Monahan PO, Löwe B. Anxiety disorders in primary care: prevalence, impairment, comorbidity, and detection. Ann Intern Med. 2007;146(5):317–25.
15. Roca M, Gili M, Garcia-Garcia M, Salva J, Vives M, Garcia Campayo J, Comas A. Prevalence and comorbidity of common mental disorders in primary care. J Affect Disord. 2009;119(1–3):52–8.
16. Sherbourne CD, Jackson CA, Meredith LS, Camp P, Wells KB. Prevalence of comorbid anxiety disorders in primary care outpatients. Arch Fam Med. 1996;5(1):27.
17. Hirschfeld R. The comorbidity of major depression and anxiety disorders: recognition and management in primary care. Prim Care Companion J Clin Psychiatry. 2001;3(6):244–54.
18. Clarke D, Currie K. Depression, anxiety and their relationship with chronic diseases: a review of the epidemiology, risk and treatment evidence. Med J Aust. 2009;190(S7):S54–60. https://doi.org/10.5694/j.1326-5377.2009.tb02471.x.
19. Malone CD, Bhowmick A, Wachholtz AB. Migraine: treatments, comorbidities, and quality of life, in the USA. J Pain Res. 2015;8:537.
20. Marrie RA, Reingold S, Cohen J, Stuve O, Trojano M, Sorensen PS, Reider N. The incidence and prevalence of psychiatric disorders in multiple sclerosis: a systematic review. Mult Scler J. 2015;21(3):305–17.
21. Bijl RV. Prevalence of mental disorders in persons with Parkinson's disease. Ned Tijdschr Geneeskd. 1998;142(1):27–31.
22. Reaven J, Blakeley-Smith A, Leuthe E, Moody E, Hepburn S. Facing your fears in adolescence: cognitive-behavioral therapy for high-functioning autism spectrum disorders and anxiety. Autism Res Treat. 2012;2012:423905.
23. Spek AA, Van Ham NC, Nyklíček I. Mindfulness-based therapy in adults with an autism spectrum disorder: a randomized controlled trial. Res Dev Disabil. 2013;34(1):246–53.
24. Lake JK, Perry A, Lunsky Y. Mental health services for individuals with high functioning autism spectrum disorder. Autism Res Treat. 2014;2014:502420.
25. Hettema JM, Neale MC, Kendler KS. A review and meta-analysis of the genetic epidemiology of anxiety disorders. Am J Psychiatry. 2001;158:1568–78.
26. Gottschalk MG, Domschke K. Genetics of generalized anxiety disorder and related traits. Dialogues Clin Neurosci. 2017;19(2):159–68.
27. Martin EI, Ressler KJ, Binder E, Nemeroff CB. The neurobiology of anxiety disorders: brain imaging, genetics and psychoneuroendocrinology. Psychiatr Clin N Am. 2009;32(3):549–75. https://doi.org/10.1016/j.psc.2009.05.004.
28. Koydemir S, Essau CA. Anxiety and anxiety disorders in young people: a cross-cultural perspective. In: Understanding uniqueness and diversity in child and adolescent mental health. New York: Academic Press; 2018. p. 115–34.
29. Metzler DH, Mahoney D, Freedy JR. Anxiety disorders in primary care. Prim Care. 2016;43(2):245–61.
30. Spitzer RL, Kroenke K, Williams JB, Löwe B. A brief measure for assessing generalized anxiety disorder: the GAD-7. Arch Intern Med. 2006;166(10):1092–7.
31. Newman MG, Zuellig AR, Kachin KE, Constantino MJ, Przeworski A, Erickson T, Cashman-McGrath L. Preliminary reliability and validity of the generalized anxiety disorder questionnaire-IV: a revised self-report diagnostic measure of generalized anxiety disorder. Behav Ther. 2002;33(2):215–33.
32. Lovibond PF, Lovibond SH. The structure of negative emotional states: comparison of the depression anxiety stress scales (DASS) with the Beck depression and anxiety inventories. Behav Res Ther. 1995;33(3):335–43. https://doi.org/10.1016/0005-7967(94)00075-U.
33. Norman SB, Hami Cissell S, Means-Christensen AJ, Stein MB. Development and validation of an overall anxiety severity and impairment scale (OASIS). Depress Anxiety. 2006;23(4):245–9.
34. Kroenke K, Spitzer RL, Williams JB, Löwe B. An ultra-brief screening scale for anxiety and depression: the PHQ-4. Psychosomatics. 2009;50(6):613.
35. Hamilton MAX. The assessment of anxiety states by rating. Br J Med Psychol. 1959;32(1):50–5.

36. Prins A, Bovin MJ, Smolenski DJ, Marx BP, Kimerling R, Jenkins-Guarnieri MA, Kaloupek DG, Schnurr PP, Kaiser AP, Leyva YE, Tiet QQ. The primary care PTSD screen for DSM-5 (PC-PTSD-5): development and evaluation within a veteran primary care sample. J Gen Intern Med. 2016;31(10):1206–11.
37. American Occupational Therapy Association. Occupational therapy practice framework: domain and process. Am J Occup Ther. 2014;68(Suppl. 1):S1–S48. https://doi.org/10.5014/ajot.2014.682006.
38. Olatunji BO, Cisler JM, Tolin DF. Quality of life in the anxiety disorders: a meta-analytic review. Clin Psychol Rev. 2007;27(5):572–81.
39. Taylor S. Treating anxiety sensitivity in adults with anxiety and related disorders. In: The clinician's guide to anxiety sensitivity treatment and assessment. New York: Academic Press; 2019. p. 55–75.
40. Erickson SR, Guthrie S, VanEtten-Lee M, Himle J, Hoffman J, Santos SF, Janek AS, Zivin K, Abelson JL. Severity of anxiety and work-related outcomes of patients with anxiety disorders. Depress Anxiety. 2009;26(12):1165–71.
41. Panayiotou G, Karekla M. Perceived social support helps, but does not buffer the negative impact of anxiety disorders on quality of life and perceived stress. Soc Psychiatry Psychiatr Epidemiol. 2013;48(2):283–94. https://doi.org/10.1007/s00127-012-0533-6.
42. Brown C, Stoffel VC, Munoz J. Occupational therapy in mental health: a vision for participation. Philadelphia: FA Davis; 2019.
43. Duncan M, Prowse C. Occupational therapy for anxiety, somatic and stress-related disorders. In: Crouch R, Alers V, editors. Occupational therapy in psychiatry and mental health. New York: Wiley; 2014. https://ebookcentral.proquest.com.
44. Shepardson RL, Funderburk JS, Weisberg RB. Adapting evidence-based, cognitive-behavioral interventions for anxiety for use with adults in integrated primary care settings. Fam Syst Health. 2016;34(2):114.
45. Hofmann SG, Asnaani A, Vonk IJ, Sawyer AT, Fang A. The efficacy of cognitive behavioral therapy: a review of meta-analyses. Cogn Ther Res. 2012;36(5):427–40.
46. Butler B, Chapman J, Forman E, Beck A. The empirical status of cognitive-behavioral therapy: a review of meta-analyses. Clin Psychol Rev. 2006;26:17–31.
47. Randall CL, McNeil DW. Motivational interviewing as an adjunct to cognitive behavior therapy for anxiety disorders: a critical review of the literature. Cogn Behav Pract. 2017;24(3):296–311.
48. Abramowitz JS, Deacon BJ, Whiteside SP. Exposure therapy for anxiety: principles and practice. New York: Guilford Publications; 2019.
49. American Occupational Therapy Association. Occupational therapy's role in medication management. Am J Occup Ther. 2017;71(Suppl. 2):7112410025. https://doi.org/10.5014/ajot.2017.716S02.
50. Cinculova A, Kamarádová D, Ociskóvá M, Praško J, Latalova K, Vrbova K. Adherence, self-stigma and discontinuation of pharmacotherapy in patients with anxiety disorders-cross sectional study. Neuroendocrinol Lett. 2017;38(6):429–36.
51. Baker KD, Loughman A, Spencer SJ, Reichelt AC. The impact of obesity and hypercaloric diet consumption on anxiety and emotional behavior across the lifespan. Neurosci Biobehav Rev. 2017;83:173–82.
52. Ho E, Siu AM. Occupational therapy practice in sleep management: a review of conceptual models and research evidence. Occup Ther Int. 2018;2018:8637498.
53. Cox RC, Olatunji BO. A systematic review of sleep disturbance in anxiety and related disorders. J Anxiety Disord. 2016;37:104–29.
54. Wolitzky-Taylor K, Krull J, Rawson R, Roy-Byrne P, Ries R, Craske MG. Randomized clinical trial evaluating the preliminary effectiveness of an integrated anxiety disorder treatment in substance use disorder specialty clinics. J Consult Clin Psychol. 2018;86(1):81.
55. McMahon K, Anand D, Morris-Jones M, Rosenthal MZ. A path from childhood sensory processing disorder to anxiety disorders: the mediating role of emotion dysregulation and adult sensory processing disorder symptoms. Front Integr Neurosci. 2019;13:22.

56. Olivares-Olivares PJ, Ortiz-González PF, Olivares J. Role of social skills training in adolescents with social anxiety disorder. Int J Clin Health Psychol. 2019;19(1):41–8.
57. Muschalla B, Heldmann M, Fay D. The significance of job-anxiety in a working population. Occup Med. 2013;63(6):415–21.
58. Maley CM, Pagana NK, Velenger CA, Humbert TK. Dealing with major life events and transitions: a systematic literature review on and occupational analysis of spirituality. Am J Occup Ther. 2016;70(4):7004260010p1–6.

Chapter 12
Arthritis

Sue Dahl-Popolizio

Introduction

The term arthritis references inflammation in one or more joints. There are many reasons for the accompanying pain, stiffness, swelling, and impaired function that typically occurs with arthritis and treatment varies based on the type of arthritis a person has. The CDC recognizes the many conditions as types of arthritis [1] which are detailed below.

- **Osteoarthritis (OA):**
  - The most common form of arthritis, it is also known as degenerative joint disease (DJD) or wear-and-tear arthritis. Though there are many factors that contribute to the development of OA, this condition tends to worsen with age and with environmental stressors, such as repetitive activities, trauma to the affected joint tissues, and the additional pressure and excessive weight bearing on the joints imposed by increased body weight (overweight/obesity). Typically, this condition is diagnosed by clinical exam, radiographs (X-ray), and sometimes lab tests such as joint fluid analysis, or blood tests to rule out rheumatoid arthritis. Movement can decrease pain/stiffness in OA [1].
  - Adults over 65 years old are at highest risk of developing OA, especially when they have engaged in repetitive occupations. Obesity, previous joint trauma, loss of upper and lower extremity strength, and genetic predisposition increase the risk of developing OA. In general, pain and stiffness are worse in the morning or after sedentary periods. Pain and stiffness decrease with warmth and activity.

S. Dahl-Popolizio (✉)
AT Still University, Mesa, AZ, USA

Arizona State University, Phoenix, AZ, USA
e-mail: sdahlpopolizio@atsu.edu

© Springer Nature Switzerland AG 2023   129
S. Dahl-Popolizio et al. (eds.), *Primary Care Occupational Therapy*,
https://doi.org/10.1007/978-3-031-20882-9_12

- **Rheumatoid arthritis (RA):**

    – Rheumatoid arthritis is an autoimmune disease where the body develops anti-bodies that attack normal healthy cells, resulting in pain and inflammation in the affected tissue, primarily joints. The joints of the hand, typically metacarpophalangeal (MCP), proximal interphalangeal (PIP), and wrists, as well as the shoulders, knees, and ankles/feet are the most commonly affected joints with RA. Chronic pain, joint deformity, impaired function, and/or disability can occur due to RA. Obesity can worsen pain and impair function, and can increase the risk of heart disease in this population as patients with RA have a higher risk of developing heart disease, diabetes, and other chronic conditions. This condition is typically diagnosed with blood tests that evaluate inflammation levels and look for the presence of biomarkers specific to RA [1]. Although not specified by the CDC as one of the arthritis types [1], psoriatic arthritis presents with symptoms similar to other arthritis types, with psoriasis being the distinguishing feature [2, 3]. Treatment by the OTP and PCP is most similar to RA [3].

    – In general, too much activity can increase pain with RA, but physical activity when paced according to patient need/condition can benefit those with RA. Consider joint condition, pain level, and patient reports regarding pain level with activity. If activity increases pain, modify the activity accordingly.

- **Childhood arthritis or juvenile idiopathic arthritis (JIA):**

    – Characterized by joint pain, swelling, stiffness, and difficulty with activities, JIA can be intermittent or the patient can experience a permanent remission. Rash, fatigue, eye inflammation, and loss of appetite are additional symptoms the patient may experience. The goal of treatment is to minimize pain, and maximize function and quality of life.

- **Gout:**

    – Gout is a painful condition that is caused by hyperuricemia or too much uric acid in the body. Characterized by painful flares that can last for days or several weeks. There are typically long periods of remission following these painful flare-ups. It typically affects one joint at a time, and the most common symptoms include pain, swelling, redness, and palpable heat. Gout is diagnosed during a flare with a clinical examination, X-rays, and lab tests that look for uric acid crystals in the affected joint [1].

- **Lupus:**

    – The CDC [4] identifies Lupus as a chronic autoimmune condition with no specific cure. It can affect any body organ so symptoms vary based on what areas of the body are affected, and symptoms can vary among people. For example, some patients report joint pain and swelling, while others report chronic fatigue or symptoms related to the organs affected, such as the kidney. Rashes, hair loss, light sensitivity, mouth sores, anemia, memory issues, or confusion are all reported symptoms of Lupus. Symptoms can be intermittent, and the condition is recognized to have periods of flares of symptoms and periods of remission. Lupus is diagnosed through medical history, family history of autoimmune conditions, physical exam looking for rashes or other indicators, blood and urine tests. The diagnosis is made as a result of many or all of these diagnostic procedures and when other conditions have been ruled out.

- **Fibromyalgia:**
  - Refer to the ***Persistent Pain*** chapter (Chap. 34) for information on diagnosis and treatment.

Role of PCP

The treatment provided by the PCP will vary based on type of arthritis.

- **Osteoarthritis (OA):**
  - The PCP typically provides symptomatic relief in the form of acetaminophen and nonsteroidal anti-inflammatory drugs (NSAID) such as ibuprofen and naproxen. NSAIDs are available at prescription and over-the-counter dosages, and the PCP will determine which dosage and type to prescribe.

- **Rheumatoid arthritis (RA):**
  - The PCP can prescribe antirheumatic drugs or "disease-modifying antirheumatic drugs" (DMARD) or a subset of DMARDs called biological response modifiers or "biologics" for RA.
  - Patients are often referred to physical therapy (PT) and OT, and if pain persists or dysfunction is more severe than is manageable at the PCP level, patients may be referred for more intense outpatient OT or PT, or for a rheumatologist or surgical consult.

- **Childhood arthritis (JIA):**
  - Treating this condition early and aggressively can help reduce the risk of disease progression. Treatment can include medications, exercise, pain management strategies, eye, and dental care. Medications can include NSAIDS, DMARDS, biologics, or corticosteroids.

- **Gout:**
  - The CDC [1] recommends a referral to a rheumatologist for diagnosis and initial treatment. A PCP can then track the condition and help the patient manage gout with anti-inflammatories, non-steroidal or steroidal. The PCP can facilitate self-management by recommending the patient change their diet and lifestyle (e.g., eat fewer foods that facilitate uric acid production, monitor medication, etc.). The patient may require drugs that reduce uric acid levels if frequent acute flares occur.

- **Lupus:**
  - This condition is medically managed by the physician with pharmacological interventions that address inflammation, pain, rashes, fatigue, and other individual symptoms [4, 5]. See the CDC website for more detailed information [4].

Common Comorbidities

According to the arthritis foundation, the following conditions can occur comorbidly with arthritis:

- Depression—PHQ-2 and PHQ-9 can easily be incorporated into an initial evaluation as they are short assessments (Chap. 18).
- Diabetes—(Chap. 19).
- Heart disease and related conditions (myocardial infarction, stroke, atrialfibrillation, hypertension (HTN), atherosclerosis, etc.)—(Chap. 26).
- Obesity (can be bi-directional)—(Chap. 30).
- Sleep problems—include questions about sleep in evaluation or complete a brief sleep assessment (Chap. 27).
- Eye inflammation (in those with JIA)—regular evaluations by an ophthalmologist are indicated.
- Trigger finger (stenosing tenosynovitis) can occur comorbidly with this population and is sometimes missed (Chap. 35).

  For more information: https://www.arthritis.org/living-with-arthritis/comorbidities/

Role of OTP

Identify how the diagnosis is impeding the patient's occupations and quality of life and provide strategies to improve both. During your initial evaluation, be sure to review the chart for common comorbidities and include basic questions/screens to determine if any of these issues are possible comorbidities that require intervention while you are working with the patient on the presenting complaint of arthritis.

There is often a relationship between arthritis and behavioral health conditions. For instance, living in chronic pain due to arthritis can lead to depression or anxiety as the patient experiences gradual progressive loss of function due to pain. The patient may be presenting to the PCP with any one of these issues as the primary complaint; be sure to assess for comorbidities.

Occupational Impact

In PC, the goal of OT is to minimize pain, maximize function, retard the progression of deformity, and address any comorbid issues that will improve the patient's quality of life. Basic management of arthritis across the lifespan can occur in PC, though if more intense or advanced treatment is indicated, a referral to outpatient OT may be required at times.

Loss of joint ROM, strength, and function, as well as joint deformity and pain are primary symptoms with OA. The hips, knees, and fingers are the most commonly affected joints, although wrists, shoulders, and the spine can be affected as well. Occupational impact varies from mild impairment to severe disability based on the level of pain and joint destruction, and which joints are affected by arthritis. Specific functional activities affected depend on the joints affected, the severity of the pain, ROM deficits, and strength loss. Fatigue, depression, and anxiety are also common symptoms that may result in reduced occupational participation.

The pain associated with arthritis can result in activity avoidance and a sedentary lifestyle. Lack of physical activity in turn leads to increased joint stiffness, pain, and general debility, which can further increase activity avoidance, creating a positive feedback loop that can foster disability and loss of occupation.

OT Areas of Emphasis

- **Pain management**—medication as prescribed or suggested by the PCP. The OTP can help the patient with medication adherence strategies, such as taking ibuprofen with meals, keeping a journal/schedule of medication times/doses. The OTP can provide non-pharmacological pain management strategies, such as progressive relaxation (focused breathing, progressive muscle relaxation), guided imagery, and mindfulness meditation.
- **Identify lifestyle modification needs**—help the patient identify specific activities that are difficult or painful and provide specific activity modification strategies. See Appendix for the ***Joint Protection Techniques Handout*** for patients. To ensure long-term sustainability of any necessary lifestyle change, be sure your suggestions are realistic for the patient based on their job responsibilities, personal goals, values, culture, resources, and specific daily routines. Provide education regarding how to maintain/regain function while protecting the integrity of the joints.
- Gout specifically may require changes in diet and weight loss. Patients with lupus may benefit from strategies to help them adhere to medical advice, including lifestyle modifications. Patients will benefit from OT to identify any barriers to these necessary changes and specific strategies to overcome these barriers.

Evaluation

Suggested Areas to Assess/Assessment Tools

Hand/wrist/shoulder pain, ROM, and strength: functional AROM and strength (can you show me how you wash your hair, tuck in a shirt, tie your shoes?). This lets you know where further task analysis is indicated. If you see specific joints that can benefit from direct treatment, complete AROM assessment of those joints. Use this concept with a basic strength assessment as well.

Overall ADL and mobility assessment: Assess transfers (sit to stand, supine to sit) simulated bathroom and kitchen mobility ambulating in room.

Pain: use the visual analog pain scale (VAS) or the numeric pain rating (0–10) free, available online (https://eportfolios.macaulay.cuny.edu/reisf16/files/2016/09/pain-scale-visual.pdf).

ROM: goniometer.

Strength
- general—manual muscle testing
- grip strength—dynamometer
- pinch strength—pinch meter

Functional Assessment

UE specific assessments:
   Quick DASH

- 11-item questionnaire indicating level of difficulty completing various tasks
- Free, available online

   Manual Ability Measure (MAM)

- 16 or 36-item questionnaire indicated level of difficulty completing various functional hand tasks
- Free, available online

   General function:
   Katz Index of Independence in Activities of Daily Living

- Brief assessment of 6 ADL areas and 8 IADL areas
- Free, available online
- Canadian Occupational Performance Measure (COPM)
- Open-ended interview assessing client's perception of their occupational performance over time

- Purchase necessary

  Assessments for co-morbid conditions outlined above.

  Assess level of deformity and determine if orthoses may retard progression of the deformity by providing external support to offset the internal joint destruction. Common issues requiring orthoses with this population that you should assess include:

- Carpometacarpal (CMC) pain, deformity, functional impairment
- Proximal interphalangeal (PIP) pain, deformity, functional impairment
- Wrist pain, deformity, functional impairment
- Triggering/trigger finger: assess for triggering and pain at the A-1 pulley/volar metacarpal phalangeal (MCP) joint

  For more assessment tools: https://www.sralab.org/rehabilitation-measures

Intervention Strategies

Orthoses

A common orthosis for this population is a CMC orthosis. PIP orthoses and volar wrist orthoses are also helpful if indicated for joint support and to reduce pain and further deformity. If a trigger finger is noted, the nodule is at the A-1 pulley at the MCP joint. If so, a PIP orthosis that allows full extension and restricts full flexion is very effective. A similar orthosis can be used for triggering at the thumb.

For patterns and pictures of orthoses, see ***Common Orthoses in Primary Care*** resource in Appendix.

Provide joint protection strategies to decrease pain and reduce the risk of causing or increasing pain with ADLs and IADLs

- Support trunk against counter for standing tasks
- Use two hands rather than one when possible
- Use built-up handles as indicated
- Use larger joints or multiple joints (e.g., carrying a bag in arms rather than with hand loop, stir with primitive grasp circling with arm rather than holding spoon in pinch and using wrist)
- Use primitive grasp rather than pinch (e.g., holding a toothbrush, pulling up socks/pants)

There are multiple sources for handouts or information to give to patients. We have provided a basic joint protection handout here. See Appendix for ***Joint Protection Techniques Handout***.

Teach the Patient to Pace Activities

- Take frequent breaks during ADLs or IADLs
- Place chairs throughout house to sit intermittently while ambulating
- Sit for activity or intermittently during activity

See Appendix for ***Joint Protection Techniques Handout***

Unless contraindicated, heat and ice can be used as needed to manage pain. Typically, heat decreases pain and stiffness. Educate patients in safe use of these modalities (e.g., avoid direct contact with skin, use temperature controlled heating pad or paraffin bath, instruct them regarding time limit, contraindications, etc.) [6].

With OA, patients can also be taught gentle joint distraction/stretching followed by AROM exercises

- finger flexion/extension
- finger abduction/adduction
- lateral and three point pinch
- shoulder elbow/wrist/hand AROM

Also with OA only, rice immersion can be used to simultaneously provide support and resistance with gentle opening/closing of fingers and gentle pinching of fingers. This can help decrease pain and increase strength. Observe the patient doing this in the clinic, and instruct the patient to do no more than 5–10 repetitions at home to avoid causing increased pain from overuse.

Adaptive Equipment

To help improve function and manage pain with ADLs and IADLs, this population often benefits from adaptive equipment commonly available through rehabilitation equipment vendors. Some things to consider include

- reacher
- long handled equipment (sponge, shoe horn, dressing stick)
- hand-held shower head
- Swedish Serrated knife (knife with gross grasp handle)
- mounted jar/bottle opener
- dycem non-slip grip material
- narrow cups/glasses
- items that allow gross grasp rather than pinch

Other Considerations and Resources

- Documentation and Billing:
  - Use the Physical Medicine and Rehabilitation CPT code that best fits your intervention. If you provide a custom or prefabricated orthosis, use the appropriate L-code or Orthotic Management and Training CPT code that reflects your intervention. See the ***Administrative and Operational Considerations*** chapter (Chap. 3).

- Suggested referrals:
  - OT in an outpatient setting for orthosis fabrication, treatment with physical agent modalities, or more intense one-on-one OT intervention.
  - PT for overall strengthening exercises.
  - Dietician or nutritionist for guidance regarding the optimal diet for the type of arthritis.
  - Orthopedic or plastic surgeon for surgery evaluation, if necessary.

- Additional resources:
  - Arthritis Foundation website: https://www.arthritis.org/
  - Occupational Therapy Toolkit for handouts: https://www.ottoolkit.com/individual

References

1. Centers for Disease Control and Prevention. Arthritis types.. https://www.cdc.gov/arthritis/basics/types.html.
2. Centers for Disease Control and Prevention. Psoriasis. https://www.cdc.gov/psoriasis/.
3. American College of Rheumatology. Psoriatic arthritis. https://www.rheumatology.org/I-Am-A/Patient-Caregiver/Diseases-Conditions/Psoriatic-Arthritis.
4. Centers for Disease Control and Prevention. Lupus. https://www.cdc.gov/lupus/index.htm.
5. OASH: Office on Women's Health. Lupus. https://www.womenshealth.gov/lupus.
6. Arthritis Foundation. Heat therapy helps relax stiff joints. https://www.arthritis.org.

Chapter 13
Chronic Obstructive Pulmonary Disease and Asthma

Tina M. Sauber

Introduction

Chronic obstructive pulmonary disease (COPD) is a group of gradually progressive diseases that cause airflow blockage and breathing-related problems [1]. It is an irreversible condition that is the result of an inflammatory process and the deterioration of pulmonary function as the disease progresses. COPD is the third leading cause of death in the United States [1]. The group of COPD diseases includes emphysema, chronic bronchitis, obstructive bronchiolitis, and asthma.

The cause of COPD includes tobacco smoke, exposure to air pollutants, genetic factors, respiratory infections, skeletal problems, such as scoliosis, obesity, or nervous system diseases that affect the muscles which assist with breathing.

Patient History Often Includes
- Long history of tobacco use
- Exposure to dust or chemicals
- Family history of respiratory issues

Signs and Symptoms Include
- Chronic cough
- Chronic sputum production
- Inhalation of smoke from cooking and heating fuels
- Reduced expiratory airflow and reduced forced expiratory volume in 1 s
- Rapid and shallow breathing using accessory muscles
- Lung hyperinflation

T. M. Sauber (✉)
Arizona State University, Phoenix, AZ, USA

Mayo Clinic, Phoenix, AZ, USA
e-mail: tinasauber@desertinet.com

© Springer Nature Switzerland AG 2023
S. Dahl-Popolizio et al. (eds.), *Primary Care Occupational Therapy*,
https://doi.org/10.1007/978-3-031-20882-9_13

- Dyspnea on exertion
- Dyspnea-related anxiety
- Progressive deconditioning
- Fatigue
- Shortness of breath and difficulty taking deep breaths

Role of the PCP

- Pathophysiological overview including diagnostic tests and thresholds

    – Spirometry test is performed to measure pulmonary function
    – Chest X-rays
    – CT scan
    – Arterial blood gas
    – Electrocardiography
    – Echocardiography
    – Pulse oximetry
    – Sputum analysis

- Overview of the role of the PCP in management

    – Vaccinations
    – Antibiotics for infections
    – Bronchodilators and steroids as needed
    – Oxygen therapy
    – Diuretics
    – Prevention of exacerbations
    – Dietary recommendations
    – Referrals to:

        Pulmonologist
        Occupational Therapy (OT)
        Physical therapy (PT)
        Respiratory therapy and or pulmonary rehabilitation programs
        Dietician/nutritionist

- Prognosis: COPD is a progressive condition that can be controlled and slowed. Lost pulmonary function cannot be restored.
- Stages of COPD according to the Global Initiative for Chronic Obstructive Lung Disease (GOLD) staging system diagnosed by the medical provider through patient-centered examination, lung function tests, exercise capacity, and ADL performance. Dyspnea and fatigue are the two most debilitating symptoms impacting a patient's general health and participation in purposeful activity [2, 3].

    – Lung function is 80% or better—Stage 1
    – Lung function is 50–80%—Stage 2

- Lung function is 30–50%—Stage 3
- Lung function is less than 30%—Stage 4

Common Comorbidities

Of COPD and asthma include
- Anxiety—GAD-7 can easily be incorporated into an initial evaluation (Chap. 11)
- Depression—PHQ-2 and PHQ-9 can easily be incorporated into an initial evaluation as they are short assessments (Chap. 18).
- Cardiovascular disease
- Osteoporosis
- Metabolic syndrome and its consequences, including diabetes (Chap. 19)

Role of OTP

Identify specific physical and behavioral health aspects of the patient's life that are impacted by the diagnosis and provide strategies and resources that the patient can use to facilitate self-management of this chronic condition. Provide ongoing support as the patient will present to PC across the lifespan.

Occupational Impact

Impaired breathing and hypoxemia (low level of oxygen in the blood) causes impairment in the ability to complete many ADLs which causes dependence in self-care skills (bathing and dressing), home management, medication adherence, functional mobility, vocational/work, social interactions, recreational/leisure activities, sleep, and cognition. Increased incidence of frequent visits to the PC office and emergency room due to physical symptoms as well as increased anxiety and depression may occur with this population. Dyspnea and fatigue are the most significant symptoms causing functional impairment.

OT Areas of Emphasis

- Assessment/evaluation and intervention
- Education
- Assist patients by modifying, pacing, and grading activities
- Environmental modifications

- Assessing adaptive equipment needs
- Promote participation in routine ADLs and IADLs
- Provide emotional and psychological support

Provide Prevention Techniques to Avoid the Condition, Retard Disease Progression, or Reduce Symptom Exacerbation
- Avoid/stop smoking
- Avoid second-hand smoke
- Avoid dust, air pollution, and work-related fumes (wear a mask as needed)
- Avoid excessive heat, cold, and high altitudes
- Early diagnosis of COPD through routine physical exams

Considerations for Treatment
- There is a risk of developing a pulmonary embolism (PE) [4, 5]. The OTP should be aware of the signs and symptoms to recognize the potential for a PE and inform the PCP
- Signs and symptoms of a PE that require emergent notification to the nurse or physician include:
- Rapid onset of tachypnea—rapid breathing (more than 60 breaths per minute)
- Anxiety—increase in frequency of intense, excessive, and persistent worrying and/or fear about routine life situations
- Lightheadedness—feeling faint or woozy (close to passing out)
- Tachycardia—fast heart rate (over 100 beats per minute)
- Chest pain—chest discomfort such as dull ache, crushing or burning feeling, sharp stabbing pain, and pain that radiates
- Dysrhythmia—abnormality of brain or heart rhythm
- Hypotension—low blood pressure (less than 90/60)
- Decreased SpO_2—oxygen saturation (normal 95–100)

Evaluation

- Vital signs

  - Blood pressure, heart rate, oxygen saturations

- Physical skills and abilities

  - Range of Motion—watch for signs of decreased range of motion
  - Manual Muscle Testing—watch for signs of diminished strength, ability to manage portable oxygen tanks
  - Endurance and Activity Tolerance—Level of exertion tolerance
  - Balance/Postural Control—Assess posture for adequate breathing and balance for falls and safety. See the Falls and Falls Prevention Chapter for additional information (Chap. 22)

- Functional Mobility—Assess use of assistive device, ability to navigate around oxygen cords and carry supplemental oxygen
- Vision
  - Assess ability to read prescription bottles and directions, lighting in the home
- Cognition
  - Assess disease awareness, memory for medication adherence, judgment and safety
  - Kokmen Short Test of Mental Status (STMS): Assesses mild cognitive impairment

    Free, available online

  - Montreal Cognitive Assessment (MOCA): Assesses cognitive impairment

    Available online

  - Cognitive Performance Test: Assesses functional cognition (ADLS and IADLs)

    Available for a fee (https://www.therapro.com/Browse-Category/ Cognitive-Assessments/Cognitive-Performance-Test.html)

- Affect and Mood
  - Look for signs of anxiety, depression, denial or passivity
  - Beck Depression Inventory-II (BDI-II): Measure to detect and measure severity of depression

    Brief self-report questionnaire may be available online (https://naviauxlab. ucsd.edu/wp-content/uploads/2020/09/BDI21.pdff)

  - Generalized Anxiety Disorder-7 (GAD-7): Screening tool for anxiety

    Brief self-report questionnaire, Free and available online (https://adaa.org/ sites/default/files/GAD-7_Anxiety-updated_0.pdf)

  - Patient Health Questionnaire (PHQ-9): Screening tool for depression

    Brief self-report questionnaire, Free and available online (https://www. apa.org/depression-guideline/patient-health-questionnaire.pdf)

- Social Support
- Activities of Daily Living Skill (ADLs)

  - Lifestyle Modifications: need for modified environment, adaptive equipment, durable medical equipment
  - Barthel Index: Assesses performance on ADLS, functional mobility and gait

    Free, available online (https://www.sralab.org/sites/default/files/2017-07/ barthel.pdf)

- Canadian Occupational Performance Measure (COPM): Assesses client's self-perception of performance in everyday living. Available for a fee (https://www.thecopm.ca/)
- Kohlman Evaluation of Living Skills (KELS): Assesses ADL function, community re-entry for independent living (https://www.sralab.org/rehabilitation-measures/kohlman-evaluation-living-skills)

- Home Management

  - Assess living situation and ability to live alone, perform home living tasks, shopping, driving, money management, home modifications

- Sleep

  - Positioning, adequate rest
  - Modified Fatigue Impact Scale: Self-report questionnaire to assess how fatigue affects a client's physical, cognitive, and psychosocial functioning (https://www.sralab.org/rehabilitation-measures/modified-fatigue-impact-scale).

- Leisure

  - Assess participation or withdrawal from social activities

- Environmental Safety

  - Assess judgment; assess home environment to decrease risk of fatigue, falls, and other safety concerns

Intervention Strategies

- Therapeutic exercise program

  - Increasing strength for bilateral upper and lower extremities
  - Increasing range of motion for bilateral upper and lower extremities

- Breathing techniques

  - Abdominal breathing
  - Pursed-lip breathing
  - Lower rib breathing
  - Relaxation breathing
  - Incentive spirometer

- Endurance training

  - Increasing tolerance to activity
  - Self-pacing

- Activity of daily living skills

  - Energy conservation/pacing
  - Basic self-care
  - Home living tasks
  - Medication management/adherence
  - Lifestyle modifications such as:

    Incorporating walks throughout the day with resting points on the way (e.g., chair in the hall on the way to the bathroom)
    Incorporating leisure activities that facilitate cognitive function but require minimal or intermittent exertion (e.g., playing chess with family member/friend)
    Modify diet to reduce the risk of mucus production (work with medical team/dietician)
    Help patient identify barriers to making lifestyle changes and help develop strategies to overcome barriers (e.g., don't like to walk for exercise, but willing to walk to the mailbox)

  - Leisure activities

- Functional mobility

  - Balance
  - Transfer training
  - Positioning needs

- Cognition and education

  - Disease awareness
  - Oxygen management
  - Symptom management
  - Fall prevention
  - Home safety
  - Community re-entry
  - Medication adherence
  - Activity management schedule
  - Recognition of hazardous materials both internal and external to the home

Other Considerations and Resources

Suggested referrals and equipment
- Pulmonary Rehabilitation Program
- Personal Training
- Pulse Ox monitor

Energy conservation resource
- https://www.bfwh.nhs.uk/wp-content/uploads/2018/02/PL721.pdf
- Home modifications—AOTA Fact Sheet: Occupational Therapy's Role with Home Modifications
- https://www.aota.org

Additional Resources

- Lippincott, Williams, and Wilkins. (2013). *Pathophysiology made incredibly easy (5th ed.)*. Philadelphia: Wolters, Kluwer Health.
- Mayo Clinic. (2017) COPD overview. Retrieved from https://www.mayoclinic.org/diseases-conditions/copd/diagnosis-treatment/drc-20353685
- Reed, K. L. (2001). *Quick reference to occupational therapy* (2nd ed.). Gaithersberg, MD: Aspen Publishers.
- Rehab Measures Database – Shirly Ryan ability lab https://www.sralab.org/rehabilitation-measures
- Smith-Gabai, Helene. (Eds.) (2011) *Occupational therapy in acute care/*Rockville, MD: American Occupational Therapy Association.
- Stephens, M.B. and Yew, K. S. (2008). Diagnosis of chronic obstructive pulmonary disease. *American Academy of Family Physicians, 78*(1), 87–92.
- Tamparo, C.D. and Lewis, M. A. (2011). *Diseases of the human body (5th ed.)*. F. A. Davis Company.
- Martinez CH, Miguel DJ, Mannino DM. Defining COPD-related comorbidities, 2004–2014. *J COPD F*. 2014; 1(1): 51–63. doi: https://doi.org/10.15326/jcopdf.1.1.2014.0119
- Martinez CH, Miguel DJ, Mannino DM. Defining COPD-related comorbidities, 2004–2014. *Chronic Obstr Pulm Dis*. 2014; 1(1): 51–63. doi: https://doi.org/10.15326/jcopdf.1.1.2014.0119

References

1. Centers for Disease Control and Prevention (CDC), National Center for Injury Prevention and Control. Basics about COPD; 2019.
2. Patel AR, Patel AR, Singh S, Singh S, Khawaja I. Global initiative for chronic obstructive lung disease: the changes made. Cureus. 2019;11(6):e4985. https://doi.org/10.7759/cureus.4985.
3. Patino M. Stages of COPD: mild through end-stage COPD. Manchester: Lung Health Institute; 2018. https://lunginstitute.com/blog/stages-of-copd-mild-through-end-stage/#:~:text=Mild%20COPD%20or%20Stage%201,and%2050%20percent%20of%20normal
4. https://www.mayoclinic.org/diseases-conditions/pulmonary-embolism/symptoms-causes/syc-20354647
5. https://www.cdc.gov/ncbddd/dvt/documents/aboutcdcswork.pdf

Chapter 14
Concussion

Tina M. Sauber and Jeri Young

Introduction

Concussions are the most common traumatic brain injury caused by a bump, blow, or jolt to the head that disrupts the normal function of the brain [1]. They are a major cause of disability including impairment in cognition, movement, sensory processing, and emotional functioning [2–4]. Concussions are typically not life threatening; however, their effects can be serious and life altering.

Signs and Symptoms

- Headache
- Dizziness
- Confusion
- Blurred vision
- Loss of consciousness
- Amnesia
- Nausea
- Sleep disturbance
- Memory loss

T. M. Sauber (✉)
Arizona State University, Phoenix, AZ, USA

Mayo Clinic, Phoenix, AZ, USA
e-mail: tinasauber@desertinet.com

J. Young
Mayo Clinic, Phoenix, AZ, USA
e-mail: Young.Jeri@mayo.edu

© Springer Nature Switzerland AG 2023
S. Dahl-Popolizio et al. (eds.), *Primary Care Occupational Therapy*,
https://doi.org/10.1007/978-3-031-20882-9_14

- Ringing in the ears
- Sensitivity to light
- Impaired balance
- Irritability
- Change in emotions (sad, crying, easily angered)
- Difficulty with attention and concentration

Role of PCP [5, 6]

The PCP will recognize common physical signs and symptoms after injury to facilitate timely diagnosis and treatment. Typically, the PCP will prescribe or recommend an active management approach to recovery while preventing secondary injury by initiating cognitive rest and symptom management before allowing the patient to return to work, play, or learning. For persons with persistent symptoms, the PCP may refer the patient for a neurology and vestibular rehabilitation (OT and physical therapy) consultation, with the goal of returning patients to full function.

Common Comorbidities

- Anxiety Anxiety—GAD-7 can easily be incorporated into an initial evaluation (Chap. 11).
- Depression—PHQ-9 can easily be incorporated into an initial evaluation (Chap. 18).
- Autonomic dysfunction

  - Variations in heart rate
  - Variations in body temperature
  - Fluctuating breathing rate
  - Blood pressure changes during digestion
  - Sensory impairments

- Prior concussions
- Chronic pain (Chap. 34)

Role of OTP

The OTP's role is to provide a holistic rehabilitation approach to facilitating return to activities of daily living including work, sleep, and leisure [7]. OT is instrumental in facilitating improved functional and cognitive outcomes post-concussion [2, 3]. The OTP is also well positioned to address any behavioral health issues related to the concussion.

Occupational Impact [2, 3]

- Decreased ability to read
- Difficulty transitioning back to school
- Impairment in driving
- Difficulty performing vocational roles
- Difficulty performing basic occupational roles
- Impairment in returning to sport or fitness activity
- Difficulty engaging in social environments and roles
- Impairment in leisure pursuits
- Decreased quality of life
- Impaired self-concept or self-image

OT Areas of Emphasis

Reduce symptoms and promote self-management [2–4, 7]
- Assist with return to work/school
- Symptom management/mindfulness and grounding techniques
- Environmental or activity adaptations
- Social and leisure pursuits

Evaluation

Therapists will use clinical judgment to include tests and measurements as appropriate and per patient's symptom tolerance. Standard concussion assessment process and specific tools are listed/explained below [2, 3].

Subjective Report (ask the patient)
- Description of symptoms
- Onset of symptoms
- Duration of symptoms
- Provoking activities
- Current medications
- Occupational profile

Physical Examination
- Note any bruising or physical injuries associated with the incident causing injury
- Assess neck range of motion and pain
- Assess dizziness and pain levels
- Assess sensation
- Assess proprioception

- Assess for nystagmus (repetitive, uncontrolled eye movements)

  - **Jerk nystagmus:** this occurs when the eyes make a quick movement in one direction and then a slowed movement in the opposite direction.

    Common with concussion, vestibular and inner ear disorders.

  - **Pendular nystagmus:** when the eye movements are of equal velocity in each direction.
  - **Past medical history:** including number of prior concussions.

Symptoms

Patient interview

Sport Concussion Assessment Tool-5th Edition (SCAT 3): Symptom rating scale (https://cdn-links.lww.com/permalink/jsm/a/jsm_23_2_2013_02_14_mccro-ryy_200872_sdc2.pdf).

Vestibular: Dix Hallpike test for Benign Paroxysmal Positional Vertigo (BPPV). (Chap. 20).

Vision Screening [3, 8]
- Smooth pursuits
- Saccades
- Visual fixation
- Dynamic visual acuity
- Convergence/divergence
- Vestibular ocular reflex (VOR)
- Gaze stabilization
- VOR cancellation

Cognition: Assess level of arousal, orientation, attention, recall, the ability to follow commands (1, 2, and 3 step commands), and new learning, problem-solving and insight into current deficits. Standardized Assessment: Montreal Cognitive Assessment (MOCA) (https://www.mocatest.org/the-moca-test/)

ADLS: Assessment of basic self-care tasks, home living tasks, sleep, leisure, and work-related tasks.

Motor: Assess Range of Motion of both upper extremities and lower extremities and cervical range of motion. Assess bilateral upper extremity and lower extremity strength through manual muscle testing.

Cardiovascular: Blood pressure, heart rate, and orthostatic tests to determine if there is correlation between symptoms and heart rate.

Balance
- Static
- Dynamic

Additional Suggested Assessment Tools (Links to Online Resource Provided When Available) [9, 10]
- Vestibular Ocular Motor Screening (VOMS)
- Dix Hallpike—(Chap. 20)
- Functional Gait Assessment (FGA)
- Modified Clinical Test of Sensory Interaction in Balance (mCTSIB)
- Modified Concussion Balance Test (mCOBALT)
- Canadian Occupational Performance Measure (COPM)
- Sport Concussion Assessment Tool-5th Edition (Step 2 symptom Evaluation)—SCAT-5
- Dizziness Evaluation and Treatment Post Concussion (http://www.azata.net/resources/Documents/2018%20Summer%20Symposium%20Handouts/Massingale%20FiNAL%20AZATA%20lecture%20without%20Video.pptx.pdf)

Intervention Strategies [2–4, 7]

- Provide adherence strategies for all lifestyle changes.
- Identify patient factors or environmental barriers that prevent full participation in everyday occupations.
- Encourage smoking cessation—work with PCP to provide a specific strategy or program once you identify what the patient is willing, and likely, to do.
- Suggest eliminating alcohol consumption as alcohol is a neurotoxin that inhibits healing.
- Provide strategies for sleep hygiene.
- Reduce environmental stimuli that increase symptoms, especially room lighting and computer brightness.
- Provide education with activity guidelines and restrictions based on individual's needs.
- Encourage appropriate rest after injury and resume activity in a sub-threshold intensity of physical and cognitive activity after 1–2 days of strict rest.
- Treatment interventions should be designed according to the client's goals, values, and assessment outcomes.
- Assist in guiding return to activity behaviors at sub-threshold levels to avoid increase in symptom severity.
- Provide strategies to minimize activity challenges through compensatory strategies and activity modifications.
- Provide guidance and dosing of appropriate visual, vestibular, and cognitive tasks according to the patient's symptom tolerance.
- Provide mindfulness, grounding, and relaxation strategies.
- Consider the most appropriate position the patient can tolerate each provocative activity or exercise and guide the client through treatment interventions of:

  - aerobic activity
  - vestibular
  - visual

– cognitive
– balance therapy interventions at sub-symptom threshold intensity

> The patient should be able to recover from symptom exacerbation after 3–5 min of rest following therapeutic activity.
> Add additional positional, visual, and cognitive demands as tolerated by the patient while working toward increased participation in occupations.

Educate patients in energy conservation and quality-of-life strategies such as

- Pacing—breaking up tasks to reduce fatigue and stress
- Delegating tasks that cause increase in symptoms
- Stress reduction

    – Mindfulness training such as relaxation techniques to reduce stress and manage debilitating symptoms and to increase tolerance to therapeutic activities.
    – Techniques for paced breathing and stress reduction, including paced-breathing applications or software on the smartphone or tablet.
    – Encourage participation in meditation, yoga, or tai chi practice to assist with adaptation to disability, increased self-efficacy, and acceptance of post-concussion symptoms throughout the recovery process.

- Provide guidance for school, vocational, and home environmental modifications.
- Provide strategies and recommendations to assist patients to return to structured activities as soon as possible for improved well-being and restoring a consistent routine.

    – Determine what modifications will reduce symptoms to allow participation in school, work, and home environments.
    – Patients can request accommodations at school and work to reduce sensory, cognitive, and fatigue challenges.
    – Recommend compensatory strategies to aid in reading performance, cognitive deficits, and limiting over stimulating environments.
    – Work with patients, teachers, and employers on strategies to manage symptoms such as creating modified workstations, modify lighting, anti-glare computer screens, and frequent rest breaks.

- Provide family training to increase understanding of the patient needs to reduce environmental stimuli in the home, to take frequent rest breaks, and to limit social and community activities as tolerated.

Other Considerations and Resources

- Documentation and billing: As there are many functional issues that are associated with a concussion, use the ICD-10 code that best matches the functional issue you are treating, and that matches your intervention and CPT code. (*see table below*) (Chap. 3)

- Suggested referrals base upon clinical findings
- Durable Medical Equipment (DME) per individual's needs
- Additional resources for provider and patient
  - Mayo Clinic—Mayoclinic.org
  - Vestibular Disorders Association—Vestibular.org
  - 360 Neuro Health—360neurohealth.com

Diagnoses and corresponding ICD-10 codes	
Treatment diagnosis	ICD-10 codes
Other abnormalities of gait and mobility	R26.89
Difficulty walking	R26.2
Unspecified abnormalities of gait and mobility	R26.9
Lack of coordination	R27.8
Dizziness	R42
Vertiginous syndrome	H81.93, unspecified
Cervicalgia	M54.2
Benign paroxysmal positional vertigo,	H81.13
Generalized visual field contraction or constriction	H53.489
Visual disturbance	H53.9

References

1. Centers for Disease Control and Prevention (CDC), National Center for Injury Prevention and Control. Report to congress on mild traumatic brain injury in the United States: steps to prevent a serious public health problem. Atlanta: Centers for Disease Control and Prevention; 2003.
2. Brayton-Chung A, Finch N, Kielty KD. Action: the role of occupational therapy in concussion rehabilitation. OT Pract. 2016;21(21):8–12.
3. Donnelly C, O'Neill C, Bauer M, Letts L. Canadian Occupational Performance Measure (COPM) in primary care: a profile of practice. Am J Occup Ther. 2017;71(6):1–8. https://doi.org/10.5014/ajot.2017.020008.
4. Finn C, Waskiewics MA. The role of occupational therapy in managing post-concussion syndrome. Phys Disabil Spec Interest Sect Q. 2015;38(1):1–4.
5. Kontos AP, Deitrick JM, Collins MW, Mucha A. Review of vestibular and oculomotor screening and concussion rehabilitation. J Athl Train. 2017;52(3):256–61. https://doi.org/10.4085/1062-6050-51.11.05.
6. Massingale S. Dizziness evaluation and treatment for athletes post concussion. Phoenix: Arizona Athletic Therapy Association; 2018. http://www.azata.net/resources/Documents/2018%20Summer%20Symposium%20Handouts/Massingale%20FiNAL%20AZATA%20lecture%20without%20Video.pptx.pdf
7. American Occupational Therapy Association. Occupational therapy practice framework: domain and process. Am J Occup Ther. 2014;68(Suppl. 1):S1–S48. https://doi.org/10.5014/ajot.2014.682006.
8. Hardison ME, Roll SC. Mindfulness interventions in physical rehabilitation: a scoping review. Am J Occup Ther. 2016;70:7003290030p1–9. https://doi.org/10.5014/ajot.2016.018069.

9. Mucha A, Collins MW, Elbin RJ, Furman JM, Troutman-Enseki C, DeWolf RM, Kontos, A. A brief vestibular/ocular motor screening (VOMS) assessment to evaluate concussions. Am J Sports Med. 2014;42(10):2479–86. https://doi.org/10.1177/0363546514543775.
10. Rehabilitation Measures Database Rehabilitation Institute of Chicago Website. https://www.sralab.org/lifecenter/resources/rehabilitation-measures-database. Accessed 27 May 2019.

Chapter 15
Dementia Care

Anna B. Harris

Introduction

Dementia is an overall term that describes a group of symptoms associated with a decline in memory or other thinking skills severe enough to reduce a person's ability to perform everyday activities [1]. Dementia is a disease that covers a wide range of specific medical conditions, including Alzheimer's disease. Disorders classified under the general term "dementia" are caused by abnormal brain changes [2]. The progression of dementia is dependent on the accompanying diagnosis and other factors.

Signs and Symptoms May Include:
- Memory loss that is disruptive to daily life
- Limited problem-solving abilities
- Difficulty planning
- Challenges with word finding
- Poor decision-making
- Poor judgment
- Poor ability to keep track of time
- Difficulty carrying on a conversation
- Challenges completing familiar tasks
- Losing or misplacing items with inability to retrace steps
- Confusion
- Difficulty concentrating
- Denial of deficits
- Disheveled appearance

A. B. Harris (✉)
CAPS, University of Arkansas & University of Arkansas Medical Sciences,
Fayetteville, AR, USA
e-mail: abh019@uark.edu

© Springer Nature Switzerland AG 2023
S. Dahl-Popolizio et al. (eds.), *Primary Care Occupational Therapy*,
https://doi.org/10.1007/978-3-031-20882-9_15

- Challenges with visual or spatial discrimination
- Social withdrawal
- Personality or mood changes

Role of PCP

The PCP should review the client's medical and psychiatric history, assess cognitive status, and behavioral changes. If a form of dementia is suspected, typically, the PCP will refer to neuropsychology and neurology for further testing, in order to formulate an official diagnosis. Prior to this referral, the PCP should rule out possible causes that may be due to a reversible dementia such as depression, low thyroid, or B-12 deficiencies. For clients with challenges disrupting daily life and/or increasing caregiver burden, the PCP should refer to other disciplines such as social work, OT, physical or speech therapy, with the goal to aid in management of the current challenges [3].

Common Comorbidities:
- Hypertension (Chap. 26)
- Cardiovascular disease
- Arthritis (Chap. 12)
- Chronic kidney disease
- Anemia
- Diabetes (Chap. 19)
- Diminished hearing and vision
- Parkinsonism
- Seizures
- Infections
- Malnutrition
- Sensory impairments
- Hip fractures
- Pressure sores
- Incontinence (Chap. 33)
- Depression (Chap. 9)
- Anxiety (Chap. 11)
- Gingivitis

Role of OT

Due to the likely progressive nature of dementia and the impact this condition can have on occupations, roles, and relationships over time, the OT in PC will generally address multiple physical, cognitive, and behavioral health aspects of the condition. This should include changes the client, their families, and caregivers experience due to the condition.

Occupational Impact

- Difficulty completing ADLs (dressing, bathing, toileting, feeding, eating/swallowing, functional mobility, hygiene and grooming, sexual activity, and personal device care) with limited or inability to initiate, process through, or complete these tasks.
- Challenges with functional mobility leading to increased fall risk.
- Difficulty completing IADLs such as driving, caring for pets or others, finances, health management, home management, meal preparation, shopping, and safety and emergency maintenance.
- Impaired social environment.
- Difficulty with social participation such as engaging in conversation and social appropriateness.
- Changing roles for client as well as the client's family, friends, and community in relation to client.
- Difficulty engaging in desired leisure activities.
- Difficulty completing work-related duties.
- Impaired sleep and rest [3–5].

OT Areas of Emphasis

The OT will aid in optimizing occupational performance and safety. The OT should provide caregiver support and education, address the social and physical environment, and challenging behaviors. OTs are essential in addressing these areas in order to promote occupational participation and engagement, well-being, and quality of life for the client and caregivers [3, 4, 6, 7].

Evaluation

Suggested Areas to Assess:
- Occupational abilities and interests
- Cognitive and mental functions
- Depression
- Environment (social & physical)
- Formal & informal caregivers (include abilities, needs, emotional status, and stress level)
- Client behaviors
- Physical abilities
- Pain
- Sensory
- Medication review with PCP

Suggested Assessment Tools (Links to Online Site for Resources Provided When Available)

Occupational Abilities/Interests:
- Occupational Profile
- Routine Task Inventory-Expanded (RTI-E)
- Interest Activity Inventory Checklist
- Disability Assessment for Dementia (DAD)
- Katz Index of Independence in Activities of Daily Living
- Barthel Index for Activities of Daily Living

Functional Cognition/Memory:
- Allen Cognitive Level Screen (LACLS)—if time allows, this is the preferred assessment
- Cognitive Assessment Tool Guide (CAT-G)
- Global Deterioration Scale (GDS)
- Functional Assessment Staging Test (FAST)
- Cognitive Performance Test (CPT)
- *Use the following in conjunction with a functional cognitive assessment* (use of a written cognitive screen without a functional cognitive measure is not best OT practice):
  - Mini-Cog
  - Mini-Mental State Examination (MMSE)
  - Montreal Cognitive Assessment (MoCA)
  - Short Blessed Test (good for visually impaired)
  - Saint Louis University Mental Status (SLUMS) Examination

Depression:
- Cornell Scale for Depression in Dementia (CSDD)
- Patient Health Questionnaire (PHQ-9 or PHQ-2) (only appropriate, at times, for clients with higher level cognitive functions). See *PHQ-9* in Appendix

Physical Environment (Provide to Caregiver for at-Home Completion):
- Home Environmental Assessment Protocol (HEAP)
- Alzheimer's Home Safety Checklist (Alzheimer's Association)

Caregiver:
- Caregiver Self-Assessment Questionnaire
- Patient Health Questionnaire (PHQ-9 or PHQ-2) (links above)
- Perceived Change Index
- Clinician assessment of caregiver readiness to change

Behaviors:
- Modified Neuropsychiatric Inventory (NPI-C)
- Caregiver report of changes in or challenging behaviors

Physical Assessment:
- Timed Up and Go (TUG)
- Functional Reach Test (standing)/Modified Functional Reach Test (sitting)

Pain:
- Standard Pain Scale
- Pain Assessment in Advanced Dementia Scale (PAINAD)
- Caregiver report

Sensory:
- Screen all senses
- Caregiver report

Intervention Strategies

Note: The OT MUST identify and continually assess which stage of dementia the client appears to be in to provide best intervention.

- Support the clients' best abilities to function in order to promote success with occupational participation and engagement [8]. Occupations include ADLs, IADLs, work, sleep & rest, social participation, education, health management, and leisure [6].
- Provide caregiver (formal and informal) support and education including, but not limited to:
  - Strategies to promote clients' occupational engagement.
  - Disease-specific education.
  - Effective communication strategies.
  - Strategies to address challenging behaviors (specific behaviors noted more in-depth below).
  - Taking care of themselves.
  - Stress management and coping strategies.
  - Strategies to continue a meaningful relationship with their loved one.
  - Support needs (support groups, respite care, resources, etc.)
  - Needs in regard to abilities and limitations as the client progresses (such as facilitating driving retirement, promoting continued independence and engagement with daily tasks, or when it is unsafe to leave the client alone).
  - Education on pursuing advance directive or living will. Ideally, in the early stages when the client can continue to aid in making end-of-life decisions [7].
  - Promote cognitive stimulation to improve social interaction and quality of life.
- Implement strategies to aid in preservation of quality hygiene (address toileting, bathing, oral care needs, nail care, etc.).
- Address incontinence, bladder and bowel management. Consider a timed toileting routine, as needed.

- Implement strategies to ensure proper nutrition and hydration.
- Promote activity engagement that is meaningful and purposeful with tailored activity programs, activity adaptation, and/or caregiver support to aid in success.
- Implement strategies to aid in decreased fall risk.

  - *Tip*: There is strong evidence to support fall monitoring devices to aid reduced fall risk for individuals with dementia [3].

- Promote physical activity for improved performance with occupations and to facilitate prevention of decline in abilities, as able.

  - *Tip*: Make this part of a routine that does not add additional duties to the caregiver [3].

- Address challenging behaviors, such as

  - Repetitive questioning
  - Shadowing
  - Wandering
  - Agitation
  - Inappropriate verbalizations (yelling, crying out, etc.)
  - Hoarding
  - Refusal of care (such as unwillingness to bathe, take medications, etc.)
  - Sleep issues
  - Paranoia
  - Aggressive behaviors
  - Restlessness
  - Harming self or others
  - Sexually inappropriate
  - Socially inappropriate
  - Worry
  - Delusions
  - Hallucinations
  - Fearfulness

- Modify the environment to ensure there are no physical safety hazards.
- Ensure the environment facilitates engagement in occupations, well-being, and quality of life.

  - *Tip:* There is strong evidence to support that enhancing the homelikeness of the environment decreases challenging behaviors for individuals with dementia [3].

- Address the social environment (formal and informal caregivers, family, friends, and community) by educating and supporting all involved with the client in order to facilitate continued success with occupational engagement and participation.
- Provide equipment, adaptations, and memory supports, as appropriate to promote occupational engagement and participation.

- Educate and facilitate use of spaced retrieval, errorless learning, cueing, and Montessori strategies, as appropriate to aid in preserving occupational independence, engagement, and participation.
- Educate and facilitate use of validation strategies with caregivers to promote quality of life, continued occupational engagement, and participation.
- Provide appropriate sensory experiences and needs to aid in quality of life, decrease challenging behaviors, and continued occupational engagement and participation.
  - *Tip*: Ambient music played, other than at mealtimes, has strong evidence that supports reduced challenging behaviors [3].
- Educate on and facilitate use of reminiscence therapy, as appropriate to aid in well-being and quality of life.
- Address durable medical equipment needs to promote safety, occupational engagement, and participation.
- Address positioning needs as they impact occupational performance, well-being, and quality of life.
- Assist in coordinating support and services for end-of-life care as appropriate.

Other Considerations and Resources

- Alzheimer's Association. (n.d.). Retrieved from: https://alz.org/
- Butler, L and Brizendine, K. (2005) *My Past Is Now My Future.* Lynchburg: Warwick House Publishing.
- Dementia Society. (n.d.) Retrieved from: https://www.dementiasociety.org/
- Family Caregiver Alliance National Center on Caregiving. (n.d.). Retrieved from: https://www.caregiver.org/
- Feil, N. and de-Klerk-Rubin, V. (2012) *The Validation Break through* (3rd ed.). Baltimore: Health Professions Press, Inc.
- Gitlin, L.N., and Piersol, C.V. (2014). *A Caregiver's Guide to Dementia: Using Activities and Other Strategies to Prevent, Reduce and Manage Behavioral Symptoms*. Philadelphia: Camino Books, Inc.
- Mace, N.L., and Rabins, P. (2017). *The 36-Hour Day*. Baltimore: Johns Hopkins University Press.
- Scott, P.S. (2018). *Surviving Alzheimer's.* San Francisco: Eva-Birch Media.

References

1. National Institute of Health. Basics of Alzheimer's disease and dementia: what is dementia? https://www.nia.nih.gov/health/what-is-dementia.
2. Alzheimer's association. What is Alzheimer's disease? https://alz.org/.

3. Piersol CV, Jensen L. Adults with Alzheimer's disease and related major neurocognitive disorders. Bethesda: The American Occupational Therapy Association, Inc; 2017.
4. Barney KF, Perkinson MA. Occupational therapy with aging adults. St. Louis: Elsevier; 2016.
5. Gitlin LN, Piersol CV. New ways for better days: tailoring activities for persons with dementia and caregivers. Baltimore: Center for Innovative Care in Aging Johns Hopkins School of Nursing; 2016.
6. American Occupational Therapy Association. Occupational therapy practice framework: domain and process (4th ed.). Am J Occup Ther. 2020;74(Suppl. 2):7412410010. https://doi.org/10.5014/ajot.2020.74S2001.
7. Gitlin LN, Piersol CV. A Caregiver's guide to dementia: using activities and other strategies to prevent, reduce and manage behavioral symptoms. Philadelphia: Camino Books, Inc.; 2014.
8. Allen Cognitive Group. https://allencognitive.com/

Chapter 16
Lewy Body Dementia

Katelyn Fell and Jyothi Gupta

Introduction

Lewy body dementia (LBD) is a disease that results due to abnormal deposits of a protein called alpha-synuclein in the brain of people with Parkinson's disease. In a healthy brain, alpha-synuclein plays a vital role at synaptic junctions of neurons; in LBD, clumps of the protein accumulate in areas of the brain that control memory and movement and disrupt functioning eventually killing the neurons. The cause for LBD is still unknown although there seems to be a link with loss of cholinergic neurons which synthesize the neurotransmitter acetylcholine and are important for memory and learning. There is also a loss of dopaminergic neurons that produce the neurotransmitter dopamine which plays an important role in behavior, cognition, movement, motivation, sleep, and mood [1].

Risk factors include age, sex (more men than women have LBD) family history of certain disease conditions particularly Parkinson's Disease (PD) and REM sleep disorders; thus far, LBD is not considered a genetic disease [2].

K. Fell (✉)
University of St. Augustine for Health Sciences, St. Augustine, FL, USA
e-mail: kfell@usa.edu

J. Gupta
The University of Texas Medical Branch, Galveston, TX, USA
e-mail: jygupta@utmb.edu

© Springer Nature Switzerland AG 2023   163
S. Dahl-Popolizio et al. (eds.), *Primary Care Occupational Therapy*,
https://doi.org/10.1007/978-3-031-20882-9_16

Sub-Types

Two related clinical disorders make up the LBD Spectrum [3]:

- Dementia with Lewy bodies also referred to as neurocognitive disorder (NCD) with Lewy bodies [4].
- Parkinson's disease dementia also referred to as neurocognitive disorder (NCD) due to Parkinson's disease [4].

The fifth edition of the *Diagnostic and Statistical Manual of Mental Disorders* further describes NCD as *major* NCD or *mild* NCD [4]. Diagnostic criteria for *mild* NCD include a modest decline in cognitive function that does not interfere with the capacity for independence in everyday activities [4]. Diagnostic criteria for *major* NCD includes significant cognitive decline which interferes with independence in everyday activities [4]. *Major* NCD is further categorized by the severity of symptoms using terms such as mild (impacting IADL performance), moderate (impacting both ADL and IADL performance), and severe (dependence in both ADL and IADLs) [4, 5].

Signs and Symptoms

LBD symptoms include a progressive decline in cognitive abilities such as planning, problem solving, and judgment. Individuals may also experience motor impairments or Parkinsonism, along with visual hallucinations and other behavior changes [6].

- Cognitive symptoms [4]:
    - Complex attention—sustained, selective, divided, processing speed.
    - Executive function—planning, decision making, sequencing, working memory, error correction.
    - Learning and memory—short-term, long-term, reasoning, comprehension, orientation.
    - Language—expressive, receptive, word finding, fluency, and rhythm.
    - Perceptual motor—visual perception, visual-constructional, praxis, proprioception, balance, postural control, hand-eye coordination, bilateral integration, fine motor control, gross motor control.
    - Social cognition—recognition of emotions, body language, understanding social norms.
- Motor symptoms [3, 6]:
    - Parkinsonism—bradykinesia (slow movement), rigidity, tremor, shuffling gait, stooped posture, reduced facial expression, dysphagia.

- Other symptoms [3, 6]:
  - Visual hallucinations
  - Sleep disturbances (REM sleep behavior disorder)
  - Depression
  - Apathy

Disease Stages

Timing and development of symptoms associated with Lewy body dementia are different for NCD with Lewy bodies and NCD due to Parkinson's disease. In NCD with Lewy bodies, cognitive symptoms typically present within 1 year of Parkinsonism and other physical changes. In NCD due to Parkinson's disease, motor symptoms are typically evident first, while cognitive symptoms present more than 1 year after the onset of Parkinsonism [1, 4].

Although some LBD symptoms are similar to that of NCD due to Alzheimer's disease (AD), the progression of the disease does vary. Unlike NCD due to AD, cognitive symptoms of LBD often fluctuate from day to day [7]. Changes in alertness, attention, and memory abilities may vary. Visual hallucinations are also distinctive features of LBD, along with sleep disturbances and changes in movement [3]. Though cognitive symptoms may fluctuate in early stages of LBD, the disease is progressive, with symptoms worsening over time. The stages of the disease may be classified as early, middle, and late stages.

Role of PCP

Condition management may be done by the PCP or neurologist. There is currently no effective treatment to cure or reverse the disease course for LBD. Medical management is focused on symptom management, maximizing function and safety, and education regarding the course of the disease. Medications are prescribed to help manage individual symptoms related to memory and cognition, Parkinsonism, and sleep. Non-pharmaceutical methods for managing hallucinations are encouraged, as use of antipsychotics can worsen symptoms of LBD [2]. A multidisciplinary approach is beneficial in addressing the needs of the individual and their caregivers.

Suggested Referrals:
- Geropsychologist
- OT
- Physical therapy (PT)
- Speech language pathologist
- Social worker
- Support groups

Common Comorbidities::
- Depression (Chap. 18)
- Anxiety (Chap. 11)
- Sleep disorder
- Stroke

Role of OTP

Due to the progressive nature and impact on cognitive, motor, and behavioral functioning, LBD greatly impacts occupational performance. In PC, the OTP will address the changes and the impact the changes have on the patient's habits, roles, routines, and relationships.

Occupational Impact

Early stages of the disease may involve only mild cognitive and motor impairments, resulting in declining IADL function while maintaining independence with ADLs. As the disease progresses, further decline in cognitive, motor, and behavioral functioning will result in decreased ability to perform ADLs, functional mobility, leisure, and social participation.

OT Areas of Emphasis

Working with individuals with LBD includes using a client-centered approach which emphasizes the client's abilities rather than focusing on impairment. OTPs facilitate continued participation in meaningful occupations and address quality of life across the disease continuum for those living both in the community and in long-term care. As the disease progresses and memory and new learning decline, incorporating the individual's past life experiences and roles through life story work may be helpful in engaging the client, enhancing participation, and encouraging better communication with caregivers [8]. Establishing a daily routine may also help to reduce behavioral outbursts and enhance participation. Specific attention to safety and falls prevention is important as motor symptoms progress. Throughout the course of the disease process, OTPs will:

- Facilitate participation in meaningful occupations
- Make recommendations for appropriate durable medical equipment (DME), adaptive equipment, or assistive devices as needed
- Consider functional mobility and community mobility needs

- Address upper extremity function/coordination
- Provide caregiver and family education/training
- Educate on community resources including support groups, transportation, and exercise/activity classes

Evaluation

A comprehensive evaluation which assesses cognition, motor function, and psychosocial components of the individual is vital. Developing an occupational profile will provide information about specific client factors and contexts which may support or hinder performance. Additionally, frequent functional reassessment is necessary as the disease progresses and the needs of the individual change.

Areas of Assessment

* Due to cognitive impairment associated with LBD, the cognitive and perceptual requirements of any given assessment must be considered by the OTP. Depending on the stage of the disease, some assessments may not be appropriate. When possible, we have included links to sites where you can access assessments. Many of these assessments can also be obtained through Shirley Ryan Abilities Lab website.

- Cognitive function (memory, new learning, executive functions, attention)

  - Montreal Cognitive Assessment (MoCA), Mini Mental State Examination, Mini-Cog©, Allen Cognitive Level (ACL), Cognitive Performance Test, Executive Function Performance Test, Cognitive Assessment of Minnesota, Routine Task Inventory-Expanded

- Fine Motor Coordination

  - 9 Hole Peg Test, Minnesota Rate of Manipulation Test, Purdue Pegboard, Jebson Hand Function Test

- Gait and Balance

  - Timed Up and Go Test (TUG), Berg Balance Scale, Tinetti, Activities-Specific Balance Confidence Scale, Five Times Sit to Stand Test, Functional Reach Test, 6 Minute Walk Test

- Psychosocial Components

  - Functional Behavior Profile, WHOQol-BREF, Patient Health Questionnaire (PHQ-9) Seep 'Appendix' for *PHQ-9*, Beck Depression Inventory, Cornell Scale for Depression in Dementia, Geriatric Depression Scale
  - Visual and auditory hallucinations

- ADLs Performance

    - Canadian Occupational Performance Measure (COPM), Barthel Index, Kohlman Evaluation of Living Skills (KELS), Assessment of Motor and Process Skills
    - ADL Situation Test, Katz Activities of Daily Living, Assessment of Motor and Process Skills (AMPS)

- IADL

    - Direct Assessment of Functional Abilities, Kitchen Task Assessment, Lawton Instrumental Activities of Daily Living Scale, Independent Living Scale

Other Considerations for Assessment

- Hearing and vision—unmanaged sensory impairments may accelerate cognitive decline leading to additional functional deficits [9, 10].
- Communication
- Feeding and swallowing
- Home modifications
- Social support systems
- Community resources
- End-of-life care

Intervention Strategies

Specific OT interventions will vary depending on the stage of the disease process and the individual needs of the client. OT intervention may include the following, as appropriate for the stage of the disease:

- Activity modification and use of adaptive equipment
- Cognitive skills; memory supports
- Routine management/establishment
- Functional mobility training
- Home exercise program (flexibility, functional strength training, endurance)
- Leisure exploration
- Family and caregiver education/training
- End-of-life care

Mild Stage

Mild memory impairment, word finding difficulties, or complex problem solving may be impaired at this stage. Unlike Alzheimer's disease, cognitive abilities may fluctuate from day to day during the early stages of LBD [7]. Routine ADLs such as dressing, bathing, and grooming are likely to remain intact, though may be impacted by motor symptoms including bradykinesia, tremors, or rigidity and require increased time, use of adaptive equipment, or activity modification. More complex IADL tasks such as managing finances, home management, driving in unfamiliar environments, or medication management may be performed with less accuracy, efficiency, or safety due to both cognitive and motor symptoms. Additionally, the presence of visual or auditory hallucinations may make concentration more difficult. Non-pharmaceutical approaches including modifying the environment to reduce clutter and distraction are recommended as antipsychotics may worsen symptoms [2].

Individuals in the mild stages of LBD may still live independently in the community and therefore benefit from training in memory strategies, establishment of routines, home safety assessments, and identification of IADL tasks such as meal preparation, shopping, and transportation that may require activity modification or assistance from caregivers and other support services. Use of environmental memory aids and visual cues such as calendars, signs, and notebooks may be effective compensatory strategies for improving occupational performance [5, 10].

Promoting physical activity including aerobic, balance, and resistance training may help to improve or maintain ADL performance, functional mobility, and sleep [5]. More specifically, movement training techniques including use of large amplitude movements and visual and auditory cueing may help to improve motor function and combat effects of parkinsonism [11].

Leisure and social participation may become more difficult during this stage of LBD. Providing opportunities and encouraging caregivers/others to initiate socialization may allow for continued participation and help the individual to maintain a positive self concept despite experiencing changes in cognitive and motor function [10].

New, complex learning may be difficult at this stage. Use of errorless learning techniques have been shown to be effective in improving occupational performance [5]. Caregiver education and training on use of simple and direct instructions may improve communication between the individual and caregiver. Establishing a support network is important as the disease progresses and the individual will likely require increased assistance from caregivers. Caregiver training and education on strategies allow the greatest levels of independence, while fostering a safe environment is a primary goal.

Moderate Stage

Individuals in this stage of LBD are not safe to live independently. The progression of cognitive impairment is likely to impact even routine ADL functions and individuals may require assistance or cueing from caregivers for accurate completion of daily tasks such as feeding, dressing, toileting, and bathing. There may also be changes in sleep and wake cycles including night-time wandering. Caregiver education on sleep hygiene, adequate physical activity during the day, reducing environmental stimuli, and addressing safety precautions related to wandering is beneficial [5].

In the moderate stage of LBD, most IADLs are too complex for the individual to complete independently, though with assistance and activity modifications, participation is still possible and should be encouraged when safe to do so. Social and leisure participation is further impaired and may be limited to activities that do not require complex problem solving, decision making, or initiation.

Safety awareness may be impaired, as well as judgment, and the ability to self correct. Falls prevention education for caregivers is important, as well as making recommendations for appropriate assistive devices and assistance with mobility, DME, and grab bar placement throughout the home. Use of unobtrusive safety measures (e.g., camouflaged doors or silent electronic locks) may be helpful in reducing exit attempts when wandering [5]. Changes in visuospatial skills including depth perception, positioning, and figure ground also increase risk for falls and accidents at the moderate stage. Removal of clutter from the environment and making important amenities (e.g., the toilet) highly visible is beneficial [5].

Communication skills are significantly impacted at this stage, making social interactions, expressing needs, and communication with caregivers even more challenging. Caregiver education on communication strategies and problem solving to help manage problem behaviors (agitation, combativeness) is vital for both the individual and caregiver [10]. Maintaining daily routines and consistencies within the environment are important for participation in overlearned tasks [10]. Routines should consist of not just ADLs and meal times but also time for exercise and physical activity, social interaction, leisure, relaxation and rest, and caregiver respite.

Severe Stage

Every aspect of cognitive functioning is impacted at this stage of the disease. Individuals require assistance with all self care and mobility. Motor skills and voluntary movement is limited, placing the individual at risk for development of contractures and pressure injuries. Caregiver education and assessment of positioning is important both for the individual's comfort and to mitigate the effects of immobility. Feeding and swallowing may also become severely impaired. Caregiver education and training on safe positioning and feeding strategies to reduce the risk for aspiration is important [10]. Communication is severely impaired and speech may be limited to only a few words, moaning, or other vocalizations. These may be expressions of discomfort, pain, or an unmet need, and should therefore be assessed. OT may be involved in end-of-life care which should focus on positioning, pain management, and quality of life.

Other Considerations and Resources

See above.

References

1. National Institute on Aging. What is Lewy Body dementia. 2018. https://www.nia.nih.gov/health/what-lewy-body-dementia.
2. Mayo Clinic. Lewy body dementia. 2020. https://www.mayoclinic.org/diseases-conditions/lewy-body-dementia/symptoms-causes/syc-20352025.
3. Lewy Body Dementia Association. About LBD. lbda.org. https://www.lbda.org/about-lbd/
4. American Psychiatric Association. Diagnostic and statistical manual of mental disorders (5th ed.); 2013. https://doi.org/10.1176/appi.books.9780890425596.
5. Piersol CV, Jensen L. Occupational therapy practice guidelines for adults with Alzheimer's disease and related major neurocognitive disorders. AOTA Press; 2017. https://doi.org/10.7139/2017.978-1-56900-408-1.
6. Mayo Clinic. Lewy body dementia: diagnosis and treatment. 2019 Mayoclinic.org. https://www.mayoclinic.org/diseases-conditions/lewy-body-dementia/diagnosis-treatment/drc-20352030.
7. Alzheimer's Society. The progression of dementia with Lewy bodies. alzheimers.org.uk. https://www.alzheimers.org.uk/about-dementia/symptoms-and-diagnosis/how-dementia-progresses/progression-dementia-lewy-bodies.
8. McKinney A. The value of life story work for staff, people with dementia and family members. Nurs Older People. 2017;29(5):25–9. https://doi.org/10.7748/nop.2017.e899.
9. Brenowitz WD, Kaup AR, Lin FR, Yaffe K. Multiple sensory impairment is associated with increased risk of dementia among black and white older adults. J Gerontol Ser A Biol Med Sci. 2019;74(6):890–6. https://doi.org/10.1093/gerona/gly264.
10. Pendleton HM, Schultz-Krohn W. Pedretti's occupational therapy: practice skills for physical dysfunction (8th ed.). Elsevier; 2018.
11. Homberg V. Motor training in the therapy of Parkinson's disease. Neurology. 1993;43(12):S45–6.

Chapter 17
Nonprogressive Neurocognitive Disorders

Steven J. Taylor and Lydia Royeen

Introduction

Nonprogressive neurocognitive disorders (NCDs) are neurocognitive disorders caused by a nonevolving event, such as stroke and traumatic brain injury (TBI). These conditions are nonprogressive (i.e., they do not progress over time), and due to the brain's capacity for recovery, individuals may have some degree of cognitive recovery [1]. NCDs are diagnosed by the severity to which they chronically limit one or more cognitive domains and capacity for functional independence [2]. Specifically, individuals with Mild NCD may complete their IADLs with increased time, adaptation, and/or environmental strategies, while individuals with major NCD cannot. Of the types of NCD that are nonprogressive, stroke and traumatic brain injury are the most common.

Stroke:
- Stroke is the major cause of neurocognitive disorder, second only to Alzheimer's disease; with 20–30% of individuals meeting the diagnostic criteria within 3-months after an ischemic or hemorrhagic event [2]. For ischemic strokes, cognitive limitations are specific to the focal area of brain injury, potentially causing deficits in one or more specific cognitive domains including attention, memory, executive reasoning, language, motor planning, or perceptual processing. Deficits are due to brain tissue injury and chronic vascular changes.

The original version of the chapter has been revised. A correction to this chapter can be found at https://doi.org/10.1007/978-3-031-20882-9_37

S. J. Taylor
Department of Occupational Therapy, Rush University, Chicago, IL, USA

L. Royeen (✉)
Texas Woman's University, Dallas, TX, USA

Traumatic Brain Injury:
- Traumatic brain injury (TBI) is responsible for functional limitations in 2% of the U. S. population, manifesting as a composite of cognitive, motor, and psychological disturbance [2]. These chronic symptoms are due to both focal and distributed lesions throughout neurological systems. Neurocognitive symptoms may be focal to one or more cognitive domains or cause global derangements in cognitive function and speed of information processing. Initial presentation at the time of injury, including the presence of a loss of consciousness, post-traumatic amnesia, disorientation, or neurological symptoms, is used for staging levels of severity, though course of recovery is variable (i.e., mild, moderate, or severe TBI) [2].

Role of PCP

The PCP is responsible for diagnosing NCDs. The PCP will order appropriate labs and imaging and may prescribe medications. In addition, the PCP identifies whether the client has decisional capacity for healthcare decisions/finances and completes the power of attorney paperwork if indicated. The PCP may also determine whether the client is safe to have a valid driver's license, though other providers including OTPs can assist with this.

Common Comorbidities

The following are common comorbidities for patients who have NCDs, based on the type of disorder.

Stroke
- HTN (Chap. 26), hyperlipidemia, diabetes (Chap. 19), other cardiac issues

Traumatic Brain Injury (TBI)
- Mental health conditions
- Disorders of the following systems: nervous, circulatory, endocrine
- Metabolic disorders
- Immune system disorders

Delirium/Altered Mental Status (AMS)
- Vascular changes
- Underlying infections (e.g., UTI, sepsis, pneumonia)
- Drug overdose or withdrawal
- Exposure to toxic substances

Role of OTP

The occupational impact of nonprogressive NCDs may vary widely. This will be an outcome of the type and site of brain injury, as well as the degree of injury severity. Individuals who meet the criteria of a Mild NCD will experience limitations with more complex occupations, including their IADL, and health management tasks. Those with a major NCD will experience some degree of pervasive deficits in all areas of occupation that can be addressed by the OTP.

Occupational Impact

Both global and specific mental functions will contribute to an individual's occupational performance. One of the most critical determinants of an injury's occupational impact is a client's level of insight into their condition and performance. Those with some degree of insight, also known as emergent awareness, will have an increased ability to monitor their performance and implement functional strategies. Therefore, a PC therapist should conduct an evaluation that allows understanding of both performance skills and client factors which at a minimum include insight (among higher level cognitive functions).

OT Areas of Emphasis

OTPs evaluate a client's functional skills and abilities to identify areas of deficit and strength. These insights help to direct appropriate decisions regarding home environment, driving, decisional capacity, and external referrals. The goal of OT is to maximize functioning for clients within the context of their environment.

The OT focus is "functional cognition" which is "the cognitive ability to perform daily life tasks, is conceptualized as incorporating metacognition, executive function, or other domains of cognitive functioning, performance skills and performance patterns." [3, p. 2]. Functional cognition addresses cognition from a holistic standpoint. Instead of solely focusing on attention or memory, a functional cognition evaluation focuses on examining the client's abilities within the context of their environment, while considering their performances, and use of habits, routines, and functional strategies [3].

Evaluation

The evaluation process should begin with a cognitive screen, either standardized or non-standardized (e.g., review of functional complaints, as well as client and caregiver interview). It is critical that this exploratory evaluation process not only determines the severity of cognitive limitations but also the client's level of insight into their performance. Clients require some level of insight into performance to benefit from direct approaches. Those who do not will require a more extensive assessment of their environment and ability to benefit from cues, as this is necessary for an indirect intervention approach.

- Cognitive Screening
  - Confusion Assessment Method (CAM)

    5 min observational assessment
  - Dys-executive Questionnaire Self and Rater Forms (DEX-S, DEX-R)

    Self and independent-rater report questionnaire, less than 5 min
  - Mini-Mental State Examination (MMSE)

    Performance Questionnaire, 10–15 min
- Cognitive Assessments
  - Contextual Memory Test (CMT)

    Structured Interview and Performance Questionnaire, 10–20 min
  - Executive Function Performance Test

    Performance measure, 30–45 min
  - Kettle Test

    Performance Measure, 10–25 min
  - Performance Assessment of Self-Care Skills (PASS)

    Performance Measure, 5–25 min
- Cognitive Batteries
  - Test of Everyday Attention (TEA)

    Structured Interview and Performance Questionnaire, 45–60 min
    Assesses Attention
  - Rivermead Behavioral Memory Test

    Structured Interview and Performance Questionnaire, 25–40 min
    Assesses Memory
  - Behavioral Assessment of the Dys-executive Syndrome (BADS)

    Structured Interview and Performance Questionnaire, 40–60 min
    Assesses Executive Reasoning

Cognitive assessments should be a part of a holistic evaluation, including assessment of motor skills and client factors.

Intervention Strategies

Direct approaches focus on promoting functional adaptations directly with the client, while indirect approaches focus on modifying their environment and providing caregiver training. Clients with some degree of accurate insight into their cognitive performance and limitations may benefit from an approach that uses both direct and indirect interventions; however, clients with more severe impairments usually require indirect interventions and task habituation.

Direct Intervention Approaches

- *ADLs and IADLs*: These occupations include activities geared toward taking care of one's own body and activities that support life within the community and household, which can be more complex in nature [4].

  - *Self-Care Management*: Addressing self-care is the OTP's unique role as part of the PC team. Often, clients with nonprogressive NCDs have co-morbidities, including chronic conditions. The OTP addressing chronic condition management with this population can improve the client's perceptions of activity performance and satisfaction, self-efficacy, independence, and quality of life [5]. This intervention approach may be beneficial for clients with nonprogressive NCDs, and these strategies that address global and task-specific deficits can be beneficial in aiding clients cognitive independence.
  - *Medication Management*: Educate the client regarding strategies that promote successful participation in medication management. A remediation intervention could address health literacy by making labels easier to read and ensure the client understands all directions [6]. Clients may miss medication for various reasons and trying to identify the root cause is important to help the client solve problem to overcome the identified barrier. The OTP can educate the client on use of visual cues, such as a reminder on the refrigerator or alarm reminders to promote medication compliance. A pill organizer is another strategy. The OTP can teach the client how to fill the organizer weekly to ensure accuracy, while using the organizer can still give the client a sense of autonomy and accomplishment. In addition, technology should be used when appropriate, such as smartphone applications that address medication management.
  - *Leisure Exploration*: Leisure activities are intrinsically motivating and are a preferred engagement activity for individuals [4]. With clients who have lost the ability to participate in their preferred leisure activities, a leisure interest checklist or motivational interviewing can be used to explore potential leisure interests and may be beneficial for re-engagement in leisure tasks that can contribute to the client's well-being. Leisure exploration is a valuable opportunity to have clients trial out cognitive strategies within a controlled environment; these skills can be translated to other more challenging or novel tasks once acquired.
  - *Vocational Training*: Educate clients and family members on vocational training recommendations if the client is no longer able to participate in their previous paid occupation. The OTP can focus on identifying the client's strengths and abilities to promote the client in identifying a vocation they may be interested in.

Indirect Intervention Approaches

- *Family Caregiver Education*: The OTP should educate family members with the results of the evaluation to ensure all stakeholders are aware of deficits. In addition, if the client has decreased insight into deficits, they can help provide carryover to the client. Several assessments allow for determination of the just-right level of cognitive and/or physical cueing. Training caregivers in this level of prompt can facilitate carryover of strategies at home and promote functional cognition.
- *Environmental Modifications*: the OTP can educate family members, alongside the client, on environmental modifications to improve ADL or IADL performance. Findings from standardized assessments are also valuable for noting potential functional safety deficits. These can be incorporated and addressed with recommendations for the client's home environment.
- *Team-based Collaborative Approach*: OTPs contribute to a team-based approach when working in the PC setting. After completion of the appropriate screen and evaluation measures, the OTP should collaborate with the appropriate team members, including the provider, to create a plan of care. Through collaboration, a client-centered and holistic plan of care can be created that best supports the client to maximize functioning within their contextual environments.

Other Considerations and Resources

Documentation and Billing

Documentation and billing are additional aspects that should be considered when an OTP is working in the PC setting. Documentation should be established prior to the OTP working within the PC setting. Ideally, the OTP will have access and is able to document into the electronic health record (EHR). Documentation should reflect the OT services rendered, including the evaluation, intervention, and care plan using therapeutic language. NCDs may be complex, and it is important the OTP properly evaluate and treat this diagnosis and reflect services rendered in the documentation.

Documentation is also important for billing purposes. Billing is another consideration that should be established prior to the OTP working in the PC clinic. Accurate and specific documentation justifies billing for OT services rendered. Evaluation charges will be used and depending on the site may have a low, medium, or high complexity. In addition, intervention charges that are used may include self-care, therapeutic exercise, therapeutic activity, cognition, and neuromuscular re-education. The OTP may have a different billing structure, but documentation is still important for other service providers to understand OT services as it relates to NCDs. Overall, documentation and billing are not mutually exclusive as proper documentation justifies billing.

Referrals

- Social Worker: Case management, especially in the case of significant cognitive impairment
- Neuropsychiatry: for additional assessment
- Vocational Training/Vocational Rehab

Additional Resources for Clients and their Caregivers

- American Stroke Association (available at www.stroke.org/en/life-after-stroke/recovery)
  - A division of the American Heart Association, this organization provides freely available resources for individuals who have functional impairments following a stroke. Numerous resources target functional limitations due to cognitive impairment. These are nicely organized by area of occupation. Support groups and regional resources are also identified.
- Brainline (available at www.brainline.org)
  - National organization providing both information and support to individuals who have sustained a TBI or concussion. Several practical resource guides are freely provided that address management of the cognitive symptoms of a TBI. Support groups and regional resources are also identified.
- American Occupational Therapy Association Stroke and TBI Tip Sheets for Recovery (available at https://www.aota.org/About-Occupational-Therapy/Patients-Clients/Adults/Stroke/RecoveringFromStroke.aspx for stroke; and, https://www.aota.org/About-Occupational-Therapy/Patients-Clients/Adults/Traumatic-Brain-Injury.aspx for TBI)
  - These brief tip sheets offer numerous functional strategies to address cognitive limitations following a stroke or TBI. They also identify the role of an OTP in treatment of these conditions. The tip sheets are brief and may serve as a valuable informative handout for clients during sessions.

For Professionals

- Functional Cognition and Occupational Therapy: A Practical Approach to Treating Individuals with Cognitive Loss

  - Authors: Wolf, T. J., In Edwards, D., & In Giles, G. M. (2019) available through AOTA Press and Amazon,
  - This text is for OTPs to guide treatment of functional limitations for clients with cognitive limitations. It offers information related to assessment, theory-driven treatment, and setting specific administrative practices. Chapters are written by content experts and offer pragmatic advice for implementation of strategies.

References

1. Dobkin B. Neurological rehabilitation. In: Daroff RB, Jankovic J, Mazziotta JC, Pomery SL, editors. Bradley's neurology in clinical practice. 7th ed. China: Elsevier; 2016. p. 784–813.
2. American Psychiatric Association. Neurocognitive disorders. In diagnostic and statistical manual of mental disorders. 5th ed. Washington, DC: American Psychiatric Association Publishing; 2013.
3. Giles GM, Edwards DF, Baum C, Furniss J, Skidmore E, Wolf T, Leland N. Making functional cognition a professional priority. Health policy perspectives—making functional cognition a professional priority. Am J Occup Ther. 2020;74:7401090010. https://doi.org/10.5014/ajot.2020.741002.
4. American Occupational Therapy Association. Occupational therapy practice framework: domain and process 3rded. Am J Occup Ther. 2014;68(Supplement 1):S1–47.
5. Garvey J, Connolly D, Booland F, Smith S. OPTOMAL, an occupational therapy led self-management support programme for people with multimoribidity in. Primary care: a randomized controlled trial. BMC Fam Pract. 2015;16:59.
6. Schwartz J, Smith R. The issue is-integration of medication management into occupational therapy practice. Am J Occup Ther. 2017;71:7104360010p1.

Chapter 18
Depression

Chantelle Rice Collins and Samantha Valasek

Introduction

Depression is defined as a mood disorder characterized by persistent feelings of sadness, hopelessness, and loss of interest or pleasure in meaningful activities. The lifetime prevalence of depression in Americans is 20% in women and 12% in men [1]. Among U.S.-born ethnic groups, rates of major depression are higher than those compared to foreign-born ethnic groups, with the highest rates of chronic depression in African Americans and Mexicans. As U.S. immigrants age, their rate of depression increases [2]. Depression occurs in children and adolescents younger than 15 at rates lower than adults and tends to peak in older adulthood [3]. Depression is the leading cause of disability worldwide and contributes significantly to the global disease burden [3]. Depression can be very serious, especially in cases where it leads to hospitalization, suicidal ideation, and death. Depression can be addressed through screening and a variety of treatment options.

Due to the pervasive nature of depression symptoms, this condition can have a wide-ranging impact on patients' lives. Patients most frequently experience a reduction in their quality of life secondary to cognitive, behavioral, social, and physiological changes [4]. Approximately 80% of adults with depression report some, moderate, or extreme difficulty with work, home, and social activities [5]. In older adults, depression symptoms are significant predictors of independence with IADLs [6].

C. R. Collins (✉)
University of Southern California, Los Angeles, CA, USA
e-mail: chantelle.rice@med.usc.edu

S. Valasek
Life Skills Occupational Therapy, Los Angeles, CA, USA
e-mail: sam@lifeskillsot.com

© Springer Nature Switzerland AG 2023   181
S. Dahl-Popolizio et al. (eds.), *Primary Care Occupational Therapy*,
https://doi.org/10.1007/978-3-031-20882-9_18

Diagnostic Criteria for Depressive Disorders by Type

Major Depressive Disorder

Major depressive disorder is a common mood disorder that significantly impacts an individual's engagement in daily activities due to changes in thinking and feeling [7]. The DSM-5 outlines the following criterion to make a diagnosis of depression:

- An individual is experiencing five or more of the symptoms listed below during the same 2-week period and at least one of the symptoms should be either [1] depressed mood or [2] loss of interest or pleasure. Of note, to receive a diagnosis of depression, there must be clinically significant distress or impairment in social or occupational function for the individual, and the cause of the symptoms cannot be a result of substance abuse or another medical condition.

    - Depressed mood most of the day, nearly every day.
    - Markedly diminished interest or pleasure in all, or almost all, activities most of the day, nearly every day.
    - Significant weight loss when not dieting or weight gain or decrease or increase in appetite nearly every day.
    - A slowing down of thought and a reduction of physical movement (observable by others, not merely subjective feelings of restlessness or being slowed down).
    - Fatigue or loss of energy nearly every day.
    - Feelings of worthlessness or excessive or inappropriate guilt nearly every day.
    - Diminished ability to think or concentrate or indecisiveness, nearly every day.
    - Recurrent thoughts of death, recurrent suicidal ideation without a specific plan, or a suicide attempt or a specific plan for committing suicide [8].

Persistent Depressive Disorder (Dysthymia)

- Dysthymia is the presence of a depressed mood for lasting most of the day, a majority of days, lasting for 2 years. During those 2 years, there may be periods of normal mood not lasting more than 2 months [8, 9].

Bipolar Affective Disorder

- Bipolar disorders are characterized by fluctuations in mood, energy, and activity level that impact one's ability to engage in daily occupations [8]. Bipolar is included here because in addition to manic episodes, characterized by high energy and feelings of elation, symptoms include depressive episodes which have similar characteristics to those listed above [10].

Other Related Diagnoses

- Postpartum Depression
- Psychotic Depression
  - Seasonal Affective Disorder

Role of PCP

The PCP will also engage in screening and assessment of depression, likely with limited time and training for counseling. They will order relevant labs and tests to screen for medical conditions that may be the primary cause of the depression. They will also prescribe and adjust medications as well as refer to mental health specialists as needed. Over the lifespan of the patient, they will provide surveillance and monitoring to identify times when depressive symptoms are relapsing or at risk for relapsing.

Common Comorbidities

Depression is one of the most common reasons for visits to PC [11], and it is estimated that 8–14% of patients in PC settings have depression [12]. Of those diagnosed with major depression, more than 75% suffer from a comorbid anxiety disorder [13]. Clinicians should be prepared to screen for anxiety when a patient has major depression, especially in the presence of symptoms such as excessive worry and fear (see Chap. 11) [14]. Effective treatment should be comprehensive and long term to prevent significant impacts on roles, routines, and quality of life.

There is a bidirectional relationship between chronic illness and depression. Adults with chronic conditions are 2.6 times more likely to also have a diagnosis of major depression and the likelihood of depression increases with the number of chronic conditions [15, 16]. It can be challenging to diagnose depression in patients with chronic illnesses since much of their focus at the time of appointments centers on their physical issues, and depression may be a secondary diagnosis. Patients with the following chronic illnesses are at an increased risk of depression:

- Cancer
- Coronary heart disease
- Diabetes (Chap. 19)
- Epilepsy
- Multiple sclerosis
- Stroke
- Alzheimer's disease (Chap. 9)
- HIV/AIDS

- Parkinson's disease (Chap. 31)
- Systemic lupus erythematosus (Chap. 12)
- Rheumatoid arthritis (Chap. 12)

Of note, certain demographic characteristics were associated with higher rates of major depression among those with chronic conditions, including younger age, female, lower income, higher body mass index (BMI), unemployment, worsening health status, and smoking [16].

Role of OTP

Understanding how underlying factors can contribute to depression will support the PC OTP in effectively collecting relevant information from the client that will enhance the OTP's clinical competence, influence treatment, and support rapport building.

Occupational Impact

As with most mental health diagnoses, the etiology of depression is complex, and it is often a combination of factors that increase an individual's risk (see table below). These factors affect the client's ability to complete all aspects of their ADLs and to function within the context of their lives.

Contributing factor	Potential impact
Family history and genetics	• Family history increases the risk of developing depression two to three times [17] • Family history can lead to developmental changes that can be seen as early as adolescence [18] • Research is beginning to learn about the role genetics might play in the development of depression [19, 20]
Brain chemistry	• Can impact the development of depression due to changes in brain regions, neurotransmitters, and their ability to communicate [21]
Stress and inflammation	• Can lead to prolonged activation of the immune system and dysregulation of the neuroendocrine system, especially when experienced in adolescence [21] • Can lead to dysregulation of neurotransmitters and physiological processes that impact the onset of depression
Traumatic and stressful life situations	• Can have a serious impact physiologically and emotionally, especially those that originate in childhood • When experienced during childhood, can also increase depression chronicity, result in earlier onset, lengthen episodes, and reduce remission and recovery [21] • Major losses, such as that of a loved one, job, or a relationship.

Contributing factor	Potential impact
Low socioeconomic status	• Is associated with depression, particularly when linked with unemployment and financial strain • When experienced in childhood, can double the lifetime risk of depression compared with those with the highest SES in childhood [22]
Resilience	• Includes positive emotions, cognitive flexibility, active coping skills, spirituality, and social support [21, 23] • Can be cultivated to prevent the onset of depression [24]

OT Areas of Emphasis

Identify issues causing or affecting depression and provide treatment to address the depression and improve the client's ability to experience improved quality of life as they complete daily occupations.

Evaluation

Screening

Due to the high rates of depression in PC settings, the OTP should be prepared to screen their patients appropriately. It is common to screen for depression in PC using the Patient Health Questionnaire-2 (PHQ 2) and Patient Health Questionnaire-9 (PHQ-9) [25]. The *PHQ-9* is available in the 'Appendix' also. The PHQ-2 is administered first. If the patient scores 3 or higher on the PHQ-2, then administer the PHQ-9. A score of 10 on the PHQ-9 indicates possible depression and the need for further evaluation [26]. The PHQ-2 and the PHQ-9 are free to access and use and can be found by visiting http://www.phqscreeners.com

Consultation

During a consultation for depression or depressive symptoms, the OTP should work with the patient to address the immediate next steps for their health, safety, and wellbeing. This discussion may include an initial gathering of details regarding the patient's background and depression symptoms, exacerbating and alleviating factors, and impact on occupational performance. The goals of this discussion may include:

• Offering the patient emotional support
• Establishing/building rapport

- Normalizing/destigmatizing the patient's experience
- Assessing the overall degree of impact on occupational performance and safety
- Assessing the need for further OT evaluation and treatment
- Assessing the need for referral to psychiatry, psychology, and social work

Evaluation

During the evaluation, the OTP will conduct interviews and assessments to identify medical and therapy history, support the development of an occupational profile and analyze occupational performance in order to develop a plan of care [27]. With the diagnosis of depression, OTPs will specifically emphasize gathering information regarding:

- Medical history including comorbidities, prescribed medications, and past and present therapy services (can be reviewed in the chart in advance)
- Pattern of depression symptoms over time, including triggering events, variation over days/weeks/months/years, variation with occupational engagement
- Impact on occupational performance, including ADLs, IADLs, work, leisure, and social participation
- Typical daily and weekly habits and routines
- Identifying barriers to participation, e.g., apathy, fatigue, decreased concentration
- Identifying action steps to begin to overcome barriers, e.g., recognize triggers, speak with a family member, engage in meaningful leisure activity
- Sources of meaning and connection, e.g., purpose, family, friends, spirituality
- Presence and severity of suicidal ideation
- Client's strengths and internal resources
- Client's stage of change
- Client's desired goals and objectives
- The need for brief psychoeducation regarding depression

Managing Suicidal Ideation

If the client reports suicidal ideation during the consultation, an immediate assessment of the client's imminent risk should be conducted, including an assessment of the desire, capability, and intent to complete suicide, as well as supports to prevent suicide [28]. Screening tools for suicidality include SAFE-T and the Columbia-Suicide Severity Rating Scale [29, 30]. The OTP should know and follow the facility protocols for care of patients demonstrating imminent risk of suicide at their clinic site. The SAFE-T Pocket Card [31] includes a five-step evaluation for determining suicide risk, including assessing risk factors, protective factors, assessing plans and intents, determining level of risk and appropriate intervention, and documentation. It is free to download for use by trained clinicians, including OTPs, and can be found along with additional resources by visiting https://www.sprc.org/resources-programs/suicide-assessment-five-step-evaluation-and-triage-safe-t-pocket-card

Intervention Strategies

Interventions in the Initial Stages of Treatment

Initial stages of treatment may focus on clients' adjustment to receiving a diagnosis of and treatment for depression. Immediate priorities, depending on the severity of the depression, include psychoeducation, behavioral activation and self-monitoring, and medication management. Building self-awareness and self-efficacy are crucial at this stage.

Techniques

Psychoeducation [32]

The PC OTP should provide clients with information that allows them to adopt the role of an expert, including:

- Common symptoms and patterns of symptoms with depression
- Possible functional impact
- Common exacerbating and alleviating factors
- Cognitive distortions and their impact on emotions and behavior
- Pathology
- Prevalence
- Treatment approaches
- Online and community resources

Behavioral Activation and Self-Monitoring [33]

The PC OTP can facilitate exploration of how clients experience depression in daily life, paying as much attention to activities and situations that provide hope, joy, relief, and comfort as to those that exacerbate depressive symptoms.

- Encourage clients to track depression-related symptoms, changes in mood, and energy levels along with daily activities

- Collaborate with clients to analyze the relationship between their health and wellbeing and their participation in daily activities
- Utilize this information to collaboratively set realistic expectations and goals for incorporating new behaviors into their routines
- Encourage clients to experiment with new behaviors and routines and notice how these changes impact their interactions with the world and their life satisfaction

Session Topics

Medication Adherence [34]

The PC OTP may need to collaborate with clients to overcome barriers and maximize supports for medication adherence.

Common barriers to medication adherence	Interventions to support medication management
• Finances	• Pill boxes
• Insurance coverage	• Alarms
• Side effects	• Checklists
• Fear of side effects	• Reminders (caregivers or phone)
• Inaccurate health beliefs	• Adaptive equipment
• Lack of motivation	• Caregiver training
• Memory impairment	• Psychoeducation regarding medication
• Fine motor deficits	• Normalization of medication needs
• Visual deficits	• Motivational interviewing
• Embarrassment or shame	• Self-advocacy skills training

Sensory Processing

Sensory processing impacts how clients respond to and interact with their external environment and internal sensation. Individuals with low registration of sensory input demonstrate the greatest likelihood to screen positively for depression and hopelessness while individuals with sensory sensitivity and sensory avoiding are more likely to screen positively for depression [35]. The PC OTP may address these sensory differences by:

- Prompting self-reflection and self-monitoring to enhance individuals' awareness of their response to the environment and their motivation to engage with it
- Providing education and recommendations for modifying the intensity, frequency, and duration of environmental stimuli and activity participation
- Providing mindfulness technique training to promote self-regulation of attention to daily activities and acceptance of internal experiences [36]

Lifestyle and Routine Modification

Given the interplay between lifestyle behaviors and mental health, it is encouraged that an OTP address as many of the topics below as sessions and time permit when treating a patient with depression. Using stages of changes, the OTP can assess which behaviors to prioritize recognizing that they build on one another.

- Forming health-promoting habit and routines

  - Utilize collaborative problem-solving to scaffold the development of habits and routine sequences to promote self-efficacy and carryover of identified action steps, e.g., utilize digital reminders, break task into smaller steps, practice compassionate self-talk

- Developing healthy eating patterns

  - A healthy diet has been shown to decrease the risk of depression. Clients should be encouraged to eat a variety of fruits, vegetables and whole grains, and lean proteins, such as fish [37].
  - Clients should reduce their intake of red meat, processed foods, and sugar [38].
  - OTPs can address eating routines through education of the principles of healthy eating, helping clients engage in meal planning and preparation, and supporting clients adopt accountability structures to support sustainability.

- Engaging in physical activity

  - Individuals with depression are more likely to live a sedentary lifestyle with little engagement in physical exercise [39].
  - Physical activity is an evidence-based treatment for depression. Aerobic exercise and mixed exercise approaches are beneficial, with moderate and intense exercises proving to be more beneficial than light exercise [40].
  - It is recommended that adults engage in at least 150 min of moderate-intensity or 75 min of vigorous-intensity aerobic physical activity each week as well as exercises for strengthening and flexibility [41]
  - OTPs can support patients as they initiate engagement in exercise, recognizing that this can be very challenging for patients with depression. The OTP should support the client in identifying activities they have enjoyed in the past or might enjoy currently. Through task analysis and scaffolding, the OTP can help the patient conceptualize how to incorporate exercise into their daily and weekly routines and facilitate participation.

- Sleeping well

  - Individuals with depression are likely to have issues with their sleep, more commonly reporting insomnia than hypersomnia [42].
  - Establish appropriate sleep/wake times, a wind-down routine, eliminate stimulating activities prior to sleep and make appropriate environmental modifications.
  - Patients at risk for insomnia should be screened and referred appropriately

- Managing time effectively

  - Developing time management skills is crucial for patients hoping to implement changes to habits and routines
  - Assess how patients approach time management and the effectiveness of systems used for scheduling and tracking time use
  - Address barriers and supports to improving time management skills

- Relaxing and managing stress

  - There is a reciprocal relationship between stress and depression in which one can increase an individual's risk of the other [43]
  - Prompt self-reflection to identify individuals' stress-related triggers and symptoms
  - Train individuals in problem-solving to promote utilization of active coping skills that target modifying situations triggering stress [44]
  - Utilize cognitive-behavioral approaches to address individuals' responses to unpleasant emotions and the consequent use of maladaptive coping strategies [44]
  - Train individuals in relaxation and mindfulness techniques to promote parasympathetic nervous system activation [45, 46]

- Quitting tobacco and substance use

  - There is a strong association between substance use and depression [47]
  - Depression significantly decreases after smoking cessation with effect sizes equal to or larger than those of antidepressant treatment [48]
  - Educate individuals regarding the impact of tobacco and/or substance use on depression, the benefits of cessation, and what physical and psychological symptoms and social and environmental challenges to prepare for in the process of quitting
  - Support individuals in developing a plan to quit smoking and/or substance use, including substitute habits and routines, coping strategies, and social support [49, 50]

Community Integration

Since social withdrawal and a lack of motivation are often experienced with depression, individuals may need support to reintegrate themselves with their families, peers, and communities. The OTP should encourage individuals to explore meaningful social connections and roles within the community context. Individuals may need to develop skills to support their engagement.

- Social Participation

  - Interventions targeting social skills and participation can be effective for decreasing depression in adults [51].

- Consider supplementing individual intervention with group sessions to provide real-time opportunities to improve social functioning [52]

- Work and School Engagement

  - Interventions targeting engagement in work and school can be effective for decreasing depression and improving function [53]
  - Prompt self-reflection to identify functional limitations, barriers, and supports to participation in work and school
  - Encourage individuals to modify factors within their control through environmental and activity modifications and assertive communication
  - Utilize cognitive-behavioral approaches to address individuals' responses to factors outside of their control and unpleasant emotions [44]
  - Collaborate with individuals to support requests for reasonable accommodations

- Spiritual Participation

  - Individuals who report high personal importance of religion or spirituality are at decreased risk of experiencing major depression [54]
  - Attending religious worship at least once per year and seeking spiritual comfort at least rarely are associated with decreased odds of suicide attempt and suicidal ideation, respectively [55]
  - Explore the importance and meaning of religious/spiritual expression and participation in the individual's daily life and within the context of their experience of depression [56]
  - Identify adaptations and compensatory strategies to overcome barriers to participation

Ongoing sessions should entail collaborative goal-setting to ensure that the client is implementing behavior changes that will support successful depression management.

Other Considerations and Resources

Discharge, Health Maintenance and Relapse Prevention, and Recovery

At the time of discharge, the OTP will re-administer any clinical assessments and outcomes, assess progress toward long-term goals, and engage the patient in planning for continued health maintenance and relapse prevention and recovery. Upon discharge, the OTP will determine the course of follow-up with the patient. One benefit of working in a PC setting is the potential for the OTP to check-in with the patient at their next PC visit to provide encouragement, accountability, and opportunities for further follow-up.

References

1. Kessler RC, Berglund P, Demler O, Jin R, Koretz D, Merikangas K, Rush J, Walters E, Wang P. The epidemiology of major depressive disorder: results from the National Comorbidity Survey Replication (NCS-R). JAMA. 2003;289:3095–105.
2. Gonzalez H, Tarraf W, Whitfield K, Vega W. The epidemiology of major depression and ethnicity in the United States. J Psychiatr Res. 2010;44(15):1043–51.
3. World Health Organization, Geneva. Depression and Other Common Mental Disorders: Global Health Estimates. Licence: CC BY-NC-SA 3.0 IGO. 2017.
4. Brown C, Stoffel VC, Munoz J. Occupational therapy in mental health: a vision for participation. Philadelphia: FA Davis; 2019.
5. Brody DJ, Pratt LA, Hughes JP. Prevalence of depression among adults aged 20 and over: United States, 2013–2016. NCHS Data Brief. 2018;303:1–8.
6. Chen SW, Chippendale T. Factors associated with IADL Independence among older adults: implications for occupational therapy practice. Am J Occup Ther. 2016;70(4_Suppl_1):7011505132p1-7011505132p1.
7. Pence BW, O'Donnell JK, Gaynes BN. The depression treatment cascade in primary care: a public health perspective. Curr Psychiatry Rep. 2012;14(4):328–35.
8. American Psychiatric Association. Diagnostic and Statistical Manual of Mental Disorders (DSM-5), Fifth edition. 2013.
9. Sansone RA, Sansone LA. Dysthymic disorder: forlorn and overlooked? Psychiatry (Edgmont (Township)). 2009;6(5):46–51.
10. Phillips ML, Kupfer DJ. Bipolar disorder diagnosis: challenges and future directions. Lancet. 2013;381(9878):1663–71.
11. Finley CR, Chan DS, Garrison S, Korownyk C, Kolber MR, Campbell S, Eurich DT, Lindblad AJ, Vandermeer B, Allan GM. What are the most common conditions in primary care? Systematic review. Can Fam Physician. 2018;64(11):832–40.
12. Craven MA, Bland R. Depression in primary care: current and future challenges. Can J Psychiatr. 2013;58(8):442–8. https://doi.org/10.1177/070674371305800802.
13. Olfson M, Fireman B, Weissman MM, Leon AC, Sheehan DV, Kathol RG, Hoven C, Farber L. Mental disorders and disability among patients in a primary care group practice. Am J Psychiatr. 1997;154(12):1734–40.
14. Hirschfeld R. The comorbidity of major depression and anxiety disorders: recognition and management in primary care. Prim Care Companion J Clin Psychiatry. 2001;3(6):244–54.
15. Dworkin SF, Von Korff M, LeResche L. Multiple pains and psychiatric disturbance: an epidemiologic investigation. Arch Gen Psychiatry. 1990;47(3):239–44.
16. Egede LE. Major depression in individuals with chronic medical disorders: prevalence, correlates and association with health resource utilization, lost productivity and functional disability. Gen Hosp Psychiatry. 2007;29:409–16.
17. Weissman MM, Berry OO, Warner V, et al. A 30-year study of 3 generations at high risk and low risk for depression. JAMA Psychiat. 2016;73(9):970–7. https://doi.org/10.1001/jamapsychiatry.2016.1586.
18. Swartz J, Williamson D, Hariri A. Developmental change in amygdala reactivity during adolescence: effects of family history of depression and stressful life events. Am J Psychiatry. 2014;172(3):276–83.
19. CONVERGE consortium. Sparse whole-genome sequencing identifies two loci for major depressive disorder. Nature. 2015;523(7562):588–91. https://doi.org/10.1038/nature14659.
20. Bigdeli TB, Ripke S, Peterson RE, Trzaskowski M, Bacanu SA, Abdellaoui A, et al. Genetic effects influencing risk for major depressive disorder in China and Europe. Transl Psychiatry. 2017;7(3):e1074. https://doi.org/10.1038/tp.2016.292Chemistry.
21. Saveanu R, Nemeroff C. Etiology of depression: genetic and environmental factors. Psychiatr Clin N Am. 2012;35(1):51–71.

22. Gilman S, Kawachi I, Fitzmaurice G, Buka S. Socioeconomic status in childhood and the life-time risk of major depression. Int J Epidemiol. 2002;31(2):359–67. https://doi.org/10.1093/ije/31.2.359.

23. Southwick SM, Vythilingam M, Charney DS. The psychobiology of depression and resilience to stress: implications for prevention and treatment. Annu Rev Clin Psychol. 2005;1:255–91.

24. Munoz R, Beardslee W, Leykin Y. Major depression can be prevented. Am Psychol. 2012;67(4):285–95. https://doi.org/10.1037/a0027666.

25. Maurer D, Raymond T, Davis B. Depression: screening and diagnosis. Am Fam Physician. 2018;98(8):508–15.

26. Levis B, Benedetti A, Thombs BD. Accuracy of Patient Health Questionnaire-9 (PHQ-9) for screening to detect major depression: individual participant data meta-analysis. BMJ. 2019;365:l1476.

27. American Occupational Therapy Association. Occupational therapy practice framework: domain and process. Am J Occup Ther. 2014;68(Suppl.1):S1–S48. https://doi.org/10.5014/ajot.2014.682006.

28. Gould MS, Lake AM, Munfakh JL, Galfalvy H, Kleinman M, Williams C, et al. Helping callers to the National Suicide Prevention Lifeline who are at imminent risk of suicide: evaluation of caller risk profiles and interventions implemented. Suicide Life Threat Behav. 2016;46(2):172–90.

29. Brodsky BS, Spruch-Feiner A, Stanley B. The zero suicide model: applying evidence-based suicide prevention practices to clinical care. Front Psychol. 2018;9:33.

30. Posner K, Brown GK, Stanley B, Brent DA, Yershova KV, Oquendo MA, et al. The Columbia-suicide severity rating scale: initial validity and internal consistency findings from three multisite studies with adolescents and adults. Am J Psychiatr. 2011;168:1266–77. https://doi.org/10.1176/appi.ajp.2011.10111704.

31. United States. (2009). SAFE-T: suicide assessment five-step evaluation and triage. Rockville: U.S. Dept. of Health and Human Services, Substance Abuse and Mental Health Services Administration. .

32. Donker T, Griffiths KM, Cuijpers P, Christensen H. Psychoeducation for depression, anxiety and psychological distress: a meta-analysis. BMC Med. 2009;7:79. https://doi.org/10.1186/1741-7015-7-79.

33. Mazzucchelli T, Kane R, Rees C. Behavioral activation treatments for depression in adults: a meta-analysis and review. Clin Psychol Sci Pract. 2009;16(4):383–411.

34. Brown C, Battista DR, Bruehlman R, Sereika SS, Thase ME, Dunbar-Jacob J. Beliefs about antidepressant medications in primary care patients: relationship to self-reported adherence. Med Care. 2005;43:1203–7.

35. Serafini G, Gonda X, Canepa G, Pompili M, Rihmer Z, Amore M, Engel-Yeger B. Extreme sensory processing patterns show a complex association with depression, and impulsivity, alexithymia, and hopelessness. J Affect Disord. 2017;210:249–57.

36. Hebert KR. The association between sensory processing styles and mindfulness. Br J Occup Ther. 2016;79(9):557–64.

37. Lai J, Hiles S, Bisquera A, Hure A, McEvoy M, Attia J. A systematic review and meta-analysis of dietary patterns and depression in community-dwelling adults. Am J Clin Nutr. 2014;99(1):181–97. https://doi.org/10.3945/ajcn.113.069880.

38. Oddy W, Allen K, Trapp G, Ambrosini G, Black L, Rae-Chi H, Peter R, Runions K, Pan F, Beilin L, Mori T. Dietary patterns, body mass index and inflammation: pathways to depression and mental health problems in adolescents. Brain Behav Immun. 2018;69:428–39. https://doi.org/10.1016/j.bbi.2018.01.002.

39. Roshanaei-Moghaddam B, Katon W, Russo J. The longitudinal effects of depression on physical activity. Gen Hosp Psychiatry. 2009;1(4):305–15.

40. Schuch F, Vancampfort D, Richards J, Rosenbaum S, Ward P, Stubbs B. Exercise as treatment for depression: a meta-analysis adjusting for publication bias. J Psychiatry Res. 2016;77:42–51.

41. U.S. Department of Health and Human Services. Physical activity guidelines for americans. 2nd ed; 2018.
42. Reimann D, Berger M, Voderholzer U. Sleep and depression—results from psychioloical studies: an overview. Biol Psychol. 2001;57(1–3):67–103.
43. Liu RT, Alloy LB. Stress generation in depression: a systematic review of the empirical literature and recommendations for future study. Clin Psychol Rev. 2010;30(5):582–93.
44. Thompson RJ, Mata J, Jaeggi SM, Buschkuehl M, Jonides J, Gotlib IH. Maladaptive coping, adaptive coping, and depressive symptoms: variations across age and depressive state. Behav Res Ther. 2010;48(6):459–66.
45. Costa A, Barnhofer T. Turning towards or turning away: a comparison of mindfulness meditation and guided imagery relaxation in patients with acute depression. Behav Cogn Psychother. 2016;44(4):410–9.
46. Hofmann SG, Sawyer AT, Witt AA, Oh D. The effect of mindfulness-based therapy on anxiety and depression: a meta-analytic review. J Consult Clin Psychol. 2010;78(2):169–83. https://doi.org/10.1037/a0018555.
47. Lai HMX, Cleary M, Sitharthan T, Hunt GE. Prevalence of comorbid substance use, anxiety and mood disorders in epidemiological surveys, 1990–2014: a systematic review and meta-analysis. Drug Alcohol Depend. 2015;154:1–13.
48. Taylor G, McNeill A, Girling A, Farley A, Lindson-Hawley N, Aveyard P. Change in mental health after smoking cessation: systematic review and meta-analysis. BMJ. 2014;348:g1151.
49. Dolan SL, Rohsenow DJ, Martin RA, Monti PM. Urge-specific and lifestyle coping strategies of alcoholics: relationships of specific strategies to treatment outcome. Drug Alcohol Depend. 2013;128(1–2):8–14.
50. Witkiewitz K, Bowen S. Depression, craving, and substance use following a randomized trial of mindfulness-based relapse prevention. J Consult Clin Psychol. 2010;78(3):362–74. https://doi.org/10.1037/a0019172.
51. Nagy E, Moore S. Social interventions: an effective approach to reduce adult depression? J Affect Disord. 2017;218:131–52.
52. Ramano EM, de Beer M. The outcome of two occupational therapy group programs on the social functioning of individuals with major depressive disorder. Occup Ther Ment Health. 2019;36:1–26.
53. Lerner D, Adler D, Hermann RC, Chang H, Ludman EJ, Greenhill A, Perch K, McPeck WC, Rogers WH. Impact of a work-focused intervention on the productivity and symptoms of employees with depression. J Occup Environ Med. 2012;54(2):128.
54. Miller L, Wickramaratne P, Gameroff MJ, Sage M, Tenke CE, Weissman MM. Religiosity and major depression in adults at high risk: a ten-year prospective study. Am J Psychiatr. 2012;169(1):89–94.
55. Rasic D, Robinson JA, Bolton J, Bienvenu OJ, Sareen J. Longitudinal relationships of religious worship attendance and spirituality with major depression, anxiety disorders, and suicidal ideation and attempts: findings from the Baltimore epidemiologic catchment area study. J Psychiatr Res. 2011;45(6):848–54.
56. Kirsch B. A narrative approach to addressing spirituality in occupational therapy: exploring personal meaning and purpose. Can J Occup Ther. 1996;63(1):55–61.

Chapter 19
Diabetes

Alyssa Concha-Chavez, Jesús Díaz, and Beth Pyatak

Introduction

Diabetes mellitus is a group of chronic metabolic conditions characterized by the body's inability to convert food into energy efficiently resulting in elevated blood glucose levels, also known as hyperglycemia. Insulin deficiency, insulin resistance, or a combination of both can lead to hyperglycemia. Chronic hyperglycemia causes long-term damage to organs, including eyes, kidneys, nerves, heart, and blood vessels. OT can be very effective in identifying barriers to disease management and facilitating lifestyle change and patient self-activation [1].

The American Diabetes Association (ADA) and the National Institute of Diabetes and Digestive and Kidney Diseases (NIDDK) classify diabetes into the following categories:[2]

- Insulin Resistance & Prediabetes
- Type 1 diabetes
- Type 2 diabetes
- Gestational diabetes mellitus
- Monogenic diabetes (Neonatal diabetes mellitus & maturity onset diabetes of the young, or MODY)
- Diabetes due to other causes, including
- diseases of the pancreas (e.g., cystic fibrosis and pancreatitis),
- drug—or chemical-induced diabetes (e.g., diabetes resulting from glucocorticoid use in the treatment of HIV/AIDS, or after organ transplantation)

A. Concha-Chavez (✉)
Independent Contractor, Phoenix, AZ, USA

J. Díaz · B. Pyatak
Chan Division of Occupational Science and Occupational Therapy, University of Southern California, Los Angeles, CA, USA
e-mail: jesus.diaz@chan.usc.edu; beth.pyatak@chan.usc.edu

© Springer Nature Switzerland AG 2023
S. Dahl-Popolizio et al. (eds.), *Primary Care Occupational Therapy*,
https://doi.org/10.1007/978-3-031-20882-9_19

Typically, a healthy body breaks down food into glucose and releases it into the bloodstream. The glucose levels in the blood trigger the pancreas to release the hormone insulin. Insulin functions almost like a key in cell walls allowing glucose to enter the body's cells to be used as energy. Therefore, without sufficient insulin, cells are starved of energy. In the context of diabetes, elevated blood glucose levels result from problems related to insulin secretion and/or insulin resistance.

These problems result from a variety of pathogenic processes. In type 1 diabetes, autoimmune destruction of the β-cells of the pancreas leads to little or no insulin secretion. Because β-cells cannot regenerate, people with type 1 diabetes require insulin therapy from the time of diagnosis for the rest of their lives. In type 2 diabetes, abnormalities lead to insulin resistance, which requires the β-cells to produce more insulin to meet the body's requirements. Over time, this results in β-cells also gradually losing the ability to produce insulin; studies have estimated that by the time a person is formally diagnosed with type 2 diabetes, they have lost about half of their ability to produce insulin. For type 2 diabetes, in addition to insulin therapy, there are effective oral and injectable treatments to reduce insulin resistance and to increase insulin secretion [1, 2].

Diagnostic Categories

Prediabetes, Type 1 Diabetes, and Type 2 Diabetes

According to the CDC, 34.2 million people or roughly 10.5% of the U.S. population has diabetes. Of those, as many as 7.3 million do not know they have diabetes. Type 1 diabetes (T1D) is much less prevalent than type 2 (T2D) diabetes, with approximately 1.6 million children and adults diagnosed [3].

Listed below are the diagnostic tests and threshold ranges recommended by the ADA for the classification and diagnosis of diabetes. See the *ADA Diabetes Risk Test*, available at the NIDDK website (https://www.niddk.nih.gov/health-information/community-health-outreach/diabetes-alert-day), that you can use for yourself or others [1, 2].

Diagnostic Tests and Thresholds

Diagnosis	A1C (percent)	Fasting plasma glucose (FPG)[a]	Oral glucose tolerance test (OGTT)[a,b]	Random plasma glucose test (RPG)[a]
Normal	Below 5.7	99 or below	139 or below	
Prediabetes	5.7–6.4	100–125	140–199	
Diabetes	6.5 or above	126 or above	200 or above	200 or above

[a] Glucose values are in milligrams per deciliter, or mg/dL
[b] At 2 h after drinking 75 g of glucose. To diagnose gestational diabetes, healthcare professionals give more glucose to drink and use different numbers as cutoffs

Role of PCP

The PCP monitors blood glucose levels, blood pressure, and lipid control and provides diagnosis according to current diagnostic guidelines. The PC team prioritizes timely and appropriate interventions for lifestyle modification and pharmacological therapy for patients with diabetes. The PCP oversees pharmacological treatment to optimize blood glucose levels, blood pressure, and lipid control in coordination with pharmacy and endocrinologists as needed. Diabetes often happens in the context of comorbidities. PCPs refer to other disciplines and specialists as needed for physical and mental health needs including but not limited to endocrinologists, pharmacists, registered dietitians, social workers, psychologists, psychiatrists, OTPs, and physical therapists. Ideally, the PC team will provide diabetes self-management education (DSME) or refer out to DSME resources.

Common Comorbidities

According to the ADA and NIDDK, the following conditions can occur comorbidly with diabetes [1, 2]:

- Heart disease (MI, A-fib, HTN, atherosclerosis, etc.)—(Chap. 26)
- Stroke
- Kidney disease
- Eye problems (Chap. 36)
- Dental disease
- Nerve damage
- Foot problems
- Depression—(Chap. 18)
- Sleep apnea
- Insomnia and other sleep problems (Chap. 27)
- Obesity—(Chap. 30)

Complications to Consider: As outlined above, chronic elevated blood glucose levels are a hallmark of diabetes. However, acute complications of diabetes can arise from acute elevated or low blood glucose. Acute elevations of blood glucose, in the absence of sufficient insulin, can lead to hyperglycemia emergencies and diabetic ketoacidosis (DKA). DKA primarily affects patients with T1D and is a serious condition that can lead to brain damage and death, and treatment usually takes place in the hospital. Depending on their pharmacological regimen, particularly if using sulfonylureas or insulin, people with diabetes may also experience hypoglycemia or low blood glucose. Hypoglycemia is also an urgent concern and, if left untreated, can lead to seizure, brain damage, and death.

1. Hyperglycemia

    (a) Common causes:

    - T1D–not enough insulin administered or ineffective insulin (i.e., insulin that is expired or has been exposed to extreme heat or freezing cold).
    - T2D–insulin resistance without effective medication to compensate (e.g., skipped or not enough diabetes pills or insulin).
    - Physical stress from an illness, such as a cold or flu.
    - Social-emotional stress, such as family conflicts or school or dating problems.
    - The dawn phenomenon (a surge of hormones that the body produces daily around 4:00 a.m.–5:00 a.m.)

    (b) Symptoms:

    - Increased thirst
    - Frequent urination
    - Dry mouth or skin
    - Tiredness or fatigue
    - Blurred vision
    - More frequent infections
    - Slow healing cuts and sores
    - Unexplained weight loss
    - High levels of sugar in the urine

    (c) Treatment:

    - Blood glucose can often be lowered by exercising. However, if blood glucose levels are above 240 mg/dL, the PCP will check urine for ketones. *If the patient has ketones, do not recommend exercise.*
    - Long-term self-management related to post-meal hyperglycemia involves behavior change related to medication management, eating patterns, and physical activity (see section "Intervention").

2. Hypoglycemia

    (a) Common causes:

    - Taking insulin or certain diabetes medications (especially sulfonylureas) without sufficient carbohydrate intake.
    - Prolonged physical activity without reduction in insulin doses or additional food intake.

    (b) Symptoms:

    - Shakiness
    - Nervousness or anxiety
    - Sweating, chills, or clamminess

- Irritability or impatience
- Confusion
- Fast heartbeat
- Lightheadedness, dizziness, and/or difficulty concentrating
- Hunger or nausea
- Color draining from the skin (pallor)
- Weakness or fatigue
- Blurred vision
- Tingling or numbness in the lips, tongue, or cheeks
- Headaches
- Coordination problems, clumsiness
- Nightmares or crying out during sleep
- Anger, stubbornness, or sadness
- Seizures

(c) Treatment

- If blood glucose is below 70 mg/dL, follow the 15–15 rule:

  - Eat or drink 15 g of carbs.

    Examples of 15 g of carbs: 4 glucose tablets, half a cup of fruit juice or full-sugar soda, 1 tablespoon of sugar or honey, or 6 large jelly beans.

  - Recheck blood glucose in 15 min.
  - Repeat until blood glucose tests above 70 mg/dL.
  - When blood sugar is stable, it is recommended that the patient eats a full meal or snack to keep it stable and prevent another low.

3. Diabetic Ketoacidosis (DKA):

(a) Causes:

- Decreased insulin
- Inability to utilize glucose for energy
- Body begins to use fat for energy, which produces ketones

(b) Early symptoms:

- Thirst or a very dry mouth
- Frequent urination
- High blood glucose (blood sugar) levels
- High levels of ketones in the urine

(c) Other Symptoms:

- Constantly feeling tired
- Dry or flushed skin

- Nausea, vomiting, or abdominal pain (Vomiting can be caused by many illnesses, not just ketoacidosis. If vomiting continues for more than 2 h, contact your healthcare provider.)
- Difficulty breathing or deep rapid breathing
- Fruity odor on breath
- A hard time paying attention or confusion

(d) Treatment:

- DKA is less likely to occur in people with type 2 diabetes. DKA is potentially fatal and often requires hospitalization. If a patient experiences unexplained nausea or vomiting, moderate or high levels of urine ketones, or blood glucose is high and can't be lowered by adjusting insulin dosing, the patient should seek care right away.

  Sources and Resources for Educational Handouts: American Association of Diabetes Educators (ADCES), American Diabetes Association ADA, NIH MedlinePlus, & Joslin Diabetes Center

Role of OTP

Since effective condition management is dependent on behavior and lifestyle modification, an OTP on the PC team can be very effective in identifying barriers to disease management and providing actionable strategies to facilitate lifestyle change and patient self-activation.

Occupational Impact

There are three processes by which diabetes can impact engagement in occupation.

- *Mandatory self-management of condition*: individuals with diabetes are typically asked to perform numerous self-management tasks, typically including taking medications, monitoring blood glucose levels, adapting their diet and incorporating physical activity into their daily routines. These tasks can be time-consuming, must be carried out on an ongoing basis, and often impact the ways in which individuals perform other daily activities.
- *Unexpected need for emergency care*: low and high blood sugar can produce acute symptoms (e.g., low blood sugar can cause tremor, rapid heartbeat, and confusion; high blood sugar can cause nausea and fatigue) that require emergent treatment (taking fast-acting glucose to correct a low blood sugar or taking insulin to correct high blood sugar). The onset of these symptoms, and their need for emergent treatment, is often unexpected and can disrupt the performance of other occupations.

- *Chronic progressive medical complications:* of diabetes (e.g., retinopathy, neuropathy, kidney disease) can produce functional impairments (e.g., visual and fine motor impairments; chronic pain; amputations) that impact how people perform various occupations.

OTPs can provide interventions to address the following *Occupational Therapy Framework Domains* [4]:

Activities of Daily Living (ADLs)
- Self-management tasks related to personal hygiene and grooming (foot/shoe inspections, wound care for diabetic foot ulcers or other slow-healing wounds)
- Personal device care (procuring and maintaining medical devices such as glucometers and lancing devices)
- Acute complications that affect mood and function in the short term (e.g., slow healing wounds, depression)
- Functional limitations secondary to chronic complications of diabetes (e.g., neuropathy, amputations, loss of vision) can also impact the performance of other ADLs and IADLs [4].

Instrumental Activities of Daily Living (IADLs)
- Medication management, meal preparation, financial management,
- Instrumental activities related to diabetes impact everyone in the patient's core social support network and often involve shared decision-making and responsibility across partners or multiple family members. For example:

  – Shared meals
  – Accessing appropriate health insurance plans
  – Budgeting for diabetes self-management

  Note: Acute complications may produce symptoms that require emergent treatment that disrupts participation in these occupations and functional limitations, such as low vision or poor fine motor dexterity, secondary to chronic complications of diabetes, can impact performance.

Rest and Sleep
- Entwined with diabetes-related health and self-management due to clear patterns between diabetes risk and sleep quality and quantity
- Sleep disruptions have a detrimental impact on metabolic health [5, 6]
- Poor diabetes self-management can lead to poor sleep and rest (e.g., low blood glucose can disrupt sleep due to need for immediate treatment, while high blood glucose can lead to an increased need to urinate at night)
- Even when diabetes is well-managed, acute events can't always be prevented and some patients need to check blood glucose or respond to glucose monitoring alarms (triggered by high or low blood glucose levels) throughout the night

Work, Education, Play, Leisure, and Social Participation
- patients may need accommodations or support to perform self-management tasks and routines embedded within these other categories of occupations.

- diabetes does not happen in a vacuum and often lifestyle change requires family and friend involvement and support (e.g., social events involve food and for many people exercise is most meaningful as a social activity, necessitating the participation of others)
- there is a stigma attached to diabetes in the larger society, which can affect social participation; in particular, navigating how and when to disclose a diabetes diagnosis to others can be difficult

OT Areas of Emphasis

The OTP can help the patient verbalize and understand how their current roles, habits, and routines impact their diabetes self-management. The OT role for diabetes treatment in a PC setting encompasses the following (see section "Intervention" for further detail).

- Identify lifestyle modification needs
- Assess and address emotional well-being needs
- Assess and address social support
- Address healthcare access and advocacy needs
- Educate on diabetes management knowledge and assess skill performance

Interprofessional Team Role—OTPs contribute valuable information about patients' beliefs, values, and roles and their impact on occupational engagement. When the interprofessional team has access to a more complete picture of the patients' life context, everyone is able to provide stronger patient-centered care. It is the OTP's responsibility to develop a clear understanding of the team make-up at any given PC practice and know the roles and scope of every team member to be able to provide relevant and concise information to the correct people at the right time and facilitate the participation of the appropriate providers.

Note: When educating patients, it is helpful to start with getting an understanding of what they already know about how diabetes works. It can be beneficial to use tools such as easy-to-understand figures and videos to explain how diabetes and insulin work. It falls on the OTP to assess literacy and Limited English Proficiency to determine what type of educational resources and handouts will be useful. OTPs will need to use their clinical judgment to gauge if education around the pathophysiology of diabetes is necessary for clients to reach their health goals. Some clients are interested and motivated by an understanding of how diabetes works, while others are not. Teach back techniques, where the OTP has the patient explain what they need to do for self-management in their own words, is very effective in ensuring the patient understands the OTP's instructions.

Evaluation

Suggested Areas to Assess
- Diabetes self-efficacy and attitudes
- Self-care practices or behaviors (formal or informal)

- Physical function
- Emotional well-being

  - Anxiety (Chap. 11)
  - Depression (Chap. 18)
  - Stress

- Fatigue
- Sleep disturbance
- Social participation
- Pain interference and severity

Suggested Assessment Tools (these can be found online)
- **Occupation**
- Occupational Profile (AOTA)
- Canadian Occupational Performance Measure (COPM)
- Balance Wheel
- **Overall Health & Wellness Assessment**
- PROMIS
- SF-36
- EQ5D
- **Diabetes-Specific Assessments**
- DSM-Q
- Summary of Diabetes Self-Care Activities Assessment (SDSCA).
- Diabetes Distress Scale
- Diabetes Self-Efficacy
- Fear of hypoglycemia
- Assess medication adherence (can do with a journal or app).
- **Mental & Emotional Wellbeing**
- GAD-7
- PHQ-9
- **Patient Engagement/Activation**
- Readiness for change ruler

Intervention Strategies

Goal-setting—facilitate patient-centered and collaborative Specific, Measurable, Achievable, Realistic, Timely (SMART) goal setting.

Identify lifestyle modification needs—analyze current habits and routines. The OTP can teach the patient to analyze the patterns in their routines and identify problem areas. OTPs can educate and guide patients to prioritize opportunities for behavior change that will have the most impact and be the most successful (e.g., cut out sugary beverages, improve accuracy of insulin dosing, etc.). Often, patients are well aware of the changes that they need or want to make and don't know how to prioritize or implement them. The OTP can help patients with:

- Habits and habit development
- Medication and monitoring
- Modifications and accommodations
- Chronic pain—neuropathy (Chap. 34)
- Sleep hygiene (Chap. 27)

Emotional Well-being—assess mental and emotional well-being and provide appropriate intervention and referrals. OTPs can facilitate sessions to improve each patient's understanding of their stressors and their emotional and physiological responses to each stressor. With improved understanding, OTPs can help patients identify and implement stress management and coping strategies. Diabetes-related stress versus general life stressors (e.g., work, school, parenting, finances, etc.) can be managed through targeted coping strategies. OTPs can also refer to other behavioral health providers as needed.

Social Support—evaluate the patient's access to social support and educate on opportunities to improve access to and quality of social support. OTPs are also well positioned to provide critical family and caregiver training around safety related to acute diabetes events, community resources (e.g., local support groups, nutrition resources/services, physical activity opportunities/education), and effective support strategies such as

- scheduling a monthly check with their nutritionist
- tracking exercise and diet through an interactive app or website
- scheduling regular outreach to check self-management success and risk of depression
- arranging regularly scheduled PCP office outreach for eye, foot, sensation checks

Access & Advocacy—assess the patient's health literacy and access to appropriate

- health care (e.g., PC and specialty care)
- community resources
- safe and supportive environments (e.g., home, school, work, etc.) to perform diabetes self-management

The OTP can educate patients on self-advocacy strategies using a variety of techniques (e.g., modeling, role play, worksheets, etc.) to strengthen patients' understanding of their rights, resources, and role on their healthcare team.

Diabetes management knowledge and skills—educate regarding basic diabetes physiology and assess a patient's ability to perform self-management skills safely and effectively. OTPs can also consult regarding appropriate accommodations and modifications to self-management processes as needed. Depending on the interprofessional team make up, the OTP may have a role in educating on basic self-management skills and device care (e.g., glucometer, insulin syringes, etc.). OTPs can become certified diabetes educators if they are filling a gap in this area for a clinical practice. OTPs can also serve as a complimentary service provider to dietitians, pharmacists, nurses, and PCPs.

Pain management—When pain is an issue, refer to Chapter on Persistent Pain (Chap. 34).

Note: The University of Pennsylvania through their PennMedicine Program offers information and resources that you can use with your patients including Apps and websites they can use to facilitate self-management.

Other Considerations and Resources

Billing and Documentation—be aware of progress note requirements for all payers. Some may require medical necessity review forms that have required templates geared primarily to orthopedic or neurological conditions. In those cases, it is important to understand the appeal system and be prepared to outline medical necessity with appropriate diagnosis and treatment codes and descriptions.

Suggested Referrals as Indicated by Patient Needs
Endocrinology
Ophthalmology
Podiatry
Social Work
Psychiatry/Psychology
Registered Dietitian
Certified Diabetes Educator
Physical therapy (PT) for strengthening exercises and pain management as needed
Peer-led diabetes self-management education (DSME) groups

Additional Resources for Provider and Patient
American Diabetes Association (ADA) https://www.diabetes.org/
Lifestyle Redesign—Life management series by University of Southern California (USC) https://chan.usc.edu/academics/continuing-education/life-management-series/intro-to-lifestyle-redesign
American Association of Diabetes Educators (AADE) https://www.diabeteseducator.org/
CDC Diabetes Prevention Program (DPP) https://www.cdc.gov/diabetes/prevention/index.html

References

1. American Diabetes Association. Diagnosis and classification of diabetes mellitus. Diabetes Care. 2009;32(Suppl. 1):S62–7. https://doi.org/10.2337/dc09-S062. PMID: 19118289; PMCID: PMC2613584
2. American Diabetes Association. Classification and diagnosis of diabetes: standards of medical Care in Diabetes 2018. Diabetes Care. 2018;41(Suppl. 1):S13–27.

3. Centers for Disease Control and Prevention. National Diabetes Statistics Report, 2020. Atlanta, GA: Centers for disease control and prevention, US Department of Health and Human Services; 2020. https://www.cdc.gov/diabetes/library/features/diabetes-stat-report.html
4. American Occupational Therapy Association. Occupational therapy practice framework: domain and process. Am J Occup Ther. 2014;68(Suppl. 1):S1–S48. https://doi.org/10.5014/ajot.2014.682006.
5. Cappuccio FP, D'Elia L, Strazzullo P, Miller MA. Quantity and quality of sleep and incidence of type 2 diabetes: a systematic review and meta-analysis. Diabetes Care. 2010;33(2):414–20. https://doi.org/10.2337/dc09-1124.
6. Nedeltcheva AV, Scheer FAJL. Metabolic effects of sleep disruption, links to obesity and diabetes. Curr Opin Endocrinol Diabetes Obes. 2014;21(4):293–8. https://doi.org/10.1097/MED.000000000000008.

Chapter 20
Dizziness

Tina M. Sauber

Introduction

Dizziness is a sensation of disturbed or impaired spatial orientation without a false or distorted sense of motion [1–6]. Sensations include lightheadedness, presyncope, or giddiness and unsteadiness. Dizziness does not involve a rotational component and is a common complaint reported to medical providers yet a vague symptom. Dizziness can range in severity from annoying to serious and debilitating (Refer to Table 20.1).

Table 20.1 Classification of dizziness

Vertigo	BPPV, Meniere's, labyrinthitis, transient ischemic attack (TIA)
Disequilibrium	Cerebellar ataxia, subcortical white matter disease, bilateral vestibular loss, sensory ataxia
Presyncope/ near-faint	Orthostatic hypotension, arrhythmias, vasovagal
Psychophysiological	Phobic postural vertigo, panic syndrome, anxiety
Physiologic/medical	Motion sickness, medication, vascular insufficiencies, lab abnormalities

T. M. Sauber (✉)
Arizona State University, Phoenix, AZ, USA

Mayo Clinic, Phoenix, AZ, USA
e-mail: tinasauber@desertinet.com

© Springer Nature Switzerland AG 2023
S. Dahl-Popolizio et al. (eds.), *Primary Care Occupational Therapy*,
https://doi.org/10.1007/978-3-031-20882-9_20

Table 20.2 Duration of vertigo

Duration of Vertigo	Likely etiology
Seconds	Benign paroxysmal positional vertigo (BPPV)
Minutes	TIA, vestibular migraine
Hours	Meniere's, vestibular migraine
Days–weeks	Vestibular neuritis, labyrinthitis, cerebrovascular accident (CVA)
Continuous	Central vertigo or psychophysiological

Description: Vertigo

Vertigo is the perception of movement or whirling in the absence of motion. This includes sensations of spinning, rocking, feeling of falling, or tilting [2, 4, 6–8]. (See Table 20.2 for details regarding Vertigo duration and etiology).

Description: Disequilibrium

Disequilibrium is a sense of unsteadiness, imbalance, or loss of equilibrium, often accompanied by disorientation while seated, standing, or walking without a directional preference [2, 6, 8, 9].

Description: Presyncope

Presyncope is the feeling of losing consciousness, fainting, or blacking out [6, 9].

Description: Lightheadedness

Lightheadedness includes vague symptoms of feeling disconnected with the environment [1, 6, 9].

Cause

Dizziness is a symptom that can be linked to a peripheral, central, or medical etiology [6] (see Table 20.3).

- Peripheral dizziness—a problem with the inner ear, which controls the balance system as well as a portion of the eighth cranial nerve. Most common Peripheral

Table 20.3 Features of central versus peripheral vestibular disorders

Feature	Central	Peripheral
Nausea	Mild–moderate	Severe
Imbalance	Severe	Mild–moderate
Hearing loss	Rare	Common
Nystagmus	May change direction with changes in gaze; poorly suppressed by fixation	Unidirectional in all directions of gaze, suppressed by fixation
Recovery	Months or longer	Days to weeks
Neuro signs	Common	Rare

Table 20.4 Posterior canal benign paroxysmal positional vertigo (BPPV)

Benign paroxysmal positional vertigo (BPPV) is a condition in which particles called otoliths detach from their normal location in the inner ear (utricle) and move into the semicircular canals (SCCs) [2–4, 6–8, 11, 12]. BPPV most commonly affects the posterior semicircular canal. Movement of the otoliths causes acute onset of dizziness, often characterized as a room spinning sensation, triggered by head motion. BPPV can occur in patients of all ages, but is most common above the age of 50. Older patients with BPPV have a higher incidence of falls, depression, and impairments of their daily activities. In most cases, BPPV is idiopathic, however, some cases have direct link to head trauma. A diagnosis of BPPV is confirmed by observation of nystagmus when the patient is placed in a provoking position.

Patient presentation:

Patient subjective report
- Room spinning dizziness lasting seconds
- Nausea or feeling 'off balance"

Reproducible provocative motions
- Rolling to one side
- Looking up or down
- Leaning forward

Presentation
- Upbeating—torsional nystagmus

vestibular disorders include benign paroxysmal positional vertigo (BPPV), see Table 20.4, vestibular neuronitis, labyrinthitis, Meniere's disease, acoustic neuroma, perilymph fistula, and semicircular canal dehiscence [4, 6, 8, 10].
- Central dizziness—a problem with the brain and the brainstem as well as the reticular activating system and the midbrain. Common medical disorders that can cause dizziness include brainstem stroke, migraine headaches, concussion, multiple sclerosis, and cerebellar degermation [6, 10, 11].
- Medical related dizziness—a medical condition causing symptoms of dizziness. Common medical disorders that can cause dizziness include cervicogenic dizziness (dizziness coming from the neck), age-related dizziness and imbalance, orthostatic hypotension, anxiety, low blood sugar (hypoglycemia), dehydration, medication reactions, Vitamin B12 deficiency, low iron levels [6, 9] (anemia).

Role of PCP

The PCP completes a full systems review/examination and provides symptomatic relief of the symptoms using Meclizine or Antivert, an antihistamine used to treat nausea and motion sickness. The PCP will determine the cause of the symptoms and will determine the approach to manage the symptoms. Laboratory testing may be based on a history of chronic medical condition(s). An electrocardiograph, Holter monitoring, and Doppler test may be requested with cardiac disease. If a neurology or central vestibular disorder is suspected, imaging may be requested [9]. If symptoms persist or worsen, the patient may be referred to an otolaryngologist or neurologist.

Common Comorbidities

- Anxiety (Chap. 11)
- Phobias
- Somatoform and affective disorders
- Migraine

Role of OTP

In PC, patients are often referred to OT for medication adherence, fall prevention, durable medical needs assessment, and vestibular rehabilitation. As behavioral health issues often co-occur with this condition, the OTP can immediately help with any behavioral health issues the patients are struggling with.

Occupational Impact

Dysfunction in many activities of daily living causes dependence in self-care skills, home management, driving, functional mobility, vocational/work, social interactions, recreational/leisure activities, sleep, and cognition. Increased incidence of falls and depression can occur with this population [13].

OT Areas of Emphasis

Provide graded activities (visual focal points, modify speed and duration of eye-head movements, various standing or walking surfaces and modify visual stimuli) and exercises (balance retraining and gaze stabilization) to facilitate head movements to reduce symptoms of vertigo and disequilibrium. Offer adapted and or compensatory techniques to improve function and safety at home and in the community (refer to interventions). Promote self-management and fall prevention strategies [13].

Evaluation

Questions asked by the PCP and OTP include:

- What medications are being taken?
- When was the onset of the symptoms?
- What is the duration of the symptoms?
- What is the type/evolution of dizziness?
- What provokes the symptoms?

  - Actions
  - Movements
  - Situations

- Blood Pressure [4] (measured in supine, sitting & standing) (https://www.cdc. gov/steadi/pdf/STEADI-Assessment-MeasuringBP-508.pdf)
- Gait is observed—observing for loss of balance, gait deviation and fall risk
- Romberg Test [5]
- Dix-Hallpike Test [3–8, 12] (refer to Fig. 20.1)

  - Important Considerations:

      Cervical Clearance [3, 4, 8],—Assess available ROM in flexion, extension, rotation, and lateral flexion before performing BPPV tests and treatment. *Dix-Hallpike Test* requires 15° cervical extension and 45° cervical rotation right and left sides

If positive, proceed to treatment with canalith repositioning maneuver (CRM or Epley Maneuver) for the affected side. See Table 20.2.

In addition to the above assessments, you will need to obtain the following information. This will be helpful also if you have ruled out BPPV with the assessment above:

Subjective Report

- Description of dizziness
- Duration of dizziness
- Onset of symptoms
- Provoking activities
- Current medications

Physical Examination [2, 5, 6, 8–12]:

- Vitals: blood pressure, heart rate
- Motor control
- Sensory
- Oculomotor assessment

- Spontaneous Nystagmus—The patient sits and looks straight forward without a fixation point. The therapist looks for spontaneous nystagmus.

  – Horizontal nystagmus that can be decreased with visual fixation is indicative of peripheral involvement. If horizontal nystagmus is present, cease further BPPV evaluation. Request transition of care to a vestibular therapist. Notify the referring physician of the patient presentation.
  – Nystagmus in a single plane that does not decrease (or increase) with visual fixation indicates potential central involvement. Cease further physical therapy (PT) intervention or OT intervention and contact physician.

Dix-Hallpike Test
Dix-Hallpike Test[3,5,7,8,10,12,13] for anterior/posterior SCC BPPV. This is the gold standard test for BPPV. There is no specific outcome measure for the condition. The Dix Hallpike test either indicates the presence or absence of BPPV. **Positive Test** - if the patient experiences dizziness with associated nystagmus. (Begin with head rotation to the right to assess for right BPPV; Begin with head rotation to the left to assess for left BPPV). 1. The patient starts in a long sitting position on the mat looking straight ahead the OTP then positions the head in 15 degrees of cervical extension. 2. While in the sitting position (with 15 degrees of cervical extension) rotate the head 45 degrees from midline in one direction; repeat this motion in the other direction. 3. The therapist then brings the patient to supine and brings the patient's head and neck into 15 degrees of extension and rotation (hold this rotated/extended position). 4. The therapist observes the patient's eyes for nystagmus and monitors the patient for reports of dizziness. **Onset of symptoms:** • Latency- how long does nystagmus last - a typical latency period ranges from 1 to 50 seconds, although it may be as long as 1 minute in rare cases. • Direction- Posterior canal BPPV results in up-beating torsional motion of the eyes toward the side being tested. • Duration- Symptoms of vertigo and nystagmus should subside within one minute.

Fig. 20.1 Dix-Hallpike test. (**a**) is steps 1 & 2 below which demonstrates the sitting position, the head position and the eye gaze position. (**b**) is steps 3 & 4 which demonstrates the supine position, head position and eye gaze position to assess for nystagmus (Image obtained from research-gate.net)

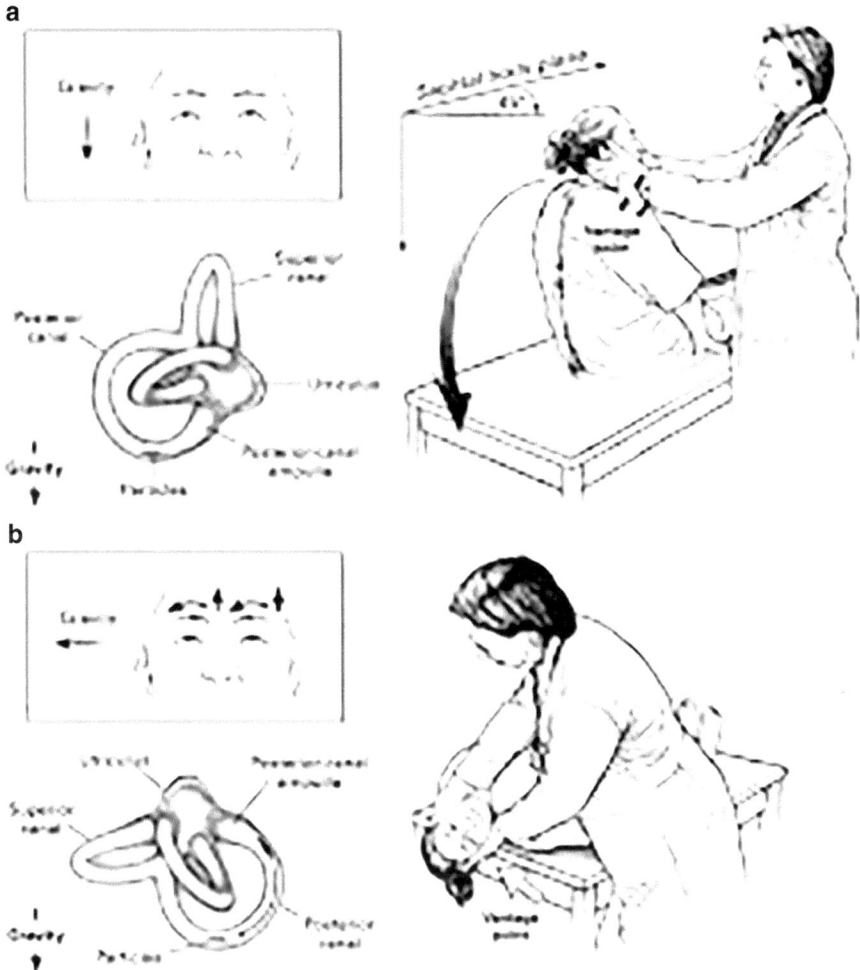

Fig. 20.1 (continued)

Ocular range of motion (ROM)—Unbalanced or incomplete movement indicates CN III, IV, or VI pathology or muscular deficits. Report findings to PCP for further assessment.

Smooth Pursuit—Have the patient follow a slow-moving object 30° in a vertical and horizontal direction looking for smoothness of eye movement. If they perform saccadic jerky movement, they may have central pathology. Abnormal Convergence (CN III)—An inability to maintain focus may indicate central nervous system impairment. Report findings to PCP for further assessment.

- Balance Assessment (refer to *suggested assessment tools*)
- Cervical ROM: Assess flexion, extension, rotation, and lateral flexion of the head/neck

Suggested Assessment Tools

- Berg Balance Scale (BERG) [5].
- Functional Gait Assessment (FGA) [5].
- Modified Clinical Test of Sensory Interaction on Balance [5] (CTSIB-M).

Intervention Strategies

- Provide adherence strategies for all lifestyle changes
- Canalith Repositioning Maneuvers (CRM/Epley Maneuver) as indicated for BPPV [12]
- Fall Prevention—Strategies for at-home and in the community [2, 13].
- Energy Conservation—Offer task modifications to minimize strain or fatigue while promoting independence [2, 6, 13].
- Habituation exercises—Repeated exposure to the movement for a reduction in symptoms [6–8, 11]
- Adaptive equipment—Recommendations of equipment to maximize functional independence [13].
- Environmental modifications—Modified approaches to maximize functional independence [2, 13].
- DME—safety equipment [13].
- Gaze stabilization—Exercises to improve vision while the head is moving [2, 6, 10, 11].
- Balance retraining—Exercises to improve coordinated movements of upper and lower extremities and posture in sitting and standing [4–8, 10].
- Medication management & adherence [9, 13].
- Patient/family/caregiver training & education [9, 13].
- Psychosocial needs [9, 13].

  - Support groups
  - Compensatory techniques

- Recommended Durable Medical Equipment (DME)

  - Cane
  - Walker
  - Shower chair

- Possible Referrals

  - Otolaryngologist
  - Neurologist
  - Vestibular Rehabilitation Therapist (OT or PT)

CRM-Specific Instructions (See Fig. 20.2)

- Before beginning CRM, the clinician should explain the movements and warn the patient that they may experience intense vertigo and nausea.

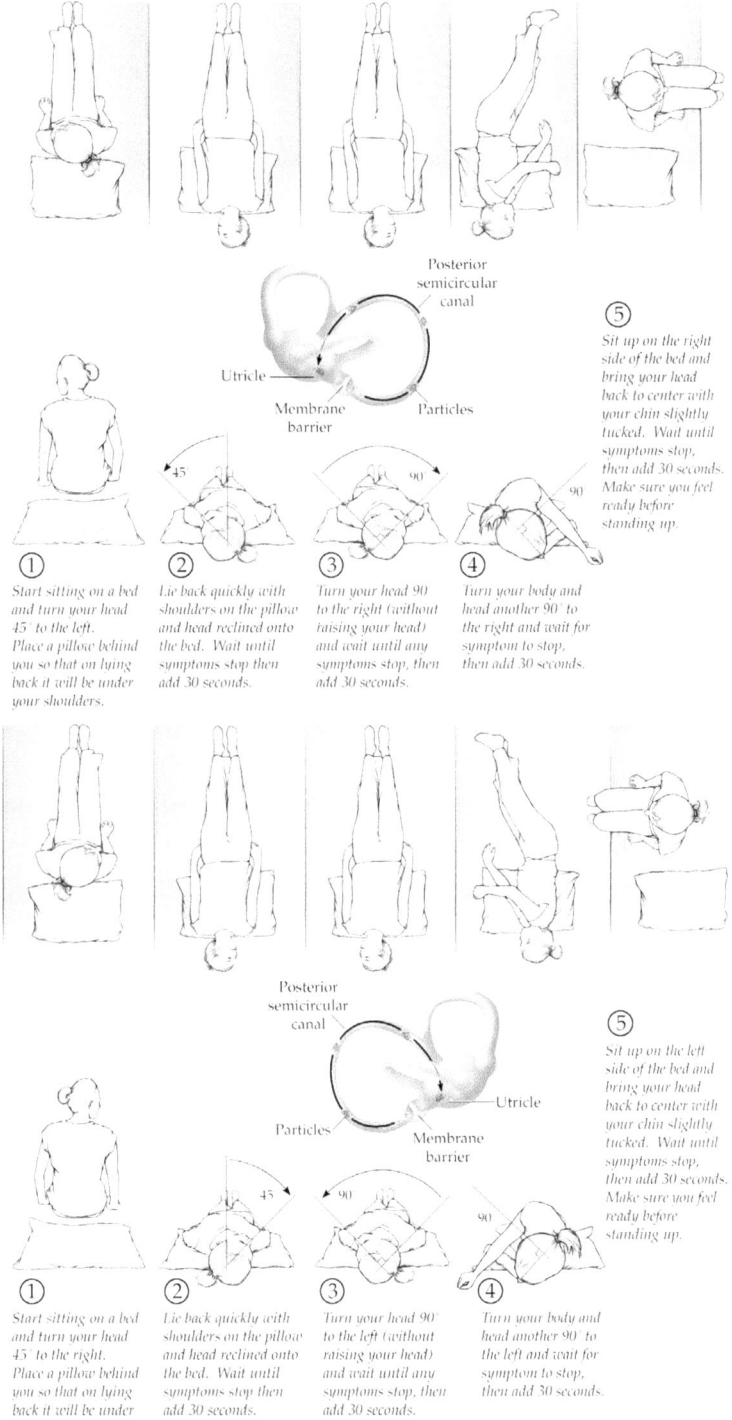

Fig. 20.2 Canalith repositioning maneuvers (CRM). **Note**: Images courtesy of Mayo Clinic. Reproduced with permission.

- The therapist should test what is believed to be the uninvolved side first, allowing the patient to become more comfortable with the procedure and the therapist to rule out the uninvolved side.
- Once the involved side is identified, proceed directly into CRM treatment.
- Patients who previously manifested severe nausea/vomiting with the Dix-Hallpike maneuver may be considered for antiemetic prophylaxis during CRM.2,
- Collaborate with the referring provider for any pre-therapy medication regimens [6, 9].
- Patients with bilateral ear involvement should have one ear treated per session. The other ear should be treated after 24 h have passed.
- BPPV as a result of traumatic injury may be more difficult to resolve, and reoccurrence is more common than with idiopathic BPPV.
- Canal switching, in which otoconia moves from the affected canal into another SCC, can occur during CRM. This can be detected most clearly by the change in movement of nystagmus upon the next round of CRM. This situation would require referral to a vestibular therapist.
- Patients should be instructed to use caution with provocative positions and activities where the risk of falls may be increased until symptoms resolve or until they are reassessed.

  - For more effective results, additional CRM are significantly more effective in achieving resolution of symptoms.

Treatment Goals
- Return otoconia to the vestibule (resolve BPPV)
- Negative positional testing
- Resolution of vertiginous symptoms
- Reduce vertigo associated with head motion
- Improve balance
- Reduce the risk of falling

Other Considerations and Resources

- Documentation and Billing: Use the *Physical Medicine and Rehabilitation* CPT codes and ICD-10 code that best fits your intervention (refer to Table 20.4).

  - Canalith repositioning (CPT code-95992)
  - Functional Therapeutic Activities (CPT code-97530)

Codes that Can Be Used for the Issues Associated with Dizziness

Medical Diagnosis: Benign paroxysmal positional vertigo, vertigo, dizziness
Therapy Diagnosis: Benign paroxysmal positional vertigo, dizziness, fall risk

Treatment diagnosis	ICD—10 Codes
Benign paroxysmal positional vertigo	H81.13
Difficulty walking	R26.2
Abnormal posture	R29.3
Lack of coordination	R27.8
Dizziness	R42
Vertiginous syndrome	H81.93, unspecified
Cervicalgia	M54.2
Abnormal gait	R26.89

References

1. Centers for Disease Control and Prevention (CDC), National Center for Injury Prevention and Control. Measuring orthostatic blood pressure: Centers for Disease Control and Prevention 2017.
2. Hamby JR. The dizzy patient. In: Smith-Gabai H, editor. Occupational therapy in acute care. Bethesda, MD: AOTA Press, The American Occupational Therapy Association; 2011. p. 639–47.
3. Helminski HO, Zee DS, Janssen I, Hain T. Effectiveness of particle repositioning maneuvers in the treatment of benign paroxysmal positional vertigo: a systematic review. Phys Ther. 2010;90:663–78.
4. Mayo Clinic Handout Benign Paroxysmal Positional Vertigo (BPPV) MC6727 [Patient Handout]. http://mayoweb.mayo.edu/sp-forms/mc6700mc6799/mc6727pf.pdf Accessed 5 Oct 2019.
5. Post RE, Dickerson LM. Dizziness: a diagnostic approach. Am Family Phys. 2010;82(4):361–8.
6. Schubert MC, Minor LB. Vestibulo-ocular physiology underlying vestibular hypofunction. Phys Ther J. 2004;84(4):373–85.
7. Bhattacharyya N, Baugh RF, Orvidas L, et al. Clinical practice guideline: Benign paroxysmal positional vertigo. J Otolaryngol Head Neck Surg. 2008;139(5 Suppl 4):S47–81.
8. Fife TD. Benign paroxysmal positional vertigo. Semin Neurol. 2009;29:500508.
9. Parnes LS, Agrawal SK, Atlas J. Diagnosis and management of benign paroxysmal positional vertigo (BPPV). CMAJ. 2003;169(7):681–93.
10. Rehabilitation Measures Database Rehabilitation Institute of Chicago Website. https://www.sralab.org/lifecenter/resources/rehabilitation-measures-database. Accessed May 20, 2019.
11. Banfield GK, Wood C, Knight J. Does vestibular habituation still have a place in the treatment of benign paroxysmal positional vertigo? J Laryngol Otol. 2000;114:501–5.
12. Disorders Association: Causes of dizziness. Vestibular.org. Accessed 15 May 2019.
13. American Occupational Therapy Association. Occupational therapy practice framework: domain and process. Am J Occup Ther. 2014;68(Suppl.1):S1–S48. https://doi.org/10.5014/ajot.2014.682006.

Chapter 21
Driving and Community Mobility

Kandy Salter

Introduction

The strong link between driving, community mobility, and other occupations provides a clear need for all OTPs to commit to addressing driving with clients. OTPs have the knowledge necessary to identify those who are medically at risk and provide necessary resources related to driving and community mobility [1]. OTPs have specialized knowledge of occupations, client factors, performance skills, performance patterns, context, and environment. In this chapter, we will discuss how this knowledge strongly positions OTPs in the PC setting to address driving and mobility concerns.

Role of the PCP

Without additional training, most PCPs are not comfortable assessing driving abilities; this supports having an OTP onsite to determine the best and safest options for the client.

Common Comorbidities

- These issues affect driving fitness [2]:

K. Salter (✉)
University of Arkansas and University of Arkansas for Medical Sciences,
Fayetteville, AR, USA
e-mail: kssalter@uark.edu

© Springer Nature Switzerland AG 2023   219
S. Dahl-Popolizio et al. (eds.), *Primary Care Occupational Therapy*,
https://doi.org/10.1007/978-3-031-20882-9_21

- Visual and auditory deficits
- Stroke
- Diabetes
- Depression
- Dementia
- Mild cognitive disorders
- Parkinson's disease
- Sleep disorders
- Cardiovascular diseases
- Musculoskeletal disorders frailty

Role of OTP

Transportation and mobility in one's community are vital to the promotion of health and well-being. The specialized knowledge OTPs have supports a professional obligation to address driving and community mobility with all clients. OTPs working in PC are uniquely positioned to provide early intervention to transportation concerns impacting patient engagement and outcomes.

Today, in the United States, driving a personal vehicle is the primary and preferred means of transportation. Many Americans view driving as a rite of passage for teenagers and maintain the view that driving is a right versus a privilege throughout their lifespan [3, 4]. These views result in strong personal feelings and values related to the ability to drive. Driving is a valued occupation that offers the freedom of spontaneity, independence, and seemingly unlimited community access.

Although driving is preferred, it is important to remind our clients that there are numerous other ways that individuals can move around in their communities. Mobility in one's community relates to personal, social, and economic well-being [5]. Public transit, passenger services (e.g., taxis, Uber, Lyft, paratransit, etc.), and personal transportation options that do not involve motorized vehicles (e.g., walking, wheelchair, bicycle, etc.) are important for the OTP to consider. Mobility allows individuals greater independence and control to participate in occupations such as work, education, leisure, self-care, and social participation.

Occupational Impact

Community mobility allows individuals across the lifespan to access health care, meet social needs, and access resources that have been shown to improve health and well-being [6, 7]. OTPs on PC teams are ideally situated to provide early intervention when community mobility concerns arise. Indicators of community mobility concerns include

- Frequently missed medical appointments.
- Inability to access health-promoting community resources.
- Challenges accessing ancillary services to assist in the care of others due to transportation issues.
- Changes in driving safety due to onset of a medical condition or
- General changes associated with aging.

OT Areas of Emphasis

OTPs have knowledge that uniquely situates them to consider the relationships between community mobility, occupational performance, and general health and well-being. They also have knowledge of available resources to provide more advanced interventions and transportation alternatives to promote community mobility. The focus of the OTP in primary care is evaluating driving safety and referring when interventions or resources are needed.

Evaluation

Regular screening of patients in the PC setting can help to achieve broader goals to improve the health of populations by assessing factors such as risk of hospital admission and readmission, adherence to care plans, and independence in occupational performances [8]. Recommended screenings are

- *Sensory:*
  - *Vision:* Visual Acuity, visual fields, contrast sensitivity, visual attention and scanning, and oculomotor function. The biVABA is a useful tool in identifying functional limitations related to visual impairment [9].
  - *Proprioception:* The OT-Driver Off Road Assessment (OT-DORA) Battery includes useful sensory assessments including vision, the Test of Proprioception-Lower Limb, and the Simulated Accelerator-Brake Test. These assessments provide information related to potential errors in targeting a vehicle's accelerator and/or brake [10].
- *Balance*: The ability to safely get in/out of a motor vehicle, manage assistive devices used for mobility (e.g., a walker or cane), and to maintain head, neck, and trunk control while seated can be quickly screened in the clinic through observation. To assess sitting balance, the therapist may sit the client on an unsteady surface (e.g., air cushion) and then apply perturbations, noting any loss of balance the patient does not independently recover from.
- The Berg Balance Scale can also provide objective assessment of fall risks. It can be found free at [11].

- *Cognition:* The OT-DORA includes two cognitive assessments, the Occupational Therapy Drive Home Maze Test and the Road Law and Road Craft Test. Other tools such as the Mini Mental Status Examination, The Saint Louis University Mental Status (SLUMS) Examination, and the Montreal Cognitive Assessment (MoCA) are used to assess cognition.
- *Motor Skills:* A functional range of motion and strength screening may reveal the need to collect additional information. Additional assessment using Goniometry and manual muscle testing can be performed to determine if range of motion and strength are adequate for entering, exiting, and operating a motor vehicle.
- *Reaction Time*: The OT-DORA includes a Right Heel Pivot Test to assess for coordination and timing of the lower extremity. There are a number of commercially available simulated brake reaction time testers. The associated costs and equipment space needs may limit access to this type of equipment in the PC setting.
- *Medication Side Effects*: Understanding potential and individualized medication side effects and effects of poly-pharmacy can help the OTP determine driving risks associated with prescription and over the counter medications. OTPs working in PC can work with physicians to determine risks and provide education to decrease risks. Physicians may be able to adjust medication dosages, timing of doses, or prescribe alternative medications that have fewer or less severe side effects.

A more thorough examination of community mobility constraints and risks can be achieved using a community mobility screening tool (see below). The OTP will explain the purpose of the screening to the patient, highlighting in what ways community mobility can impact health care and overall well-being. Information is gathered through observation, self-report, and/or family/caregiver report.

Community Mobility Screening Tool

Name:_____ DOB/Age:_____

Past Medical History:_____

Primary Complaint:_____

Prior Level of Function/ Recent Functional Changes:_____

Optometrist/Opthamologist:_____

Most Recent Formal Vision Test:_____

Does the individual use a mobility device? Yes____   No____

Mobility Device (s):   Cane____ Walker____ Manual Wheelchair____ Motorized Wheelchair____

                        Other (please list):_____

Activity	Independent	1 to 25% Assist	26 to 50% Assist	51 to 75% Assist	75% Assist or Greater	N/A
Navigates parking lot (car <> building)						
Crosses street at crosswalk with signal						
Crosses street without signal						
Coordinates own transportation (personal or public)						
Utilizes public transportation app						
Gets in/out of car						
Drives motor vehicle						
Rides Bicycle/Tricycle/ non-motorized						

Intervention Strategies

The American Occupational Therapy Association (AOTA) and the Association of Driver Rehabilitation Specialists (ADED) have valuable online resources, including a directory of driver rehabilitation specialists. This information is free and available to the general community. Practitioners may contact a driver rehabilitation specialist in the community or region to help identify local resources.

Patient engagement in care can be disrupted due to multiple factors, including transportation. The OTP in a PC setting can identify patterns in healthcare utilization and promote patient engagement in care. This can be done through the creation of an occupational profile that includes habits and routines of community mobility.

When to Refer Offsite

In a typical PC setting, an OTP may not have the time, resources, or expertise to complete comprehensive evaluation to determine fitness to drive. A referral is recommended when a more comprehensive evaluation of abilities and limitations specific to driving are needed. A professional who has completed additional training in the field of driver rehabilitation is best suited to complete this evaluation. Professionals with advanced training have the necessary knowledge of driving laws, remediation, training, adaptive equipment, and vehicle modifications to make evidence-based recommendations. The American Occupational Therapy Association (AOTA) and the Association of Driver Rehabilitation Specialists (ADED) provide valuable online resources, including a directory of driver rehabilitation specialists.

Other Considerations and Resources

Legal Considerations

Driving is a privilege awarded by each state. While many driving laws are common to all states, there are specific functional requisites that vary from state to state. For example, an unrestricted driver's license in Arkansas requires a minimum uncorrected visual acuity of 20/40, while Kansas only requires visual acuity of 20/40 in one eye, and California allows 20/40 in one eye and at least 20/70 in the other eye.

Each state's organizational structure is unique, yet each state has a department that is solely responsible for managing licensing to operate motor vehicles. For example, the Kansas Department of Revenue Division of Vehicles manages drivers licensing, while the Office of Driver Services is responsible in Arkansas. Inconsistencies between states can create challenges for OTPs who do not have advanced training in driver rehabilitation. A local or regional driver rehabilitation specialist can be a good resource in finding state-specific information.

References

1. American Journal of Occupational Therapy. Occupational therapy practice framework: domain and process. Am J Occup Ther. 2020;74:7412410010. https://doi.org/10.5014/ajot.2020.74S2001.
2. Falkenstein M, Karthaus M, Brüne-Cohrs U. Age-related diseases and driving safety. Geriatrics. 2020;5(4):80. https://doi.org/10.3390/geriatrics5040080.
3. Anstey KJ, Wood J, Lord S, Walker JG. Cognitive, sensory and physical factors enabling driving safety in older adults. Clin Psychol Rev. 2005;25(1):45–65. https://doi.org/10.1016/j.cpr.2004.07.008.
4. Dickerson A, Reistetter T, Davis E, Monahan M. Evaluating driving as a valued instrumental activity of daily living. Am J Occup Ther. 2011;65(1):64–75. https://doi.org/10.5014/ajot.2011.09052.
5. McGuire M, Davis E, editors. Driving and community mobility occupational therapy strategies across the lifespan. Bethesda, MD: American Occupational Therapy Association Press; 2012.
6. Heatwole Shank KS, Presgraves E. Using geospatial mapping of late-life Couplehood: dimensions of joint participation. Occup Ther J Res. 2018;39:176. https://doi.org/10.1177/1539449218808277.
7. Yang S, Zarr RL, Kass-Hout TA, Kourosh A, Kelly NR. Transportation barriers to accessing health Care for Urban Children. J Health Care Poor Underserved. 2006;17(4):928–43. https://doi.org/10.1353/hpu.2006.0137.
8. Halle A, Mroz T, Fogelberg D, Leland N. Occupational therapy and primary care: updates and trends. Am J Occup Ther. 2018;72(3):7203090010. https://doi.org/10.5014/ajot.2018.723001.
9. visABILITIES Rehab Services, Inc. (2014). Brain injury visual assessment battery for adults. http://www.visabilities.com/bivaba.html
10. Unsworth C, Pallant J, Russell K, Odell M. Occupational therapy driver off-road assessment battery. Bethesda, MD: American Occupational Therapy Association Press; 2011.
11. The Shirley Ryan Ability Lab. (n.d.) The Berg Balance Scale. https://www.sralab.org/rehabilitation-measures/berg-balance-scale

Chapter 22
Falls and Falls Prevention

John V. Rider

Introduction

Falls are the leading cause of both fatal and non-fatal injuries among community-dwelling older adults aged ≥65 years and incur significant healthcare costs [1]. One out of four older adults fall annually, with the likelihood of falls increasing with age [1]. Additionally, falling once doubles your chance of falling again [2]. Falls threaten older adults' safety and independence. Unfortunately, less than half of older adults that experience a fall tell their PCP about the fall, indicating that the PCP or other provider needs to directly ask the patient about falls, and screen for fall risks.

A combination of risk factors causes most falls. The more risk factors a person has, the greater their chances of falling. The most common risk factors include, but are not limited to

- Age-related changes.
- Lower body and core weakness.
- Difficulty with walking, posture, or balance.
- Vitamin D deficiency.
- Vision problems.
- Foot pain or poor footwear.
- Inner ear problems.
- Home hazards.
- Use of medications that can affect balance or cause dizziness.
- Fear of falling.

J. V. Rider (✉)
School of Occupational Therapy, Touro University Nevada, Henderson, NV, USA
e-mail: jrider@touro.edu

© Springer Nature Switzerland AG 2023
S. Dahl-Popolizio et al. (eds.), *Primary Care Occupational Therapy*,
https://doi.org/10.1007/978-3-031-20882-9_22

- Poor balance confidence.
- Cognitive deficits.
- Sensory deficits.
- Acute illnesses.
- Chronic conditions.
- Neurodegenerative diseases or neurological disorders.

Fall risk factors can also be categorized into *physical risk factors* (changes in the body that increase fall risk), *behavioral risk factors* (things people do or don't do that increase fall risk), and *environmental risk factors* (hazards in the home or community).

Role of PCP

The PCP will typically perform a fall risk assessment, which includes asking about fall history, reviewing medications, and performing a brief physical assessment. The PCP typically reviews all medications likely to increase fall risk and modifies prescriptions as appropriate. The PCP also assesses vitamin D intake and makes recommendations for vitamin D supplements, if needed.

Current guidelines from the Center for Disease Control and Prevention (CDC) recommend that PCPs screen and assess for fall risks annually after the age of 65 or after any acute fall. The CDC recommends appropriate referrals to OT, physical therapy (PT), ophthalmologist/optometrist, podiatrist, etc., for evaluation and continued treatment.

Common Comorbidities

Common comorbidities that may increase fall risk include

- Postural hypotension.
- Musculoskeletal impairments (gait, balance, trunk and lower body weakness).
- Vestibular impairments.
- Visual impairments.
- Chronic health conditions with increased risk of falls:

    - Myocardial infarction
    - Cerebrovascular accident
    - Asthma (Chap. 13)
    - Cancer
    - Chronic Obstructive Pulmonary Disorder (Chap. 13)
    - Chronic Kidney Disease
    - Arthritis (Chap. 12)

- Depression (Chap. 18)
- Diabetes (Chap. 19)
- Osteoporosis
- Peripheral neuropathy
- Parkinson's Disease (Chap. 31)
- Dementia (Chap. 15)
- Chronic pain (Chap. 34)
- Urinary incontinence (Chap. 33)

- Medications that increase the risk of falls [3]:

  - Psychoactive Medications

      Anticonvulsants
      Antidepressants
      Antipsychotics
      Sedative hypnotics
      Benzodiazepines

  - Other Medications:

      Anticholinergics
      Antihistamines
      Muscle relaxants
      Antihypertensives
      Nonsteroidal anti-inflammatory drugs
      Diuretics
      Opioids

Role of OTP

The OTP evaluates fall risk factors and avoidance behaviors and provides interventions to reduce fall risk, fear of falling, and avoidance behavior and increase safe participation in meaningful occupations.

Occupational Impact

Occupational impact varies from mild to severe impairment, depending on comorbidities and level of fall risk. Some people become so afraid of falling, even if they have not fallen, that they stop engaging in preferred activities of daily living (ADLs) and instrumental activities of daily living (IADLs), which leads to the cessation of daily activities [4, 5]. This results in further physical, social, and mental decline, which ultimately increases fall risk and decreases quality of life. Fear of falling or increased fall risk impacts occupations that require functional mobility or that challenge balance. Additionally, living situations play a significant role in the impact of fall risk and the necessity of intervention. For instance, does the patient live alone? Does the patient live in a multilevel home? Are there other issues in their environment that affect fall risk or fear of falling?

OT Areas of Emphasis

The OTP will perform a comprehensive evaluation to determine fall risk (low, moderate, or high), identify modifiable risk factors, occupational performance barriers, and develop an intervention plan. In PC, the OTP will focus on providing client education for evidence-based fall prevention strategies, including but not limited to, home modifications, adaptive equipment, durable medical equipment, balance strategies, strengthening, activity modifications, behavioral interventions, and recommendations for evidence-based community fall prevention programs available locally.

Evaluation

Suggested areas to assess:

- Global screening of fall risk should be done annually after the age of 65, after any acute fall or near fall, or when fall risk factors are present
- Fall Risk Checklist
- Patient's physical risk factors, including balance, strength, and mobility
- CDC's STEADI (Stopping Elderly Accidents, Deaths, and Injuries) Fall Risk Screening Tools (*you can search each tool on the CDC website, STEADI page, or search them independently*)

  - 30-second Chair Stand Test
  - 4-stage Balance Test
  - Timed Up and Go Test (TUG)
  - Orthostatic Blood Pressure

- Observation of functional mobility and balance

  - Seated vs. standing balance
  - Static vs. dynamic balance

- Additional balance assessments
  - Berg Balance Scale

Assesses balance during mobility tasks
- Tinetti Performance-Oriented Mobility Assessment

Assesses seated, standing, and walking balance
- Functional Reach Test

Assesses dynamic balance
- Timed Up and Go Test (Manual and Cognitive versions)

Assesses fall risk during functional mobility (Manual version includes walking while holding a cup of water and the Cognitive version includes counting backward by threes)
- Mini-BESTest

Assesses dynamic balance, functional mobility, and gait
- Environmental risk factors, including home safety and accessibility screening
- Rebuilding Together Safe at Home Checklist (Free, available online)
- HOME-FAST (Free, available online)
- Fear of falling avoidance behavior, balance confidence, and falls efficacy
- Activities-Specific Balance Confidence Scale (Free, available online)
- Fear of Falling Avoidance Behavior Questionnaire (Free, available online)
- Falls Efficacy Scale—International (Free, available online)
- Additional areas to screen include
- Proprioception or vestibular involvement.

  - Assesses sensory contributions to balance (Free, available online)

- Vision: acuity, peripheral vision, visual fields, depth awareness, visual perception
- Footwear: ensure proper fitting, secure, non-slip

Intervention Strategies

Evidence-based interventions should be multi-factorial and must address physical, behavioral, and environmental risk factors. In PC, the OTP will focus on education and training on fall prevention strategies for identified risk factors, as well as recommendations for community-based fall prevention programs or skilled therapy services.

- Home Modifications
- Client education on common home safety hazards and modifications to increase safety during daily routines (e.g., throw rugs, loose carpet, poor lighting and glare, pets, uneven sidewalks, clutter, thresholds, unstable or nonexistent handrails, etc.).
- Home Exercise Program

- Provide the client with a written home exercise program to address physical deficits contributing to fall risk. Recommendations can include exercises and activities to improve endurance, strength, and/or flexibility. The OTP must provide education and training in the clinic to ensure the client can complete the exercises and activities safely. Strengthening exercises should focus on balance strategies and lower body strength (e.g., ankle: toe raises and heel raises; knee: knee extension and flexion; hip: abduction, adduction, flexion, and extension; compound: squats, walking side-to-side, walking heel-to-toe, walking in figure-eight pattern, etc.). Exercises can be completed in a seated position and then graded up to a standing position. Balance exercises can also be graded based on the amount of upper extremity support or by adding ankle weights.
- Additional resources for home exercise:
  - Otago Exercise Program Activity Booklet

    https://www.med.unc.edu/aging/cgwep/courses/exercise-program
    Free patient handout offering exercises for fall prevention from the University of North Carolina (UNC)
  - Stepping On

    https://www.steppingon.com
    Evidence-based community fall prevention program
  - Tai Ji Quan: Moving for Better Balance

    https://www.betterbalance.net
    Evidence-based community balance training program
  - A Matter of Balance - Programs

    Evidence-based community program to reduce fear of falling and improve activity levels
    https://mainehealth.org/healthy-communities/healthy-aging/matter-of-balance
    https://www.ncoa.org/article/evidence-based-program-a-matter-of-balance

- Adaptive Equipment and Durable Medication Equipment
- Client education and training on appropriate adaptive equipment and durable medical equipment to increase safety and independence with ADL/IADLs (e.g., shower chair, tub transfer bench, long-handled sponge and shoehorn, sock aid, grab bars, ambulation aids, emergency alert systems, etc.)
- Balance Strategies and Body Mechanics
- Client education and training on balance strategies and body mechanics during performance of ADL/IADLs (e.g., increasing base of support with a wider stance or use of cane or walker, staggered stance when reaching in cupboards, touching a stable surface, maintaining eye gaze on a fixed object during functional mobility, etc.)

- Activity Modifications
- Client education and training on activity modifications for preferred ADL/ IADLs to increase safety while encouraging occupational engagement (e.g., rearranging commonly used items in the kitchen to a shelf within reach, pacing techniques during activity, modifications to increase physical activity and leisure engagement, negotiating the environment in a supportive or protective way, etc.)
- Behavioral Interventions
- Client education and training to improve falls self-efficacy and balance confidence during ADL/IADLs and address activity avoidance behavior (e.g., cognitive adaptations such as paying attention to changes in balance and level of alertness when trying a new medication, using defensive walking strategies such as walking away from crowds, avoiding risky situations, increasing awareness of hazards, anticipating problems and finding solutions, etc.).
- Using new fall prevention strategies often requires changes in daily routines and habits. The OTP should help patients identify new routines and habits that are safe and work well for them, as well as strategies to remember when to change behavior.
- Community-Based Fall Prevention Programs
- Additionally, the OTP should provide a referral to an appropriate community-based fall prevention program for adults with any fall risk. Evidence-based community fall prevention programs include, but are not limited to (access through links above)

  - Stepping On.
  - Tai Ji Quan: Moving for Better Balance.
  - A Matter of Balance.
  - The Otago Exercise Program.

Other Considerations and Resources

Documentation and Billing

Depending upon a client's insurance provider, risk of falling may or may not be a reimbursable diagnosis for OT services. Often, diagnoses that contribute to risk of falling (such as peripheral neuropathy, dementia, Parkinson's disease, cerebrovascular accident, or osteoarthritis of the lower extremities) do trigger reimbursement. Review reimbursement policies of clients' most common insurance providers to understand when a charge is likely to be reimbursed or not. Be sure to select the CPT code that best represents the needs of your client and skilled services provided. When necessary, advocate with insurance providers to promote reimbursement for OT services related to falls and fall prevention.

Additional Resources

- National Council on Aging
  - https://www.ncoa.org/healthy-aging/falls-prevention/
- CDC STEADI program
  - https://www.cdc.gov/steadi/index.html
- National Institute on Aging
  - https://www.nia.nih.gov/health/topics/falls-and-falls-prevention
- American Geriatrics Society
  - http://stopfalls.org/

References

1. Bergen G, Stevens M, Burns E. Falls and fall injuries among adults aged ≥65 years-United States, 2014. MMWR Morb Mortal Wkly Rep. 2016;65(37):993–8.
2. O'Loughlin J, Robitaille Y, Boivin J, Suissa S. Incidence of and risk factors for falls and injurious falls among the community-dwelling elderly. Am J Epidemiol. 1993;137(3):342–54.
3. Woolcott J, Richardson K, Wiens M, Patel B, Marin J, Khan K, Marra C. Meta-analysis of the impact of 9 medication classes on falls in elderly persons. Arch Intern Med. 2009;169(21):1952–60.
4. Rider J, Longhurst J, Navalta J, Young D, Landers M. Fear of falling avoidance behavior in Parkinson's disease: most avoided activities. OTJR (Thorofare N J). 2022.
5. Choi N, Bruce M, DiNitto D, Marti C, Kunik M. Fall worry restricts social engagement in older adults. J Aging Health. 2020;32(5-6):422–31.

Chapter 23
Gastrointestinal Disorders

Myka Persson and Laura Cox

Introduction

Gastrointestinal (GI) disorders account for about 10% of the work of PCPs [1]. These disorders have a close relationship to lifestyle factors such as physical activity and stress management, and must be treated holistically. A bio-psychosocial model has been proposed that links stress to somatic symptoms of FGID, and stress management is a specific component of a holistic treatment plan.

The emerging role of OT in PC may expose more practitioners to this population, and the profession has a large role to play in lifestyle modification for GI disorders.

Chronic GI Disorders

- *Dyspepsia* is an upper GI disorder that is common, and involves heartburn, bloating, nausea, vomiting, or burping. Peptic ulcers or *H. pylori* infection may cause dyspepsia; however, the majority of dyspepsia cases are considered functional dyspepsia, which is not due to any underlying pathology. Dyspepsia is diagnosed by symptoms and endoscopy and testing for *H. pylori* infection should be done. Lifestyle factors and eating routines can benefit individuals with dyspepsia.

M. Persson (✉)
Chan Division of Occupational Science and Occupational Therapy, University of Southern California, Los Angeles, CA, USA
e-mail: mpersson@chan.usc.edu

L. Cox
University of Southern California, Los Angeles, CA, USA
e-mail: Laura.Cox@med.usc.edu

© Springer Nature Switzerland AG 2023
S. Dahl-Popolizio et al. (eds.), *Primary Care Occupational Therapy*,
https://doi.org/10.1007/978-3-031-20882-9_23

- *Gastroesophageal reflux disease (GERD)* is highly prevalent, and involves reflux of stomach contents into the esophagus or beyond. GERD is diagnosed based upon symptoms and often confirmed when proton pump inhibitor (PPI) treatment is successful. Endoscopy may be performed as well.
- *Inflammatory Bowel Disease (IBD)* includes both ulcerative colitis and Crohn's disease, and is often diagnosed in young adulthood. It is a lifelong and chronic condition. Specific characteristics of pain and diarrhea are common clinical presentations of IBD. PCPs will make a diagnosis based on endoscopic and histological results.
- *Irritable Bowel Syndrome (IBS)*, a common functional GI disorder, has no consistent biological marker. Diagnosis is based on symptoms, and clusters of symptoms may lead to diagnosis with a subgroup of IBS. Common symptoms include abdominal pain and discomfort, diarrhea and/or constipation, and bloating and gas. IBS may be diagnosed by symptomatology without testing. Dietary changes and lifestyle modifications can improve symptoms.

Other GI Disorders

- *Celiac disease (CeD)* is an autoimmune gastrointestinal disease that is often under- or misdiagnosed. In celiac disease, ingestion of gluten leads to inflammation and damage in the small intestine. Symptoms include diarrhea, fatigue, and pain. Diagnosis involves gastroscopy with duodenal biopsies following a positive serological test. With dietary management, symptoms can be well managed.
- *Chronic constipation (CC)* is a common condition, particularly in older adults, relating to colonic motor disorders.
- *Fecal incontinence (FI)* is the inability to control bowel movements, and is more common in older adults.

Role of PCP

- *Malignant GI disorders*:
  The PCP is actively involved in screening for cancers of the GI system, and imaging such as endoscopy should be done before prescribing medication by gastroenterologists. The PCP will collaborate with oncologists for cancer treatment.
- *Dyspepsia*:
  The PCP can prescribe proton pump inhibitors (PPIs) for dyspepsia. For H. pylori infection, eradication procedures should be done. Functional dyspepsia should be managed using a multifaceted approach with dietary and lifestyle interventions and psychotherapy.

- *Gastroesophageal reflux disease (GERD)*:

  The PCP commonly prescribes proton pump inhibitors (PPI) and monitors symptoms. Patient education on medication adherence and positive communication are important, as symptoms may often be overlooked although they significantly impact quality of life.

- *Inflammatory Bowel Disease (IBD)*:

  The PCP works closely with a multidisciplinary team, particularly gastroenterology, and often serves as gatekeeper to provide referrals during times of flare-ups. The PCP should screen for symptoms and help to monitor a medication plan. The PCP can also be involved in patient education and support for psychosocial problems related to IBD diagnosis.

- *Irritable Bowel Syndrome (IBS)*:

  The PCP provides a positive diagnosis, patient education, and support. Medications may be prescribed, such as anti-bulking agents or antispasmodics. However, non-pharmacological interventions seem to demonstrate the most efficacy [1]. Monitoring a food and symptom log is recommended and dietary therapies are often used.

- *Celiac disease (CeD)*:

  The PCP should consider celiac disease as a differential diagnosis when symptoms are apparent, and conduct a serological test and gastroscopy. If CeD is diagnosed, the PCP should refer the patient to a dietician to support the patient to follow a strict gluten-free diet.

- *Chronic constipation* (CC):

  Blood work and colonoscopy should be performed to rule out colorectal cancer. Treatment may involve supplemental dietary fiber, laxatives, stool softeners, biofeedback, and surgery.

- *Fecal incontinence* (FI):

  PCPs take a detailed history and conduct a rectal examination. Lifestyle modifications, including dietary modifications and bulking supplements to improve stool consistency, should be provided. Pharmacology or surgery may also be considered.

Common Comorbidities

- Depression (Chap. 18),
- Anxiety (Chap. 11).

Role of OTP

During the initial evaluation, the therapist should review the chart and include basic questions or screens to determine if the common comorbidities of depression and anxiety also require treatment alongside intervention for the presenting complaint of gastrointestinal symptoms. A holistic approach is recommended, which includes lifestyle modification.

Occupational Impact

Gastrointestinal disorders are chronic and debilitating, and patients exhibit a poorer quality of life, visit the doctor more frequently, miss more workdays, and are hospitalized more frequently than patients without FGID [2]. Population surveys show a strong correlation between anxiety, depression, and functional gastrointestinal disorders (FGID) [3]. Social participation is often affected due to pain, fear of not having a bathroom easily accessible, or symptoms such as gas or burping.

OT Areas of Emphasis

OTPs can address several aspects of symptom management and prevention for this population.

- Lifestyle modification is extremely important, including building and maintaining regular habits and routines concerning sleep, eating, and exercise.
- A psycho-educational behavioral approach has been shown efficacious to decrease symptom severity and improve quality of life.
- OTPs should train patients on strategies to manage stress, anxiety, and depression.
- The OTP can help the patient to identify lifestyle factors that impact symptoms, and then create an individualized plan to manage symptoms.
- OTPs work to empower clients with GI disorders and improve their self-efficacy to manage symptoms of these chronic and complex disorders.

Evaluation

Suggested Areas to Assess:

- *Pain and other symptoms:* Practitioners should assess pain levels and symptoms (type, frequency, contributing factors).
- *Lifestyle factors impacting symptoms:* the use of a food, occupation, and symptom diary should be used to identify factors impacting symptoms.

Suggested Assessment Tools:

Symptoms: IBS Symptom Severity Scale
Pain: use the visual analog pain scale or the numeric pain rating (0–10).
General Function and Quality of Life: Canadian Occupational Performance Measure (COPM)
RAND SF 36 Quality of Life survey
Assessments and screenings for comorbid conditions outlined above

Intervention Strategies

Symptom Monitoring

- Educate client about their GI disorder and common triggers
    - For example, IBS education can include [4]:
        Prevalence to normalize client's condition
            Approximately 10–15% in North America
        Chronic nature of the condition
            Requires lifelong management
        The pathophysiology of the condition
            Largely uncertain, but is thought to involve hypersensitivity and disturbances of the motility of the large and small intestines
        Common symptoms
            For example, abdominal pain, bloating, increased gas, diarrhea, and/or constipation
        Common triggers
            For example, certain foods/beverages, stress
- Encourage client to track their symptoms in order to increase insight regarding their potential triggers
    - Clients can use mobile phone apps such as Cara Care, Bowelle, or MyGiHealth
    - Clients can use a paper-based tracker, if preferred. See the example template below

GI SYMPTOM TRACKER						
Date & Time	Foods/Beverages consumed	Symptoms (pain, bloating, gas, diarrhea, constipation, nausea, heartburn)	Duration	Level of Discomfo rt (scale of 0-10)	Possible Triggers (food, activity, mood, stress, sleep, hormones,	Other Notes

Stress Management

- Educate client regarding the neurobiology of the stress response and its connection to gut symptoms

  - Activation of the sympathetic nervous system in response to stress (cascade of stress hormones)
  - Cortisol (the "stress hormone") triggers inflammation and exacerbates pain
  - Intestinal barrier weakens when stressed, allowing gut bacteria to enter the body [5]

    Triggers an immune response to take care of this bacteria, thus increasing inflammation

  - Stress can delay or speed up stomach emptying and passage through the intestines, resulting in abdominal pain and altered bowel habits [4]

- Identify client's triggers of stress
- Identify client's signals of stress
- Train client in techniques for eliciting relaxation response

  - Techniques include: diaphragmatic breathing, meditation, progressive muscle relaxation, body scan, imagery/visualization, and more.
  - YouTube videos

    Diaphragmatic Breathing
    Meditation with Diaphragmatic Breathing

  - Mobile Apps

    Calm
    Headspace
    Insight Timer
    Stop, Breathe, and Think

- Collaborate with client to develop a stress management plan he/she can integrate into daily routine

Coping with Pain (Chap. 34)

• Educate client regarding chronic pain and the pain pathway.
• Train client in techniques for coping with the pain (e.g., attention diversion, cognitive restructuring, transformation imagery, coping self-statements, meditation, visualization, diaphragmatic breathing).

Eating Routines

• Educate client regarding common dietary triggers [4, 6]
  – Cramping- or diarrhea-causing foods:

    Coffee, caffeine, alcohol, sorbitol, fructose, fatty foods

  – Gas producing foods

    Beans, legumes, cabbage, broccoli, cauliflower, onion, brussels sprouts, raisins, bagels

  – Intolerances

    Lactose
    Fructose
    FODMAPs   (Fermentable   Oligosaccharides,   Disaccharides, Monosaccharides, and Polyols)

  – Mobile apps to assist with "safe" food identification

    MyHealthyGut
    FODMAP Helper—Diet Companion
    Fast FODMAP Lookup and Learn

• Problem-solve food modifications as necessary to reduce consumption of dietary triggers
• Establish an eating routine that has consistent timing of meals and snacks to promote stable blood sugar levels and metabolism

  – Identify non-triggering and enjoyable snacks with the client

• Discuss optimal water intake and strategies to increase consumption

  – Several factors impact the recommended daily water intake, such as exercise, weather, caffeine consumption, sex, weight, etc.
  – General recommendations are [7]:

    15.5 cups for men
    11.5 cups for women

– Strategies to increase consumption

> Pair it with meals
> Flavor it with fruits, veggies, and/or herbs
> Have a reusable bottle to bring anywhere (work, errands, etc.)
> Set reminders
> Track intake. See mobile apps below.
>
> > Waterlogged
> > Drink Water Reminder N Tracker
> > Plant Nanny

Sleep Routines

- Educate client regarding sleep hygiene strategies

  – Avoiding screen use 1–2 h before bedtime
  – Creating a dark, cool, and quiet sleep environment
  – Physical activity (but at least 3 h before bed)

- Collaborate with client to develop an individualized wind-down routine
- Determine optimal sleep routine (i.e., bed time, wake time)

  – Consider having the client track their sleep using a sleep diary. See below.

SLEEP DIARY								
Date	What did you do before bed?	What time did you go to bed?	How long did it take to fall asleep?	How many times did you wake?	What time did you wake up?	How many hours of sleep did you get?	How would you rate your sleep quality (very poor, poor, fair, good, excellent)	Notes: (include any naps, caffeine or alcohol intake, and exercise)

- Discuss sleep positioning strategies to increase comfort

Physical Activity Routines

- Educate client regarding the connection between exercise and stress reduction, constipation relief, and pain relief
- Discuss types of exercise that won't aggravate symptoms
- Identify enjoyable forms of physical activity for the client
- Identify barriers to engagement in physical activity and problem-solve to overcome barriers

Medication Management

- Identify barriers to medication regimen adherence
- Discuss strategies to improve adherence
  - Pill organizers
  - Reminders
  - Auto-refill from pharmacy

Self-Advocacy

- Determine strategies for communicating symptoms and needs with friends, family, co-workers, etc.
- Train client in assertive communication strategies

Social Participation

- Discuss barriers (e.g., fear, embarrassment) to social participation
- Problem-solve strategies for social engagement
  - Prior research to identify nearest restrooms
  - Examine menus or call restaurants to ensure food modifications can be made
  - Identify pain coping strategies to use if pain flares while in social settings

Other Considerations and Resources

Documentation and Billing—Use the *Physical Medicine and Rehabilitation* CPT code that best fits your intervention.

Suggested referrals if you are unable to help patient sufficiently in PC:

- OT in an outpatient setting for lifestyle modification and behavior change.
- Dietician or nutritionist for guidance regarding the optimal diet for the type of GI disorder.
- Gastroenterologist for advanced treatment and monitoring of symptoms.
- Mental health counselor and/or psychiatrist to support management of depression or anxiety.

References

1. Gikas A, Triantafillidis JK. The role of primary care physicians in early diagnosis and treatment of chronic gastrointestinal diseases. Int J Gen Med. 2014;7:159–73.
2. Saha L. Irritable bowel syndrome: pathogenesis, diagnosis, treatment, and evidence-based medicine. World J Gastroenterol. 2014;20(22):6759–73.
3. Simpson CA, Mu A, Haslam N, Schwartz OS, Simmons JG. Feeling down? A systematic review of the gut microbiota in anxiety/depression and irritable bowel syndrome. J Affect Disord. 2020;266:429–46.
4. International Foundation for Gastrointestinal Disorders (2016). *What is IBS?* International Foundation for Gastrointestinal Disorders, Inc. (IFFGD). https://www.aboutibs.org/what-is-ibs-sidenav.html
5. van Tilburg M. Stress effects on the body. American Psychological Association; 2018. https://www.apa.org/helpcenter/stress/effects-gastrointestinal#:~:text=S tress%20can%20affect%20digestion%2C%20and,bacteria%20to%20enter%20the%20body
6. Wald, A. (2019). Clinical manifestations and diagnosis of irritable bowel syndrome in adults. UpToDate. https://www.uptodate.com/contents/clinical-manifestations-and-diagnosis-of-irritable-bowel-syndrome-in-adults#H14.
7. Mayo Clinic Staff (2017). Water: how much should you drink every day? Mayo Clinic. https://www.mayoclinic.org/healthy-lifestyle/nutrition-and-healthy-eating/in-depth/water/art-20044256#:~:text=So%20how%20much%20fluid%20does,fluids%20a%20day%20for%20women.

Chapter 24
Guillain-Barré Syndrome

Lara Taggart and Gillian Porter

Introduction [1–3]

The exact cause of Guillain-Barré Syndrome (GBS) is unknown. GBS is an acute inflammatory demyelinating polyneuropathy that results in axonal demyelination of peripheral nerves. Triggers can be a viral or microbial infection, most commonly a Campylobacter jejuni infection followed by a Cytomegalovirus infection, the flu, Epstein Barr virus, and the Zika virus. Rarely, people have developed GBS in the days or weeks after receiving certain vaccines.

- *Risk Factors*:
    GBS can develop in anyone. In the United States, GBS is more common in men and adults older than 50.

- *Types of GBS:*
    There are several forms of GBS, with the three main types:

    - Acute Inflammatory Demyelinating Polyradiculoneuropathy (AIDP)—weakness starts in the lower body and ascends superiorly
    - Miller Fisher Syndrome (MFS)—paralysis starts in the eyes and is associated with unsteady gait
    - Acute Motor Axonal Neuropathy (AMAN) and Acute Motor-Sensory Axonal Neuropathy (AMSAN)

L. Taggart (✉)
Northern Arizona University, Flagstaff, AZ, USA
e-mail: Lara.Taggart@nau.edu

G. Porter
Northern Arizona University, Flagstaff, AZ, USA

Carefree Physical Therapy, Carefree, AZ, USA
e-mail: gp288@nau.edu

© Springer Nature Switzerland AG 2023
S. Dahl-Popolizio et al. (eds.), *Primary Care Occupational Therapy*,
https://doi.org/10.1007/978-3-031-20882-9_24

Signs and Symptoms [1, 2]

- Characteristics include

  - Quickly progressing, symmetrical paresthesias and muscle weakness
  - Ascending paralysis starting with the feet
  - Pain in the legs
  - Absence of deep tendon reflexes
  - Mild sensory loss in glove-and-stocking distributions; cranial nerve dysfunction with possible facial palsy and swallowing problems
  - An autonomic nervous system response of postural hypertension and tachycardia
  - Respiratory muscle paralysis
  - Pain
  - Fatigue
  - Urinary dysfunction

- Cognition, however, remains mostly intact

  - Subtle cognitive deficits in executive functions, short-term memory, and decision making may occur

- GBS has three phases:

  - *Onset/acute inflammatory phase*—manifests as weakness in at least two limbs that progresses and reaches its maximum in 2–4 weeks accompanied by increasing symptoms

       Mechanical ventilation is required for 20–30% of individuals

  - *Plateau phase*—no significant change which lasts for a few days or weeks, when the greatest disability is present.
  - *Progressive recovery*—remyelination and axonal regeneration occur and may last for up to two years, although the average length is 12 weeks

       Recovery starts at the head and neck and proceeds distally (extent varies)
       Approximately 50% of patients have complete return of function, and another 35% experience some residual weakness that may not resolve
       Remaining 15% experience more significant permanent disability
       Fatigue is the most common residual problem for 93% of patients

Role of PCP [2, 4]

Because of the severity of GBS, immediate hospitalization and treatment are required to promote best outcomes. Patients may be seen in the PC office after hospitalization as they are progressing through the phases of the condition.

- Comprehensive medical exam to assess muscle weakness/paralysis, as these are the earliest signs of GBS. Reflexes may be decreased or missing, and breathing may be compromised by paralysis of breathing muscles.
- Other tests may include:

  - Spinal tap
  - ECG
  - EMG
  - Nerve conduction velocity
  - Pulmonary function tests

- Treatment focuses on reducing symptoms, addressing complications, and promoting recovery:

  - Apheresis or plasmapheresis may be administered to reduce proteins that attack nerve cells
  - Intravenous immunoglobulin (IVIg)
  - Other treatments to reduce inflammation
  - Breathing support may be required
  - Pain management
  - Blood thinners
  - Body positioning or feeding tube to prevent choking or provide nutritional support
  - Therapies to maintain strength, mobility, and participation in self-care

Common Comorbidities

There are no specific common comorbidities, but there are medical complications that can occur in people with GBS.

Role of OTP

In PC, the role of the OTP is to ensure the patient remains as functional as possible throughout the long recovery process. This includes recommending referral for more intense treatment when necessary, providing adaptive strategies and devices as indicated, connecting patients with resources, communicating concerns to other team members, and providing emotional support to the patient and family as indicated through behavioral health interventions and referrals.

Occupational Impact

GBS is devastating as the onset is rapid and results in loss of function throughout the body. All aspects of the patient's life are affected.

OT Areas of Emphasis [1]

In ADL and IADL, the OTP assists the client to maintain independence in priority activities, use specialized equipment, and participate using energy conserving methods such as:

- Assisting in setting priorities
- Education in areas such as how the disease process affects motor or cognitive changes
- Recommendation of environmental modifications at home to promote safety and independence
- Range of motion (ROM) and strength exercises to facilitate occupations like bathing
- Behavior modification such as use of energy and time management techniques
- Use of smart phone and electronic tablet technology for grocery lists and to provide reminders
- Balancing independence with assistance from others

Evaluation

Evaluation and Assessment in the Acute Phase
- Referral to OT is common when the course of GBS is moderate to severe.
- Approximately 40% of all GBS patients require rehabilitation services.
- Assessment at the onset of the plateau phase typically occurs in the intensive care unit, when the individual is undergoing extensive medical procedures and pain can be significant.
- Therapists should complete an interview to understand the client's feelings and fears and evaluate communication, control of the environment, comfort, and level of anxiety.
- A sensory assessment is essential because marked sensitivity is typical of acute GBS.
- The guiding principle is to ask permission prior to touching the client.
- Therapists should also be aware of the 7-point GBS disability scale that primarily assesses ambulation and the need for a ventilator.

Evaluation and Assessment in the Progressive Recovery Phase

- During the recovery phase, therapists evaluate self-care, communication, leisure, as well as mobility, sensation, strength, Range of Motion (ROM) and, as appropriate, reintegration into the workplace.
- Patients with GBS should not be pushed to fatigue, because recovery will be prolonged, and fatigue may slow the rehabilitation process.
- During this phase, OT services can be provided in an inpatient rehabilitation facility, through an outpatient program, and/or at home or work.

Assessment [5]

- Canadian Occupational Performance Measure (COPM)
- Functional Testing
  - Self-care (ADLs)
  - IADLs
  - Leisure activities
  - Mobility/transfers

    Assistive device assessment
    Wheelchair evaluation

  - Home evaluation

    Durable medical equipment (DME)
    Caregiver training

- 7-point GBS disability scale
  - Rates overall functional abilities of people with GBS

- Vitals
  - Blood Pressure
  - Heart Rate
  - Blood Oxygen Level (SpO2)
  - Signs of cardiopulmonary distress, such as lightheadedness, dizziness, headache

- Joint ROM
- Strength testing
- Manual muscle testing, upper and lower extremities
- Grip/pinch strength
- Fine motor assessment

  - Nine Hole Peg test

- Sensory assessment

  - Upper and lower extremity dermatomes
  - Light touch
  - Sharp/dull
  - 2-point discrimination
  - Pain assessment (Visual Analog Scale)

- Orthotics
- Fatigue

  - Borg Rate of Perceived Exertion
  - Vital capacity and inspiratory force assessment
  - Patient/caregiver education on importance of avoiding fatigue to promote optimal recovery

- Fall Risk

  - Falls Efficacy Scale
  - See chapter on falls and falls prevention (Chap. 22)

- Cognitive Screen

  - Montreal Cognitive Assessment (MoCA)

Intervention Strategies [1, 5]

Primary focus of intervention is to

1. Promote a patient's optimal use of strength and pain-free ROM to complete daily activities while avoiding fatigue.
2. Educate and train the use of supportive equipment and functional adaptations to resume activity level resembling prior level of function.
1. Acute/Plateau Phases

   During the acute phase, the OTP's role may be more consultative in providing patient/caregiver education about maintaining comfort in bed and protecting against bed sores. The patient may be actively involved in directing care because they are often less able to physically participate in therapy.

   - Modifications during the acute and plateau phase should be considered temporary and may include

     - Communication tools, such as sign or picture board or voice-activated devices, if appropriate.
     - Access to the nurse call button, TV, and lights by remote control, as appropriate.

- Use of hands-free telephone.
- Modification of lying and sitting positions for optimal function and comfort.
- Positioning trunk, head, and upper extremities for stability and comfort.

    Skin integrity inspection.
    Be watchful for deep vein thrombosis (DVT).

- Introducing strategies to reduce anxiety.

2. Progressive Recovery Phase
    Recovery-phase interventions are initially completed with few repetitions, punctuated with rest. The number and complexity of tasks should be increased gradually.
- Interventions include

    - Providing activities and dynamic splints to maintain ROM, particularly of wrists, fingers, and ankle (hinged drop-foot orthosis).

        Skin integrity inspection.
        Be watchful for deep vein thrombosis (DVT).

    - Instructing both caregiver and client in safe mobility and independent transfers.
    - Providing a sensory stimulation or desensitization program, as appropriate.
    - Training in modified self-care techniques and adapting other daily activities.
    - Using smart devices to facilitate communication and conserve energy.
    - Modifying and encouraging reengagement in routine activities, as appropriate.
    - Adapting equipment for in home, leisure, and work activities.
    - Instructing in energy conservation and fatigue management strategies.
    - Modifying employment roles, tasks, and environment, as indicated.
    - Recommending a fine-motor program to enhance strength, coordination, and sensation.
    - Completing a home assessment and modifications, as appropriate, to facilitate return to home.

Other Considerations and Resources

For patients and providers: GBS/CIDP https://www.gbs-cidp.org/

References

1. Radomski MV, Trombly Latham CA. Occupational therapy for physical dysfunction. 7th ed. Philadelphia, PA: Lippincott Williams & Wilkins; 2008.
2. Mayo Clinic. Guillain-barre syndrome. 2020. https://www.mayoclinic.org/diseases-conditions/guillain-barre-syndrome/symptoms-causes/syc-20362793.
3. Centers for Disease Control and Prevention. Guillain-Barre syndrome. 2019. https://www.cdc.gov/campylobacter/guillain-barre.html.
4. Minagar, A. Guillain-Barre syndrome. 2019. https://www.mountsinai.org/health-library/diseases-conditions/guillain-barr-syndrome.
5. GBS/CIDP Foundation International. Guidelines for physical and occupational therapy. 2019. https://www.gbs-cidp.org/wp-content/uploads/2019/12/GBSCIDP-Guidelines-for-PT-and-OT-Booklet_Final.pdf.

Chapter 25
Huntington's Disease

Katelyn Fell and Jyothi Gupta

Introduction

Huntington's Disease (HD) is a progressive and fatal neurological disorder that is acquired by inheriting a dominant gene that codes for the Huntingtin (Htt) protein. The mutation results in an elongated stretch of glutamine near the amino terminus of Htt, that causes the protein to misfold and form toxic aggregates throughout the body [1]. Neuropathologically, HD is characterized by degenerating medium spiny neurons (MSN) in the striatum of the basal ganglia and the cerebral cortex.

Sub-type

- Juvenile onset HD occurs when the condition develops before the age of 20 and usually has a more rapid progression [2].

    - Juvenile onset HD symptoms may present differently and include [3]:

        Stiffness of the legs
        Scissoring gait
        Toe walking
        Decreased gross motor coordination of limbs
        Early swallowing and speech difficulties

K. Fell (✉)
University of St. Augustine for Health Sciences, St. Augustine, FL, USA
e-mail: kfell@usa.edu

J. Gupta
The University of Texas Medical Branch, Galveston, TX, USA
e-mail: jygupta@UTMB.EDU

Bradykinesia
Cerebellar signs
Tremors

Signs and Symptoms

HD symptoms include progressive cognitive, motor, and behavioral impairments.

- Cognitive symptoms [2–4]:

  - Memory—new learning, memory retrieval
  - Attention—divided attention, sustained attention, concentration
  - Executive functions—planning, initiating, decision making, goal-directed behaviors
  - Lack of mental flexibility, perseveration
  - Lack of insight into functional limitations

- Motor symptoms [2–4]:

  - Choreiform movements and athetosis impact fine and gross motor control

    Chorea: involuntary, irregular, or writhing muscle movements
    Athetosis: slow, involuntary writhing muscle movements

  - Disturbances in balance; ataxic (staggering) gait pattern; postural control
  - Oculomotor control; slowed saccadic eye movement and ocular pursuits
  - Tics
  - Dysarthria
  - Dysphagia
  - Motor impersistence
  - Rigidity (late stages)
  - Dystonia (late stages)

- Behavioral symptoms [2–4]:

  - Anxiety
  - Apathy—difficulty with initiation and a decrease in goal-directed behavior
  - Anosognosia
  - Depression—increased risk for suicide
  - Irritability
  - Obsessions and compulsions
  - Poor impulse control
  - Poor emotional regulation

Disease Stages

HD progresses through five stages identified by the Unified Huntington's Disease Rating Scale (UHDRS), a standardized rating system used to quantify the severity of HD symptoms, including motor function, cognitive function, behavioral abnormalities, and functional capacity. Management of HD varies based on the stage of the disease. The five stages include: Stage I (presymptomatic); Stage II (early); Stage III (middle); Stages IV and V (late) [3–5].

Role of PCP

There is currently no effective treatment to cure or slow the progression of HD. Medical management is focused on symptom management, maximizing function, and education regarding the course of the disease. Medications are prescribed to help manage symptoms of depression and chorea. A multidisciplinary approach is beneficial in addressing the varied and diverse symptoms of HD [4, 6].

Suggested Referrals:

- Psychotherapy
- Physical therapy (PT)
- OT
- Speech language pathologist
- Nutrition counseling
- Social worker
- Genetic counseling
- Support groups

Common Comorbidities [2, 3]

- Depression (risk of suicide) (Chap. 18)
- Anxiety (Chap. 11)

Role of OTP

Facilitating participation in meaningful occupations while providing opportunities for the individual to maintain a sense of control over their environment is important at each stage of the disease [4].

Occupational Impact

Due to the progressive nature and impact on cognitive, motor, and behavioral functioning, HD greatly impacts occupational performance. Early stages of the disease may involve only mild cognitive and motor impairments, resulting in declining IADL function while maintaining independence with ADLs. As the disease progresses, further decline in cognitive, motor, and behavioral functioning will result in decreased ability to perform ADLs, functional mobility, leisure, and social participation [3, 4].

OT Areas of Emphasis

A client-centered approach, which focuses on the client's values, roles, and autonomy, should guide OT intervention.

Throughout the course of the disease process, OTPs will

- Facilitate participation in meaningful occupations and role fulfillment.
- Make recommendations for appropriate durable medical equipment (DME), adaptive equipment, assistive devices, or assistive technology as needed.
- Consider functional mobility and community mobility needs.
- Address upper extremity function/coordination.
- Provide caregiver and family education/training.
- Educate on community resources, including support groups, transportation, and exercise/activity classes.

Evaluation

A comprehensive evaluation which assesses cognition, motor function, and psychosocial components of the individual is vital. Developing an occupational profile will provide information about specific client factors and contexts which may support or hinder performance. Additionally, frequent functional reassessment is necessary as the disease progresses and the needs of the individual change.

Areas of Assessment

- Cognitive function (memory, new learning, executive functions, attention/concentration)
  - Montreal Cognitive Assessment (MoCA), Mini Mental Status Examination (MMSE), St Louis University Mental Status (SLUMS) Examination, Trail Making Tests, Executive Function Test, Cognitive Performance Test
- Motor function (fine motor coordination, gross motor coordination, gait, balance, choreiform movements, lack of voluntary motor control, eye movement irregularities, dysarthria, dysphagia, rigidity)

 – Fine Motor Coordination

   9-Hole Peg Test, Minnesota Rate of Manipulation Test, Purdue Pegboard, Jebsen Hand Function Test

 – Gait and Balance

   Timed Up and Go (TUG), Berg Balance Scale, Tinetti, Activities-Specific Balance Confidence Scale, Five Times Sit to Stand Test, Functional Reach Test

 – Tone

   Modified Ashworth Scale

• ADL performance

 – COPM, Barthel Index, KELS, Assessment of Motor and Process Skills

• Psychosocial components (emotional regulation, depression screening, coping skills)

 – Patient Health Questionnaire (PHQ-9), WHOQoL-BREF, Beck Depression Inventory

• Vision (saccades, ocular pursuits)

 – *See Vision Chapter* (Chap. 36)

Other Areas to Consider:

• Communication
• Caregiver support
• Workplace modifications
• Home modifications
• Social support systems
• Community resources

Intervention Strategies

Specific OT interventions will vary depending on the stage of the disease and the individual needs of the client. OT intervention may include the following, as appropriate for the stage of the disease:

• Activity modification and use of adaptive equipment
• Cognitive skills; memory supports
• Routine management/establishment
• Functional mobility training
• Home exercise program (flexibility, functional strength training, endurance)
• Leisure exploration

- Environmental controls
- Family and caregiver education/training

Early-Stage

- Choreiform movements may be subtle, or limited only to the hands in the early stages of the disease. Impairments in fine motor coordination may result in difficulty with managing buttons or snaps on clothing, manipulating small items, or typing [3, 4].
- Cognitive symptoms include memory impairment and decreased concentration. Individuals at this stage of HD may still be employed, and therefore benefit from strategies that include establishment of daily routines, use of checklists, planners, and reminders in the workplace [3, 4]. Reducing external stimuli may help to improve concentration.
- Home and workplace evaluations should be conducted at this stage in order to maximize participation and allow for skill development and habit formation utilizing new adaptive equipment, assistive devices, or activity modification [4].
- Developing and establishing healthy lifestyle routines and habits, including exercise and a healthy diet, is beneficial during the early stages of the disease [3].
- Addressing the emotional responses to a new diagnosis of HD may also be appropriate, both for the individual and caregivers [4].
- Providing education on the disease process, support groups, coping strategies, and encouraging social participation is beneficial.

Middle-Stage

- Motor impairment becomes more pronounced during this stage of the disease, impacting gait and balance. The individual may require use of a walker or wheelchair for safe mobility and ADLs such as dressing and bathing may need to be performed in a seated position [4].
- Chorea may impact various parts of the body, including limbs and trunk as well as speech and swallowing functions. Use of additional cushions, padding, railings, and positioning aids may be necessary if excessive choreiform movements place the individual at risk for injury or falling out of the wheelchair or bed [4].
- Due to excessive movements associated with chorea, fatigue may become a factor along with higher energy expenditure. Education on energy conservation and activity modification may help to reduce energy demands.
- Dietary adjustments and weight monitoring may be needed in order to avoid weight loss [3, 4]. Impairment in oculomotor control may impact saccades and smooth pursuits required for functional vision tasks, reading, and scanning the environment [3, 4].
- Progressive cognitive decline at this stage results in the decreased ability to complete sequential tasks or learn new information. Providing simple visual or written cues to instruct or remind the individual may facilitate continued participation in self-care and simple household activities [4].
- The individual may experience a progression of behavioral symptoms, including irritability and depression, at this stage of HD. Providing opportunities to participate in meaningful activities and leisure pursuits is important [3].

Late-Stage

- Some individuals experience a decrease in chorea during the late stages of HD, leading to rigidity [3, 4]. Assistance for all self-care, positioning, and feeding is needed at this stage. Positioning, splinting, and prevention of contractures is important.
- The individual may require the use of a feeding tube due to the risk for aspiration during these late stages of the disease [3].
- Providing the individual with adaptive switches and controls for the environment, including lights, television, communication, and call buttons, are strategies that promote autonomy and client control over the environment, when possible [4].
- Promoting a sense of autonomy and maintaining consistent daily routines may help to reduce behavioral outbursts during the late stages of the disease.
- OT may be involved in end-of-life care, which should focus on client values and quality of life at this stage.

Other Considerations and Resources

- The Huntington's Disease Society of America website is an excellent source of information: http://hdsa.org
- This free downloadable guide for physical and occupational therapy is available through the Huntington's Disease Society of America: http://hdsa.org/wp-content/uploads/2015/03/PhysicalOccupationalTherapy_FamilyGuide.pdf

References

1. Schulte J, Littleton JT. The biological function of the huntingtin protein and its relevance to Huntington's disease pathology. Curr Trends Neurol. 2011;5:65–78.
2. Mayo Clinic. Huntington's disease. 2020. Mayoclinic.org https://www.mayoclinic.org/diseases-conditions/huntingtons-disease/symptoms-causes/syc-20356117.
3. Kostyk S. Huntington's disease: a primer for community-based occupational therapists. [Lecture notes, PowerPoint slides]. AOTA Press; 2019.
4. Pendleton HM, Schultz-Krohn W. Pedretti's occupational therapy: practice skills for physical dysfunction. 8th ed. Amsterdam: Elsevier; 2018.
5. Liou S. The HD measuring stick: assessment standards for Huntington's disease. hopes.stanford.edu. 2010. https://hopes.stanford.edu/assessment-standards-for-huntingtons-disease-severity/#unified-huntingtons-disease-rating-scale-uhdrs-physical-and-mental.
6. Nance MA. Comprehensive care in Huntington's disease. Brain Res Bull. 2007;72(4):175–8. https://doi.org/10.1016/j.brainresbull.2006.10.0271.

Chapter 26
Hypertension

Sue Doyle and Sue Dahl-Popolizio

Introduction

According to the CDC and the American College of Cardiology, approximately 45% of the adults in the United States have hypertension [1, 2]. Approximately 24% of those with hypertension (HTN) have their condition under control [1]. In 2018, HTN was a primary or contributing cause of death for nearly half a million people in the United States [1]. It is estimated that HTN costs the United States economy over $131 billion each year [1]. With medication and other treatment costs as well as lost productivity due to related complications, the cost to the economy is quite high. High blood pressure is often referred to as the silent killer as frequently there are no signs or symptoms until there are serious complications [3].

Risk factors for HTN include [3, 4]

- Unmodifiable risk factors

  - Family history in close blood relatives.
  - Age. In Western cultures blood pressure increases with age.
  - Sex. 64 years and under men are more likely to get high blood pressure, over 65 years of age women are more likely.
  - Race. African Americans have a higher risk of HTN. Blood pressure in this population also tends to be more severe and respond less to medications.
  - Chronic Kidney Disease.

S. Doyle
OT Lifestyle Solutions PLLC, Vancouver, WA, USA
e-mail: sdoyle@otlifestylesolutions.com

S. Dahl-Popolizio (✉)
Arizona State University, Phoenix, AZ, USA

AT Still University, Mesa, AZ, USA
e-mail: Sue.Dahlpopolizio@asu.edu; sdahlpopolizio@atsu.edu

© Springer Nature Switzerland AG 2023   261
S. Dahl-Popolizio et al. (eds.), *Primary Care Occupational Therapy*,
https://doi.org/10.1007/978-3-031-20882-9_26

- Modifiable/lifestyle risk factors

  - Decreased physical activity.
  - Diet high in sodium (salt), saturated and trans-fats, processed foods and sugars.
  - Overweight and obesity.
  - High cholesterol.
  - Alcohol consumption.
  - Sleep apnea, sleep deprivation, and sleep impairments.
  - Smoking and tobacco use.
  - Ongoing high levels of unmitigated stress.
  - High caffeine intake or other stimulants.

HTN, also known as high blood pressure, is a condition in which blood pressure is persistently elevated. Blood pressure is measured using two numbers: systolic (the pressure when the heart muscles contract) and diastolic (the pressure when the heart muscles relax). Measurements are given in mmHg, or millimeters of mercury. The definition of HTN has been modified. Table 26.1 below outlines the most recent diagnostic thresholds for HTN.

- Primary versus Secondary HTN

  - Primary HTN is the most common and is seen as HTN that develops without another medical condition as the likely cause.
  - Secondary HTN develops as a result of another condition, e.g., kidney damage, pregnancy, heart defects, long term diuretic use.

Role of PCP

- Identifying high blood pressure (includes at home monitoring program)
- Identifying at-risk patients for closer monitoring
- Screening and diagnosis
- Pre-pharmaceutical intervention
- Medication management
- Monitoring medication side effects and effectiveness
- Monitor drug interactions
- Referral to specialist

Table 26.1 Blood pressure measures [2]

Normal Blood Pressure	Systolic: less than 120 mmhg Diastolic: less than 80 mmHg
Elevated	Systolic: 120–129 mmHg diastolic: <80 mmHg
Stage 1 Stage 2 Hypertensive crisis	Systolic: 130–139 mmHg or diastolic: 80–89 Systolic at least 140 mmHg; diastolic at least 90 mmHg Systolic >180 and or diastolic >120. Immediate medication changes, hospitalization if signs of organ damage

Common Comorbidities

Chronic HTN can lead to

- Blood vessel damage

    - Artery narrowing and damage.
    - Aneurysms.

- Heart damage

    - Coronary artery disease.
    - Enlarged left heart.
    - Heart Failure.

- Kidney damage

    - Kidney failure.
    - Kidney scarring (glomerulosclerosis).
    - Kidney artery aneurysm.

- Brain damage

    - Transient Ischemic Attacks.
    - Cerebral vascular accident.
    - Dementias.
    - Mild Cognitive Impairment.

- Eye damage

    - Retinopathy.
    - Choroidopathy—fluid buildup under the retina.
    - Nerve damage.

- Other potential complications [5, 6]

    - Erectile dysfunction.
    - Female decreased sexual arousal, vaginal dryness, and difficulty achieving orgasm.
    - Bone loss.
    - Obstructive sleep apnea.
    - Pulmonary edema.
    - Benign prostatic hyperplasia.

- Anxiety (Chap. 11)

    - Though it has not been found to be a cause of HTN, there is evidence supporting a relationship between anxiety and HTN, suggesting that HTN can worsen during periods of anxiety [7].

- Depression (Chap. 18)

  - There are mixed reports regarding a relationship between depression and HTN. Some studies suggest there is an association with lower systolic blood pressure and depression [8, 9], but some blood pressure medications (noradrenergic and serotonergic medications) are associated with higher diastolic and systolic blood pressures [8]. Persons taking tricyclic antidepressants were more likely to have stage 1 and stage 2 HTN [8].

Role of OTP

OTPs will evaluate medication adherence, and identify any barriers to adherence to medical advice. As this condition is asymptomatic, the OTP will provide education to ensure patients understand hypertension and why adhering to medical advice through medication management and lifestyle modification is critical. The OTP will develop realistic, actionable strategies to facilitate effective condition self-management.

Occupational Impact

- Invisible or no impact

  - Usually HTN does not produce signs or symptoms. In these cases, clients do not experience any observable occupational impact. Lack of tangible impact may reduce clients' likelihood to seek out or adhere to medical interventions.
  - Because of the lack of symptoms, patients experience health risks due to lack of management of their condition (e.g., stroke, myocardial infarction, death). The occupational impact is most apparent when the condition is not effectively treated.

- Physical activity

  - Severe HTN may cause symptoms that impact a client's daily occupations, such as fatigue, headache, or shortness of breath.
  - These will vary significantly between clients, and can impact many areas of occupation.
  - Due to the patient's overall physical health that has led to HTN, they may have physical activity limitations imposed by their health (obesity, shortness of breath, etc.), or imposed by their provider because of their underlying health status.

- Economic impact
  - HTN is one of ten most expensive diagnoses in the workplace. It impacts absenteeism, productivity, and overall healthcare costs. On average, people with HTN miss up to 4.2 additional days of work compared to those without HTN [10].
- Cognitive impairment
  - Midlife HTN impacts cognitive function and is associated with the development of Alzheimer's Disease [11, 12].
  - Cognitive impairments can appear early and the cognitive impairments need to be managed early to reduce later progression [12].
  - Reduced cognitive capacity can result in difficulties performing job responsibilities, and progress to impeding ADLs, IADLs, or participating in cognitively challenging leisure pursuits.

OT Areas of Emphasis

- Reducing occupational impact
  - Adaptations for any functional impact related to HTN such as vision changes, cognitive changes, and other body function impairments that impact occupational performance.
- Promote condition self-management
- Educate the patient and their support system regarding:
  - Overall health literacy
  - The asymptomatic nature of HTN
  - The health risks associated with HTN
  - The importance of improving self-management
- Medication management and adherence (identify barriers and provide adherence strategies)
- Lifestyle modifications
  - Identify patient needs regarding lifestyle modification, and develop strategies to sustain lifestyle modifications once the patient makes the necessary lifestyle changes.
  - This includes lifestyle issues that increase risk of developing/worsening of the condition such as obesity, smoking, alcohol use, poor diet choices, etc.
- Address behavioral health issues, including depression, anxiety, and other mental health concerns that can be addressed in PC. Recommend referral to a specialty practice, if necessary.

Evaluation

- Medication Adherence
    - Brief Medication Questionnaire 2—identifies adherence and barriers. Designed specifically for blood pressure medications.
    - Self-efficacy for Appropriate Medication Use Scale (SEAMS). Designed for use in chronic disease management and across a range of literacy levels.
- Overall functional and occupational performance
    - PROMIS Profile 29

        Free, available online

    - Canadian Occupational Performance Measure (COPM)
- Anxiety and Stress
    - General Anxiety Disorder 7 item Scale (GAD-7)

        Free, available online

- Depression
    - Patient Health Questionnaire (PHQ-9) The *PHQ-9* is also available in the Appendix

        Free, available online

- Cognitive Status
    - St Louis University Mental Status (SLUMS) Examination

        Free, available from slu.edu

    - Montreal Cognitive Assessment (MOCA)

        Free, available online

    - Trail Making Tests Parts A & B (normal <20 s) & B (normal <30 s)

        Free, available online

- Vision
    - Visual acuity Feinbloom chart or Snellen Chart
    - Contrast sensitivity ETDRS Low-contrast charts
    - Visual fields confrontation testing
    - Motor Free Visual Perception Test (MVPT)
    - *See Vision Chapter for additional assessments* (Chap. 36)
- Lifestyle Behaviors
    - CAGE Alcohol use questionnaire

        Free, available online

- Tobacco Use Assessment

    Free, available online

- International Physical Activity Questionnaire (IPAQ)

    Free, available online

Intervention Strategies

- For all of these interventions, work closely with the PCP and other team members. As this condition is asymptomatic, the patient needs consistency of message and reinforcement across providers and all team members who interact with the patient.
- The American Heart Association (https://www.heart.org/) offers resources for patients and for providers. It provides detailed recommendations and can help the therapist tailor a program to each patient's individual needs.
- Education
    - Regarding lifestyle modifications:

        Diet—work with PCP or dietician recommendations to reduce salt intake and change diet (guide patients with specific instructions, recipes, etc.) Specific instructions are critical to ensure maximal carry over and sustainable lifestyle change.
        Alcohol—educate patients regarding the effect alcohol has on blood pressure (it increases blood pressure), and instruct them how to reduce alcohol consumption.
        Smoking—encourage patients to quit smoking. Work with PCP to determine if the patient will benefit from a cessation program/medication and help patients adhere to the prescribed regimen.

    - Regarding impact of work environments and modifications.

        Avoid: prolonged cold, stress, hot and humid work environments, heavy physical load.

- Manage stress with actionable techniques:
    - Meditation/prayer
    - Jacobson relaxation techniques
    - Visualization
    - Anger coping strategies
    - Guided imagery (include visually and auditorily calm environment)
    - Mindfulness
- Exercise/physical activity

- If blood pressure is greater than 180/100, exercise must be monitored by health professionals and maybe lowered with medication first.
- Avoid activities with short intense periods, e.g., weightlifting, sprints, bursts.
- Identify activities that the patient enjoys and will realistically do.
- Increase participation in active IADLs and routines, e.g., mowing, vacuuming.
- Exercise such as walking, bicycling, swimming, dancing, or any other activity the patient enjoys.
- Avoid some activities without medical approval (e.g., scuba, skydiving, flying a plane).
- Typical recommendation for adults is 30 min per day, 5 days per week of moderate-intensity exercise.

- Medication self-management

  - Identify barriers to medication adherence—these are some example barriers:

    Don't like side effects
    Pills are too hard to swallow
    Forget to take medication
    Don't want to take medication at work—it's embarrassing

  - Once you identify the barriers, work with patients to develop strategies that will improve medication adherence such as:

    Using a smartphone app to track medication and provide reminder notifications.
    Log any side effects.
    Work with PCP to change a medication that is too expensive or not well tolerated by the patient.
    Develop strategies to address difficulties, if possible (e.g., if the pill is too big, can it be crushed and taken with applesauce?)
    Provide a strategy (app, log book, schedule on the refrigerator, etc.) to track when medication is due, and when the patient took the medication.

- Lifestyle Modification

  - Lifestyle Redesign Program®.
  - This is a program that you can purchase to strategically address multiple aspects of lifestyle modification.
  - Address habits, roles, and routines that can impact HTN and underlying risk factors.

- Sleep

  - Sleep hygiene
  - Sleeping with CPAP machine

- Education and self-management strategies addressing all of the above issues.

Other Considerations and Resources

Documentation and Billing

- Focus on impact on ADLs and IADLs and skilled level of service.
    - Use wording from the Occupational Therapy Practice Framework related to:

        Occupations: Rest and sleep, Work, Leisure, ADLs, IADLs, Play, e.g., sleeping less than 6 h per night on average.
        Client factors: Values, Beliefs, Body functions, Body structures, e.g., beliefs that HTN is inherited and nothing can be done to change it.
        Performance Patterns: Habits, Roles, Routines, Rituals, e.g., habits of drinking alcohol prior to bedtime, not exercising.
        Environment: Physical, Cultural, Personal, Temporal, e.g., Work environment is cold, stressful, and there are temporal stressors related to time management.

    - Note their association with risk factors and the impact on health management behaviors.
- You can find more information on billing resources at most health insurance company websites. CMS has a section on therapy services that can be found on CMS.gov and then type therapy services in the search box. This is updated regularly and provides information related to billing Medicare/Medicaid.
- Lifestyle redesign and lifestyle change programs provided by University of Southern California (USC) Chan OT faculty practice have been successfully billed to insurance. USC Chan website and faculty have provided discussions related to billing that are available when searched online.

Suggested Referrals or DME

- Mental health referral for stress management
- Nutrition/dietician
- Physical therapy (PT) for guided exercise
- Optometrist or Ophthalmologist

Additional Resources

- Sleeping with a CPAP machine

- – https://www.resmed.com/au/en/consumer/diagnosis-and-treatment/sleep-apnea/sleep-apnea-treatment/falling-asleep-on-cpap.html
- – https://www.tuck.com/choose-cpap-mask-by-sleeping-postion/

• American Heart Association (https://www.heart.org) offers resources for patients and for providers. It provides detailed recommendations and can help the therapist tailor a program to each patient's individual needs.

- – Lifestyle Change Chart
- – Blood Pressure Tracking Chart
- – How to Measure My Blood Pressure Chart
- – Additional handouts for blood pressure management
- – Why Should I be Physically Active Handout
- – Making Physical Activity a Way of Life Handout
- – Physical Activity Log
- – The American Heart Association (https://www.heart.org/)

• Stress management strategies.

- – https://www.helpguide.org/articles/stress/stress-management.htm?pdf=15118

• Managing stress and anxiety handout

- – https://medicine.umich.edu/sites/default/files/content/downloads/Relaxation-Skills-for-Anxiety.pdf

References

1. Centers for disease control website. https://www.cdc.gov/bloodpressure/facts.htm.
2. American College of Cardiology. New ACC/AHA high blood pressure guidelines lower definition of high blood pressure. 2017. https://www.acc.org/latest-in-cardiology/articles/2017/11/08/11/47/mon-5pm-bp-guideline-aha-2017.
3. American Heart Association. https://www.heart.org.
4. Rakotz M, Bakris G, Woolsey S. Treating hypertension in primary care: a comprehensive process. Healio primary care. 2017. https://www.healio.com/family-medicine/cardiology/news/online/%7B86109a85-5f52-44fe-860a-06f93d06656b%7D/treating-hypertension-in-primary-care-a-comprehensive-process.
5. Mayo Clinic. High blood pressure dangers: hypertension's effects on your body. 2019. https://www.mayoclinic.org/diseases-conditions/high-blood-pressure/in-depth/high-blood-pressure/art-20045868.
6. CDC. Effects of high blood pressure. 2014. https://www.cdc.gov/bloodpressure/effects.htm.
7. Sheps S, Mayo clinic. Anxiety: a cause of high blood pressure? 2019. https://www.mayoclinic.org/diseases-conditions/high-blood-pressure/expert-answers/anxiety/faq-20058549.
8. Licht CMM, de Geus EJC, Seldenrijk A, van Hout HPJ, Zitman FG, van Dyck R, Penninx BWJH. Depression is associated with decreased blood pressure, but antidepressant use increases the risk for hypertension. Hypertension. 2009;53:631–8. https://doi.org/10.1161/HYPERTENSIONAHA.108.126698.

 9. Hildrum B, Romild U, Holmen J. Anxiety and depression lowers blood pressure: 22-year follow-up of the population based HUNT study, Norway. BMC Public Health. 2011;11:601. https://doi.org/10.1186/1471-2458-11-601.
10. Penso J. How addressing hypertension creates a healthier more productive workplace. Benefits Magazine. 2015. http://www.ifebp.org/inforequest/ifebp/0166852.pdf.
11. Iadecola C, Yaffe K, Biller J, Bratzke LC, Faraci FM, Gorelick PB, Gulati M, Kamel H, Knopman DS, Launer LJ, Saczynski JS, Seshadri S, Al Hazzouri AZ, American Heart Association Council on Hypertension, Council on Clinical Cardiology, Council on Cardiovascular Disease in the Young, Council on Cardiovascular and Stroke Nursing, Council on Quality of Care and Outcomes Research and Stroke Council. Impact of hypertension on cognitive function: a scientific statement from the American Heart Association. Hypertension. 2016;68(6):e67–94. https://doi.org/10.1161/HYP.0000000000000053.
12. Jimenez-Balado J, Riba-Llena I, Abril O, et al. Cognitive impact of cerebral small vessel disease changes in patients with hypertension. Hypertension. 2019;73:342. https://doi.org/10.1161/HYPERTENSIONAHA.118.12090.

Chapter 27
Insomnia

John V. Rider and Katie Smith

Introduction

Insomnia is characterized by trouble falling asleep or staying asleep. A key distinction between insomnia and sleep deprivation is that sleep deprivation may be due to limited opportunity for sleep. In contrast, insomnia includes an opportunity for a full night of sleep, despite sleep disturbances. Insomnia is typically persistent, and most cases are initially seen in PC [1]. Historically, insomnia has been viewed and treated as a symptom rather than a disease due to its frequent association with underlying comorbidities and many other contributory factors (e.g., shift work, age, infection, seasonal variations, etc.). There has been much debate about insomnia and its classification. While there is no single test for insomnia, physicians utilize published criteria, along with patient reports, to make a diagnosis. Currently, the Diagnostic and Statistical Manual of Mental Disorders, Fifth Edition (DSM-5), and the International Classification of Sleep Disorders, Third Edition (ICSD-3) provide diagnostic criteria for insomnia.

- The DSM-5 classifies insomnia as a Sleep-Wake Disorder with a predominant complaint of dissatisfaction with sleep quantity or quality, associated with one (or more) of the following symptoms:

  - Difficulty initiating sleep.
  - Difficulty maintaining sleep, characterized by frequent awakenings or problems returning to sleep after awakenings.

J. V. Rider (✉)
School of Occupational Therapy, Touro University Nevada, Henderson, NV, USA
e-mail: jrider@touro.edu

K. Smith
Revolutionary Alignment, LLC, Detroit, MI, USA
www.RevolutionaryAlignment.com

© Springer Nature Switzerland AG 2023
S. Dahl-Popolizio et al. (eds.), *Primary Care Occupational Therapy*,
https://doi.org/10.1007/978-3-031-20882-9_27

- Early morning awakening with inability to return to sleep.
- The sleep difficulty must be present for at least 3 months and occur at least three nights a week despite adequate sleep opportunities.

• Additional criteria include the following:

- The sleep disturbance causes clinically significant distress or impairment in social, occupational, educational, academic, behavioral, or other important areas of functioning.
- Insomnia is not better explained by and does not occur exclusively during the course of another sleep-wake disorder (e.g., narcolepsy, a breathing-related sleep disorder, a circadian rhythm sleep-wake disorder, a parasomnia).
- Coexisting mental disorders and medical conditions do not adequately explain the predominant complaint of insomnia.
- Insomnia is not attributable to the physiological effects of a substance (e.g., a drug of abuse, a medication).

• The ICSD-3 consolidates all insomnia diagnoses under a single, chronic insomnia disorder. The criteria include:

- A report of sleep initiation or maintenance problems.
- Adequate opportunity and circumstances to sleep.
- Daytime consequences.
- Additionally, these symptoms must be present at least three times per week for 3 months [2].

In summary, the following criteria are used to diagnose insomnia:

• *Unhappiness with the quality or quantity of sleep*, which can include trouble falling asleep, staying asleep, or waking up early and being unable to get back to sleep.
• The sleep disturbance causes *significant distress or impairment in functioning*, such as within the individual's working or personal life, behaviorally or emotionally.
• Difficulty sleeping *occurs at least three times a week* and is present for at least *3 months.*
• The problem *occurs despite ample opportunity to sleep.*
• The difficulty *cannot be better explained by other physical, mental, or sleep-wake disorders.*
• The problem *cannot be attributed to substance use or medication.*

Another important distinction is whether the primary concern is falling asleep or staying asleep. When it takes an average of 30 minutes or more before falling asleep, it is commonly referred to as sleep-onset insomnia. When wake time after falling asleep averages 30 minutes or more, it is commonly called sleep-maintenance insomnia. As interventions vary based on the aspect of sleep affected, it is important to clarify the type of insomnia the client is experiencing to identify the most appropriate interventions.

Role of PCP

PCPs are on the forefront of insomnia care, as most cases of insomnia are first addressed in the PC setting [1]. The PCP will typically ask patients about their sleep quality and further investigate the need for prescription medications (e.g., Eszopiclone (Lunesta), Zolpidem (Ambien), Temazepam (Restoril), etc.), supplements, or referrals (e.g., sleep medicine specialist, OTP, psychologist, etc.). Often, patients don't discuss their sleep problems with their PCP until they become severe, and at that point, they are desperate for treatment. PCPs play an important role in identifying sleep disorders early to help prevent significant problems associated with insomnia. PCPs often use a variety of techniques to support a diagnosis of insomnia disorder, such as patient interviews, self-report assessments such as a sleep diary (see *Weekly Sleep Log* in Appendix), and standardized assessments such as the Epworth Sleepiness Scale. The PCP will review current medications to identify if any prescription or nonprescription drugs may be contributing to increased wakefulness or poor sleep quality. A physical examination and blood work may also be performed to rule out other common disorders. The PCP may also investigate conditions such as Restless Legs Syndrome, Periodic Limb Movement Disorder, and Obstructive Sleep Apnea, by referring patients to a sleep specialist. Additionally, due to the strong association of insomnia with mental health disorders, the PCP may ask questions about mood and anxiety disorders, to determine if additional evaluation and treatment is warranted.

Common Comorbidities

Psychiatric disorders represent the most common comorbidities in insomnia. Multiple medical and neurological disorders have also been associated with insomnia. Comorbidities is the most appropriate term because the direction of causality is not always clear when insomnia is present. Below are common comorbidities that OTPs should consider when evaluating and treating an individual with insomnia [3, 4].

• Psychiatric disorders

  – Mood disorders
  – Anxiety disorders (Chap. 11)
  – Substance use disorders (Chap. 8)
  – Posttraumatic stress disorder

• Medical disorders

  – Congestive heart failure, which may cause paroxysmal nocturnal dyspnea or orthopnea
  – Chronic obstructive pulmonary disease, which may cause dyspnea (Chap. 13)

- Gastroesophageal reflux disease, which may cause epigastric pain, burning, and sudden nocturnal awakenings (Chap. 23)
- Prostatic hypertrophy, which may cause frequent nocturia
- Diabetes (Chap. 19)
- Chronic pain (Chap. 34)
- Peripheral neuropathy
- Migraines or headaches
- Endocrine disorders
- Pregnancy

• Neurological Disorders

- Major neurocognitive disorders
- Parkinson's disease and parkinsonian syndromes (Chap. 31)
- Huntington's chorea (Chap. 25)
- Dystonia
- Tourette's syndrome
- Epilepsy

• Additional Sleep disorders

- Obstructive sleep apnea syndrome
- Restless legs syndrome
- Periodic limb movement disorder
- Circadian rhythm sleep disorders

Caffeine consumption, increased stress, daily routines, and poor sleep hygiene habits have also been associated with insomnia. Insomnia is reported more often in women and tends to increase with age.

Role of OTP

The OTP will evaluate the functional impact of the sleep disorder, and provide interventions to maximize function and quality of life. It is important to understand that persistent or chronic insomnia disorders are typically associated with maladaptive cognitions and behaviors that become contributing and perpetuating factors [2] to the continuation of insomnia. These factors must be skillfully addressed by OTPs to achieve successful long-term outcomes.

Occupational Impact

Insomnia is the most common sleep complaint across all stages of adulthood and for many, the problem is chronic [4]. The CDC (2005) highlighted insufficient sleep as a public health problem, citing the link of insufficient sleep to numerous health concerns (e.g., increased health care utilization, chronic diseases such as hypertension, diabetes, depression, obesity, cancer, early mortality), safety concerns (e.g., motor vehicle crashes, industrial accidents), decreased work productivity, and overall reduced quality of life [5]. Insomnia, and associated poor sleep, has the potential to impact every area of occupation. Restorative sleep is necessary to support healthy and active engagement in activities of daily living (ADLs) and instrumental activities of daily living (IADLs). OTPs in PC should consider the negative impact insomnia has on performance skills (e.g., motor and process skills) and how this affects ADLs, IADLs, health management, education, work, play, leisure, and social participation. For example, interpersonal interactions can become more challenging or tense due to lack of tone regulation and/or emotional regulation. Work can be challenged by decreased cognitive flexibility and memory. Planning and sequencing can become disrupted for ADLs, especially if the need to problem-solve a change in routine takes place. Motor control may be impaired increasing the risk for falls and injuries.

OT Areas of Emphasis

The importance of adequate and restful sleep has always been recognized by OTPs. Sleep is categorized as a distinct occupation in the Occupational Therapy Practice Framework [6]. Sleep is a necessary part of life and provides a foundation for optimal occupational performance. The PC setting is often the first place a client seeks care, providing a unique opportunity for OTPs to be on the front line of sleep evaluation and intervention. The OTP will perform a comprehensive evaluation to examine rest and sleep. This includes activities related to obtaining restorative rest and sleep that support healthy and active engagement in other occupations [6]. A comprehensive evaluation should include an occupational profile, and an evaluation of environmental, physical, and behavioral factors that impact sleep, and daily routines (especially current sleep preparation and hygiene routines). The OTP will identify occupational performance barriers imposed by ineffective sleep. Using this information, the OTP will develop a client-centered intervention plan that will address sleep problems framed from the perspective of health maintenance and health promotion through self-management. The OTP will provide evidence-based education and training to

- Increase the client's knowledge of rest and sleep and awareness of how their current routines and thoughts about sleep impact sleep participation.
- Assist the client in developing behaviors and beliefs to improve sleep preparation and participation.

Evaluation

- Suggested areas to assess
  - Physical environment.
  - Temporal environment.

– Current sleep patterns.

How many nights and how long the client is experiencing sleep-onset insomnia, sleep-maintenance insomnia, awakenings, etc.

– Cognitive and behavioral factors.

It is important to assess the client's understanding of how their thoughts and behaviors contribute to their sleep participation.

– Lifestyle and environmental factors.
– Sleep medication use (e.g., type, dose, and frequency).
– Additional medical and mental health problems that may be contributing to insomnia.

• Suggested assessment tools

– A sleep diary can help identify any potential causal elements and habits, as well as variability in sleeping patterns. See *Weekly Sleep Log* in the Appendix.
– The Epworth Sleepiness Scale determines how drowsy a person feels in situations like waiting at traffic signals, watching television, or reading.

Intervention Strategies

Suggested intervention strategies:

1. Education on sleep misconceptions and expectations (e.g., the appropriate amount of sleep needed per night, what to do when you can't sleep, the negative impact of mood and thoughts on sleep and daytime performance, "core" sleep, perceived vs. actual sleep duration, etc.). For example, the following information can be used to initiate a discussion with the client to improve their health literacy surrounding sleep and manage expectations. The OTP can then continue the discussion into ways to modify activities related to obtaining restorative rest and sleep to support healthy, active occupational engagement, with specific education on sleep preparation and participation strategies.

    (a) Adults sleep an average of 7 hours per night with a typical range of six to 8 hours. Seventy-five percent of adults sleep less than 8 hours per night.
    (b) People who sleep 7 hours per night have been shown to live longer on average than people who sleep 8 hours per night.
    (c) Most people who experience insomnia underestimate the duration of their wakefulness.
    (d) Five and a half hours has been shown to be sufficient for core sleep. Impact on daytime performance typically happens when individuals get less than five and a half hours of sleep.

(e) Negative mood and negative sleep thoughts related to insomnia can impact daytime performance [7].

2. Daily routine modification (e.g., initiating a formal sleep preparation routine, establishing predictable routines, etc).

3. Environmental and physical factors (e.g., preparing the physical environment for periods of sleep, modifying noise, light, or temperature in the bedroom, etc.) (see *Sleep Hygiene* handout in Appendix).

4. Management of pain, fatigue, anxiety, or depression.

5. Food/drink intake with relation to sleep (e.g., limiting caffeine, heavy meals, etc., before bedtime).

6. Activity modifications (e.g., modifications to personal care, mobility, or toileting in relation to sleep preparation).

7. Encouragement of health and wellness behaviors (e.g., smoking cessation, adequate exercise, sunlight exposure during the day, etc.).

8. Sleep positioning/ergonomics.

9. Sensory disorder management.

10. Caregiver training.

11. Behavioral interventions.

(a) Cognitive behavioral therapy for insomnia (CBT-I) is currently the "gold standard" for treatment of insomnia and recommended as the standard, first-line treatment for insomnia [8]. CBT-I strategies can be provided in the PC setting and, if warranted, a referral to a CBT-I trained provider can be recommended. OTPs are qualified to deliver CBT-I interventions and can seek additional training if there is a need and interest.

- CBT-I covers topics such as stimulus control (e.g., using the bed for sleep and for sex and avoiding other activities in bed to associate the bed only with sleeping), sleep restriction (e.g., setting strict limits on the time spent in bed each night), relaxation training and biofeedback (e.g., progressive muscle relaxation, diaphragmatic breathing, visual imagery, and biofeedback monitoring), and sleep hygiene training (e.g., creating a cool, dark sleep environment and a bedtime routine). Additional topics covered may include food and substance use, the biological clock/circadian rhythms, sleep-interfering arousal/activation, the use of sleep diaries, and restructuring thoughts and behaviors.

  Cognitive restructuring enables patients to recognize, challenge, and replace negative sleep thoughts (NSTs) (e.g., "I won't be able to function tomorrow if i don't get to sleep now") with positive sleep thoughts (PSTs) (e.g., "Sleep loss does not always have a significant impact on my daytime functioning") which improve sleep by reducing emotional arousal, and negative cognitive appraisal of sleep. Multiple examples of CBT-I, including worksheets, handouts, and resources can be found online.

12. Medication management and tapering (e.g., certain medications have been shown to cause daytime sleepiness and the OT can assist patients with taking medications at the appropriate time to avoid side effects that may interfere with sleep and support the PCP in modifying routines and preparing for withdrawals during medication tapering).
13. Sleep scheduling.

- Sleep diaries to determine baseline patterns, and track progress.
- Reduce daytime naps after 2 pm.
- Set a consistent wake time within 30 min.
- 20/20 rule

  Avoid lying in bed if you have been awake for 20 minutes or longer, whether after lights out, waking up in the middle of the night, or in the morning before rising.
  Get out of bed, leave the bedroom, and do a different, calming activity for at least 20 minutes before returning to bed.

- Reduce time allotted for sleep to increase sleep efficiency. (For example, if you are only getting 6 hours of sleep throughout a 9 hours sleep window, reduce the sleep window to increase the hours of sleep within the allotted sleep window).

14. Relaxation techniques (e.g., deep breathing, progressive muscle relaxation, visualization, etc.)

Other Considerations and Resources

If the sleep problems require further evaluation outside the scope of OT, recommendations may be necessary for evaluation by a Board-Certified Sleep Medicine Physician or a Behavioral Sleep Medicine Specialist. Specialized sleep centers can perform additional tests (e.g., in-lab sleep study, multiple sleep latency test, maintenance of wakefulness test) and physicians can order home apnea tests to provide a more comprehensive understanding of the sleep disorder. Additionally, behavioral health providers, such as psychologists, psychiatrists, counselors, and OTPs, can specialize in CBT-I and may be more appropriate when long-term intervention is needed.

References

1. Billiard M, Bentley A. Is insomnia best categorized as a symptom or a disease? Sleep Med. 2004;5(Suppl 1):S35–40. https://doi.org/10.1016/s1389-9457(04)90006-8. PMID: 15301996
2. Sateia M. International classification of sleep disorders-third edition: highlights and modifications. Chest. 2014;146(5):1387–94. https://doi.org/10.1378/chest.14-0970.
3. Khurshid KA. Comorbid insomnia and psychiatric disorders: an update. Innov Clin Neurosci. 2018;15(3–4):28–32.
4. National Institutes of Health. National Institutes of health state of the science conference statement on manifestations and management of chronic insomnia in adults, June 13–15, 2005. Sleep. 2005;28(9):1049–57. https://doi.org/10.1093/sleep/28.9.1049.
5. Centers for Disease Control and Prevention. Insufficient sleep is a public health problem. 2015. https://www.cdc.gov/features/dssleep/.
6. American Occupational Therapy Association. Occupational therapy practice framework: domain and process (4th ed.). Am J Occup Ther. 2020;74(Suppl. 2):07412410010. https://doi.org/10.5014/ajot.2020.74S2001.
7. Jacobs G. CBT training manual for insomnia-solo clinicians. 2021. https://www.cbtforinsomnia.com.
8. Hauk L. Treatment of chronic insomnia in adults: ACP guideline. Am Fam Physician. 2017;95(10):669–70.

Chapter 28
Multiple Sclerosis

Lara Taggart and Gillian Porter

Introduction [1]

The *multiple* in multiple sclerosis refers to both time and location of MS lesions and relapses. The *sclerosis* refers to the hardened or sclerotic plaques that are the scar tissue resulting from autoimmune attacks on the Central Nervous System (CNS) (axons and myelin covering). Axonal transection is considered as significant as the demyelination process found in MS. At least temporarily, demyelinated axons may remyelinate and provide conduction of nerve impulses. Transected axons are permanently destroyed and lose all potential for conduction. There is also evidence that disease activity continues even during periods that are clinically quiet or when no change in symptoms is apparent. Inflammation occurs with demyelination and axonal damage, which may explain the rapid improvement often seen in treatment of relapses with corticosteroid anti-inflammatory agents.

The precise cause of MS remains unknown. The present theory is that an environmental trigger or an infectious agent initiates the autoimmune response in people with genetic susceptibility. MS is the most commonly diagnosed neurological disease that can cause disability in young adults. An estimated 400,000 people in the United States have MS, and worldwide that number is 2.5 million. MS causes severe disability in some people, but many continue to lead active, productive lives and are not severely disabled

There are four types of MS: Relapsing-Remitting, Secondary Progressive, Primary Progressive, and Progressive Relapsing.

L. Taggart (✉)
Northern Arizona University, Flagstaff, AZ, USA
e-mail: Lara.Taggart@nau.edu

G. Porter
Northern Arizona University, Flagstaff, AZ, USA

Carefree Physical Therapy, Carefree, AZ, USA
e-mail: gp288@nau.edu

© Springer Nature Switzerland AG 2023   283
S. Dahl-Popolizio et al. (eds.), *Primary Care Occupational Therapy*,
https://doi.org/10.1007/978-3-031-20882-9_28

- *Relapsing-Remitting*
    - The relapsing-remitting course, the most common at the time of diagnosis, produces clearly defined relapses of acute worsening of neurological function followed by partial or complete improvement and then stable periods of remission between attacks

- *Secondary Progressive*
    - People with secondary progressive MS start with a relapsing-remitting course of up to 10–15 years
    - The secondary progressive course is typically diagnosed when there is continued neurological deterioration

- *Primary Progressive*
    - People with primary progressive MS have continuously declining neurological function from onset.

- *Progressive Relapsing*
    - The progressive-relapsing course is much less common and characterized by continued disease progression with superimposed relapses
    - Clinically isolated syndrome or the first neurological episode that may result in an MS diagnosis is important to identify so that treatments to minimize disease progression can be provided

Risk Factors [1, 2] Include
- 15–50 years old, although children are increasingly being diagnosed
- Peak age of onset is at 20–30 years
- Women are two to three times as likely to have MS
- Caucasians of northern European descent have the greatest risk of developing MS, whereas groups like the Norwegian Lapps, Inuit, and New Zealand Maoris who live in similar latitudes have no incidence of MS
- Living geographically further from the equator
- Vitamin D deficiency
- Smoking

Signs and Symptoms

- *Fatigue* is the most common symptom, with various types of fatigue:
    - Primary MS fatigue—caused by MS disease process
    - Secondary MS fatigue—fatigue from untreated MS issues
    - Physical fatigue—fatigue experienced in the limbs, trunk, head, and neck
    - Cognitive fatigue—mental fatigue
    - Local or focal fatigue—motor fatigue caused by ineffective nerve conduction to a selected area of the body.

– Generalized fatigue—complete exhaustion that is physical and cognitive.
– Normal fatigue—fatigue experienced by excessive energy output.

- *Weakness*
  – Weakness may occur in all parts of the body, resulting in referral to therapy.
  – Weakness that increases after repeated muscle contractions or fatigue of the same muscle(s) is known as "nerve fiber fatigue".
  – The cause is unknown but likely related to the conduction impairment in demyelinated nerves.

    An example is increased dorsiflexion weakness resulting in foot-drop after walking which may increase stumbling, especially on uneven surfaces. Coupled with decreased balanced and gait impairment, the risk of falls is increased by 58. After resting, conduction and muscle contraction are improved.

- *Cognition*
  – Up to 65% of people with MS have cognitive problems that vary considerably in severity that appear related to

    Loss of brain volume (particularly grey matter)

  – It is estimated that 5–10% of those with MS have cognitive problems that interfere with participation in everyday occupations.
  – Cognitive problems are seen at all stages of the disease and are significant in leading to unemployment in MS.
  – Common problems include

    Memory (acquiring and retaining new information)
    Word functioning
    Attention
    Concentration
    Executive functioning
    Slowed information-processing speed
    Visual–spatial

  – Cognitive issues in MS do not correlate with physical disability, but are influenced by depression, stress, anxiety, and fatigue and vary during the day, increasing in the afternoon or when sustained mental concentration is required.
  – Both individuals and their families may be unaware that cognitive problems such as reduced insight and inflexible thinking are related to the disease and should not be mistaken for personality or psychological issues.

- *Visual–Spatial Problems*
  – Perceptual-cognitive problems may also occur such as visual–spatial impairments that might result in a tendency to get lost or a history of motor vehicle accident.

- *Pain*

    - Pain is estimated to occur in 40–60% of people with MS, with 48% reporting chronic pain.
    - Pain negatively impacts quality of life and independence and is not related to age, length of time with MS, or degree of disability, although twice as many women report having pain than men.
    - Pain in MS can be localized as in trigeminal neuralgia, Lhermitte's sign (a stabbing, electric shock along the spine when neck forward flexes), or pain as a result of spasticity.
    - Pain directly caused by the neurological lesions is considered primary to MS and is treated with medications.
    - Pain secondary to MS is often due to posture, gait, and positioning problems and can be relieved by therapy and proper mobility equipment.

- *Spasticity*

    - Spasticity in MS is usually greater in the lower extremities and may be source of pain, interrupted sleep, and activity limitations.
    - Up to 30% of patients eliminate or modify activities because of spasticity.

- *Tremors and Ataxia*

    - Tremors

        Intention tremor is the most common tremor seen in MS and is one of the most difficult problems to manage.

        - Intention tremor occurs in the upper extremities, but may also manifest in the lower extremities, torso, and neck.

        As an activity progresses and the extremity approaches the target (a point when the greatest precision is required), the tremor is at its worse.
        A comprehensive OT assessment was developed, the Multidimensional Assessment of Tremor (MAT), which measures both the severity and functional impact of intention tremor.

    - Ataxia

        Ataxia presents in the trunk and lower extremities where postural responses tend to occur before upper extremity movements.
        The functional challenges of ataxia are further magnified because of the multiple joints involved in the ataxic movement.

- *Dysphagia*

    - Difficulty with swallowing.

- *Sensory Impairment*

    - Thermosensitivity.
    - Loss of sensation/paresthesias.

- *Respiratory Weakness*
  - Dyspnea
  - Risk for aspiration
- *Integumentary Issues*
  - Increased risk for decubitus ulcers
  - Hygiene issues due to sensory/motor impairments
- *Balance and Vestibular Impairments*
  - Abnormal gait impairment secondary to postural and lower extremity weakness
  - Vestibular hypofunction
  - Vertigo, nystagmus, diplopia, nausea

Role of PCP

PCP's should be aware of the warning signs/symptoms that indicate MS and refer patients to a neurologist [3]. As patients will still be seen at the PC practice throughout the course of their lives, the PCP will be involved in some of these tasks.

1. Diagnostic testing [4]

   - There is no single test that can specifically diagnose MS
   - Common diagnostic testing includes:

     - MRI
     - Spinal tap
     - Evoke potential test (EMG)
     - Blood tests

2. MD's should be aware of:

   - The symptoms of MS
   - Stages of MS
   - The importance of wellness prevention
   - Disease modifying therapies

     - The most significant clinical medical advances that have consumed enormous research efforts and impacted clinical practice are the advent of disease modifying therapies (DMTs)
     - There are five self-injectable immune-modulating medications approved for use in the United States

       interferon beta-1a (Avonex)
       interferon beta-1b (Betaseron)
       interferon beta-1b (Extavia)

glatiramer acetate (Copaxone)
interferon beta-1a (Rebif)

- These drugs have been shown to reduce the number of lesions evidenced on MRI and the frequency and severity of relapses, although a recent study suggests that the beta interferons do not impact long-term disability.
- Natalizumab (Tysabri), a monthly injectable, is administered by qualified practitioners and is approved for relapsing-remitting MS.
- Mitoxantrone (Novantrone), an immunosuppressant rather than an immunomodulator, is rarely used because of significant side effects.
- Fingolimod (Gilenya) is the only DMT that is taken orally and is generally used when the response to injectable DMTs has diminished.
- Another class of medications, neurofunctional modifiers, targets underlying pathophysiology and MS symptoms.

  Of these drugs, dalfampridine has been shown to improve walking ability in people with any type of MS.

- Clients may want to discuss their medications with therapists, asking their opinion about the efficacy of medications.

  This is true particularly for DMTs because they are designed not to reverse disability, but to slow disease progression.
  The therapist's responsibility is to understand and explain the importance of taking medications because the benefits may further contribute to maintaining employment and participating in high-priority occupations for a longer period.

- Medication side effects [5]

  - Abnormal lab results (liver function)
  - Diarrhea
  - Hair loss
  - Pain
  - Headache
  - Nausea

3. MD's should consider ordering referrals

- Neurologist specializing in MS
- OT, PT, SLP
- Social services

Common Comorbidities

- Depression (Chap. 18)
- Anxiety (Chap. 11)

- Vascular and cerebrovascular disease
- Aautoimmune diseases
- Chronic lung disease
- Gastrointestinal disease
- Renal disease
- Visual disorders
- Hypertension
- Hyperlipidemia
- Diabetes

Role of OTP

Identify issues impeding function, and affecting quality of life across all aspects of the patient's ADLs, IADLs, family and work roles, and community function.

Occupational Impact

Signs and symptoms fluctuate and can vary widely throughout the lifespan. Aspects of motor and cognitive function can be affected to varying degrees, which will impact the patient's ability to work, complete ADLs and IADLs, and can affect their family roles and relationships. The OTP will evaluate and provide interventions for the patient's presenting issues and the level of deficit.

OT Role and Focus [6]

Evaluate and treat musculoskeletal, cognitive, visual, sensory, and psychosocial systems and the impact of MS on occupational performance in the home, work, and community.

- Assist with daily activities.
  - Increase independence and perform daily tasks with more efficiency with energy conservation and work simplification techniques.
  - Bladder management.
  - Home evaluation to assess and recommend modifications to reduce fall risk.
  - Orthotic management.
  - Educate on sleep and hygiene.
- Educate on energy conservation (see Handout in Appendix X).
  - Temperature regulation.

- Use of adaptive devices (to improve task performance) and assistive devices (to improve mobility) in the work, home, and school.
- Improve strength and coordination.
- Cognitive rehabilitation.

  – Evaluate memory, concentration, problem-solving, organization, and planning.
  – Develop compensatory techniques for degenerative changes.

- Address psychosocial challenges.

  – Stress management.
  – Relaxation techniques.

Evaluation

- Musculoskeletal Exam

  – Postural Control

      Trunk Control Test
      Trunk Impairment Scale
      Functional Reach Test

  – ROM/PROM assessment

      Assess contractures

  – Manual Muscle Testing
  – Grip/Pinch Strength

- Fine Motor Coordination

  – 9-Hole Peg Test
  – Box and Blocks
  – Timed functional task with self-report of perceived exertion (e.g., buttoning, writing, donning LE clothing)
  – Borg Rating Scale of Perceived Exertion

- Neurological Exam

  – Spasticity

      Modified Ashworth Scale
      Multiple Sclerosis Spasticity Scale (MSSS-88)

  – Ataxia

      Scale for the Assessment and Rating of Ataxia (SARA)

  – Deep Tendon Reflexes

- – Clonus
- – Babinski

- Sensory/Dermatome Exam

  - – Light touch

    Semmes-Weinstein Monofilaments

  - – Proprioception/Kinesthesia
  - – Temperature
  - – Pain—Sharp/Dull Discrimination

- Quality of Life

  - – Canadian Occupational Performance Measure (COPM)
  - – MS Quality of Life (MSQOL-54)
  - – MS International Quality of Life Questionnaire (MusiQoL)
  - – Multiple Sclerosis Impact Scale (MSIS-29)
  - – Functional Assessment of Multiple Sclerosis

- Fatigue/Endurance

  - – Modified Fatigue Impact Scale (MFIS)
  - – Multi-component Fatigue Scale
  - – Patient-specific Functional Scale
  - – Fatigue Descriptive Scale
  - – 6 Min Walk Test
  - – 5 Time Sit-to-Stand

- Pain

  - – Visual Analogue Scale

    Consider recording scores during particular positions/activities

- Cognition

  - – Montreal Cognitive Assessment (MOCA).
  - – Trail Making Tests A & B
  - – Executive Function Performance Test
  - – Multiple Errands Test

- Balance/Mobility

  - – Tinetti Performance Oriented Mobility Assessment (POMA)
  - – Tinetti Falls Efficacy Scale
  - – Timed Up and Go (TUG)

    Complete TUG under dual-task conditions:

    - Functional task
    - Cognitive task

- Motor task

  – Functional Gait Assessment
  – Four Square Step Test
  – Dynamic Gait Index
  – Clinical Test for Sensory Interaction on Balance (CTSIB)
  – Berg Balance Scale
  – Balance Evaluation Systems Test (BESTest).
  – Activities-specific Balance Confidence Scale

- Vestibular

  – Motion Sensitivity Test
  – Dizziness Handicap Inventory.

Intervention Strategies [1]

- *Fatigue* is the most common symptom of MS.

- Factors that contribute to fatigue include comorbid medical conditions, sleeping issues, depression, stress, anxiety, pain, deconditioning, side effects to medications, poor nutrition or caloric intake, mobility issues.

  – Interventions for fatigue

    The fatigue intervention begins with the OTP providing explanations of each relevant underlying type and factor of fatigue impacting the individual. The client then completes a detailed activity diary that can be done on well-selected apps and makes a list of goals and priorities.
    The therapist and client use the diary to systematically analyze daily work, home, and leisure activities and understand rest–activity ratios.
    Identifying activity and environmental modifications, equipment, and technology to address fatigue issues then follows.
    Education on energy conservation strategies.
    Research has demonstrated the effectiveness of a face-to-face OTP–led group intervention (in energy conservation).
    A teleconference format and an online version of this energy conservation program have also been shown to be effective.

- *Energy Conservation Techniques*
- Designed to save, conserve, or reduce consumption or expenditure of energy. An individual's conservation of energy and optimization of endurance during participation in occupations refers to efficiently using available energy while decreasing unnecessary expenditure; see this Energy Conservation Handout available online. Use high, low, and smart technology appropriately.

- Use smart devices and helpful apps to save steps, such as voice options to replace touch typing.
- Decrease prolonged standing and walking by modifying tasks to be done sitting.
- Maintain a cooler body temperature by using, for example, an air conditioner, cooling wraps fitted comfortably at wrist or on neck or a cooling vest when active.
- Reduce the energy required to walk by using an ankle–foot orthosis, cane, or walker.
- Obtain seating systems for trunk support in wheelchairs.
- For work, use a fitted ergonomic chair with armrests, correct height, and back support.

- Plan approaches to occupation and daily schedule.

  - Do important activities in the morning.
  - Break large time-consuming activities into smaller tasks and do one task at a time.

- Problem-solve using a step-by-step approach.
- Use techniques to maintain cooler body temperature, for example, layer clothing, have warm versus hot showers, and avoid electric blankets or down comforters when sleeping.
- Delegate necessary highly energy-consuming occupations.
- Manage environmental controls and modifications.

  - Adjust heights of work surfaces to avoid strain.
  - Avoid stairs in daily activities.

- Simplify or eliminate tasks.

  - Avoid multitasking.
  - Have tools required for the task readily available at arm's reach.

- Educate others about your energy limits.

  - Teach others about increased body temperature and effects on reduced function and energy.
  - Work with others to accomplish a task, sharing the energy expenditure.

- Punctuate activities with rest.

  - Alternate activity with intervals of rest, such as walking, sitting, and then walking.

- Numerous screening measures for fatigue in MS include the Fatigue Severity Scale, the Modified Fatigue Impact Scale, and the Rochester Fatigue Diary.
- The Comprehensive Fatigue Assessment Battery for MS (CFAB-MS) was developed to identify factors contributing to MS fatigue and to guide clinicians'

treatment decisions. Interventions are then directed at mitigating these factors as well as managing the primary MS fatigue.

Weakness
- Weakness may occur in all parts of the body, resulting in referral to therapy
- Weakness that increases after repeated muscle contractions or fatigue of the same muscle(s) is known as "nerve fiber fatigue".
- The cause is unknown, but likely related to the conduction impairment in demyelinated nerves.

  – An example is increased dorsiflexion weakness resulting in foot-drop after walking which may increase stumbling, especially on uneven surfaces.
  – Coupled with decreased balance and gait impairment, the risk of falls is increased by 58. After resting, conduction and muscle contraction are improved.

- Exercise routines will also be incorporated to help the individual perform valued occupations and activities through optimal energy management techniques.
- OTPs should collaborate with physical therapists who treat fatigue through obtaining gait equipment, recommending appropriate aerobic exercise routines, and educating on the difference between energy expenditure during functional activities and exercise to increase endurance.

  – Use caution with exercise intensity to avoid fatigue/weakness that interferes with functional performance.

- Written recommendations and summaries should be provided which outline the frequency, duration, and self-monitoring of fatigue levels with any of these interventions.

Cognition
- OT intervention for clients with cognitive problems focuses on compensation for deficits and inefficiencies in order to manage everyday life.
- Treating fatigue often improves self-reported cognitive performance.
- Caution should be exercised in disclosing cognitive issues to employers, with careful consideration given to each circumstance.
- Education of clients and families about cognition is often beneficial. Awareness that these problems are due to MS and not personality eases stress and optimizes receptivity to modifications.
- Interventions that include group therapy, stress management, personal digital assistants, electronic memory aids, and cognitive-behavioral therapy have been shown to have positive effects on cognitive function in MS.
- Examples of cognitive techniques, strategies, and modifications include

  – Scheduling work responsibilities and cognitively demanding tasks to reduce the influence of the cognitive problems; for example, planning to do these in the morning or after breaks.
  – Maintaining a paper, smart phone, or electronic diary as a memory aid and to help identify the timing of cognitive and fatigue problems as well as the environment in which these problems occur.

- Changing the environment to reduce distractions and interruptions and promote organization.
- Using problem-solving strategies for decision-making rather than emotion-focused strategies.
- Supporting involvement of social network to assist with problem solving.
- Using step-by-step written home and/or work directions.
- Doing one activity at a time and avoiding multitasking.
- Incorporating assistive technology to improve function in high-order IADL, such as money management and bill payment, family schedules, and transportation options.
- Increasing time allotted for an activity and reducing the number of activities planned or undertaken.
- Delegating difficult tasks to others.
- Using repetition in the learning process.
- Assessing driving safety and recommending appropriate testing and interventions.

Visual—spatial problems
- Perceptual-cognitive problems may also occur such as visual–spatial impairments that might result in a tendency to get lost or a history of motor vehicle accident.
- Intervention may include compensatory strategies (scanning techniques), assistive technologies (GPS), and occupational modifications. See Vision Chapter for additional information (Chap. 11).

Pain
- For pain related to weakness or spasticity, interventions such as posture training, ergonomic seating, stretching, supportive splinting, and focal heat modalities on muscle trigger points may be effective.
- An ergonomic workstation (such as ergonomic chair with armrests, headsets, and mouse and keyboard trays) tailored to the individual can be beneficial.
- Exercise and mobility equipment to correct gait problems may also assist to minimize pain.

Spasticity
- The appropriate intervention for spasticity depends on the severity and the extent to which it interferes with function and impacts quality of life.
- In addition to stretching exercises, adapted dressing techniques may prove helpful, such as using a stool to maintain hip flexion to decrease extensor spasm and/or using dressing sticks to compensate for inability to reach the feet.
- A standing home program may also be employed, using a standing frame for 30–60 min per day.
- Other interventions include resting splints and posture and positioning techniques, such as bringing the hips into 90° or more of flexion to decrease extensor tone in the lower extremities.

- Therapists should be familiar with the standard medications for spasticity, such as baclofen and tizanidine, and their side effect of drowsiness that may increase fatigue.

  - Botox® (onabotulinumtoxin), a neurotoxin, results in relaxation of the targeted muscle and can last up to 3 months.
  - Intrathecal baclofen pump has been shown to reduce pain and improve function and quality of life for people with MS with moderate to severe spasticity.
  - Should a baclofen pump be indicated, the therapist may be involved in assessment prior to pump implantation and reevaluation following implantation.

Tremors and Ataxia
- The hallmarks of OT intervention for tremor and ataxia are proximal stabilization or support, modified approach to occupations, and adapted equipment and orthoses.
- Proximal stabilization includes supporting the trunk and larger joints of the upper and lower extremities are.

  - For example, at mealtime, position the client's torso against the table with arms resting on the table.
  - Because the position is sitting, the lower extremities are supported, the trunk is stabilized by leaning against the table, and the shoulders and elbows are supported.

- A modified approach may be the use of hand-over-hand guidance for writing or dialing a cell phone.

  - If one hand is unaffected by tremor, consider retraining the unaffected hand as tolerated.
  - Orthoses might include a cervical collar to reduce the travel of the head and neck or wrist splints to minimize travel and number of joints in motion.

- Weights on the wrist, for example, may also serve to dampen tremor but may contribute to fatigue.
- Peripheral cooling of the forearm has been shown to reduce tremor amplitude and frequency and increase functional capacity for up to 30 min.
- An OT intervention program, the Step-wise Approach to the Treatment of Intention developed specifically for MS was pilot tested and has shown some promising results.

Dysphagia
- OTPs should routinely screen for choking, aspiration, and swallowing difficulties.

Other Considerations and Resources

For additional information and resources for patients and providers, visit the National Multiple Sclerosis Society website: https://www.nationalmssociety.org/

References

1. Radomski MV, Trombly Latham CA. Occupational therapy for physical dysfunction. 7th ed. Philadelphia, PA: Lippincott Williams & Wilkins; 2008.
2. Anderson L. New oral agents for multiple sclerosis: a healthcare professional's guide. 2020. https://www.drugs.com/slideshow/oral-agents-for-multiple-sclerosis-1216.
3. Coyle P, Bermel R, Cohen B. What the PCP needs to know about MS diagnosis, treatment, and adherence. Healio. 2019. https://www.healio.com/news/primary-care/20180522/what-the-pcp-needs-to-know-about-ms-diagnosis-treatment-and-adherence.
4. Melinosky C. Multiple sclerosis diagnosing. Webmd. 2020. https://www.webmd.com/multiple-sclerosis/multiple-sclerosis-diagnosing.
5. Melinosky C. Treatment for multiple sclerosis. Webmd. https://www.webmd.com/multiple-sclerosis/ms-treatment.
6. Cafasso M. Multiple sclerosis and occupational therapy. Healthline. 2019. https://www.healthline.com/health/multiple-sclerosis/occupational-therapy#understanding-occupational-therapy.

Chapter 29
Nerve Impingement

John V. Rider and Sue Dahl-Popolizio

Introduction [1, 2]

Nerve impingement/compression is a condition in which a peripheral nerve is trapped or pressed by a nearby structure. This pressure disrupts the nerve's function, commonly causing pain, tingling, numbness, or weakness. The impingement can be caused by broken bones, swollen tendons or muscles, bone spurs, ruptured discs, or edema and can occur anywhere in the body.

Peripheral nerve injury is commonly divided into three classifications: neuropraxia, axonotmesis, and neurotmesis [1]. Most nerve impingement syndromes are type 1 (neuropraxia) injuries, causing mild to moderate sensory symptoms, or type 2 (axonotmesis) injuries that also include motor impairment. In PC, you will likely not have this level of detail in your prescription, but you may be told it was a crush, stretch, or laceration injury. You may see early mild compression injuries or old injuries with residual symptoms. If the patient needs more intense therapy than you can provide in the PC setting, you can refer to a specialty outpatient therapy clinic. These patients often need intermittent follow-up after they have completed their outpatient OT or physical therapy (PT) treatment regimen.

The most common nerve impingement conditions an OTP is likely to encounter in PC include carpal tunnel syndrome, cubital tunnel syndrome, thoracic outlet syndrome, and radial nerve palsy. Radial tunnel syndrome and ulnar tunnel syndrome are less common, but may present to PC as well.

J. V. Rider (✉)
School of Occupational Therapy, Touro University Nevada, Henderson, NV, USA
e-mail: jrider@touro.edu

S. Dahl-Popolizio
Arizona State University, Flagstaff, AZ, USA

AT Still University, Mesa, AZ, USA
e-mail: Sue.Dahlpopolizio@asu.edu; sdahlpopolizio@atsu.edu

© Springer Nature Switzerland AG 2023
S. Dahl-Popolizio et al. (eds.), *Primary Care Occupational Therapy*,
https://doi.org/10.1007/978-3-031-20882-9_29

- *Carpal Tunnel Syndrome*: This condition occurs when the median nerve is compressed by the contents of the carpal tunnel. Nerve compression results in pain, paresthesias (e.g., abnormal sensations such as "pins and needles"), primarily on the lateral side of the hand (thumb, index, middle, and ring fingers), and can result in weakness of the affected hand, especially when gripping objects. In severe cases, atrophy of the thenar eminence occurs.
- *Cubital Tunnel Syndrome*: This occurs with compression or stretching of the ulnar nerve as it passes superficially between the medial epicondyle of the humerus and the olecranon of the ulna at the elbow (commonly called the funny bone). Activities that require prolonged elbow flexion are the most common cause of symptoms. External compression at the elbow such as pressure from resting the elbow on a hard surface, physical trauma, fractures, or dislocations can also cause cubital tunnel syndrome. Pain will be primarily on the medial side of the forearm with decreased sensation, numbness, tingling, or a feeling of coldness in the ring and little fingers. In severe cases, atrophy of the hypothenar muscles and intrinsic muscles of the hand may occur.
- *Thoracic Outlet Syndrome (TOS)*: This is a group of disorders caused by compression of the neurovascular structures (brachial plexus, subclavian artery, or subclavian vein) in the thoracic outlet and is one of the most difficult upper extremity compressive neuropathies to manage. There are three areas of the thoracic outlet where compression can occur: between the scalene muscles, between the clavicle and the first rib, and between the coracoid process of the scapula and the pectoralis minor. Common causes of thoracic outlet syndrome include physical trauma, repetitive injuries, poor posture, anatomical defects (cervical rib), and pregnancy. Often, the exact cause is unknown. Most patients complain of pain or aches in the neck, shoulder, or hand, fatigue throughout the arm with activity, weak grip strength, and numbness or tingling in the fingers. Patients with TOS often present with hand symptoms, resulting in diagnoses unrelated to the shoulder girdle. The OTP must evaluate to determine if the etiology of these symptoms is proximal to the wrist and hand. In PC, the issues related to posture can be addressed expediently and effectively.
- *Radial Nerve Palsy*: As the radial nerve traverses around the spiral groove of the humerus (approximately mid-humerus), it is vulnerable to injury and compression. High radial nerve palsy, often called Saturday Night Palsy, may be caused by compression or humeral shaft fractures. The most common cause is mid-humeral fractures, but compression in the axilla from crutches can also result in radial nerve palsy. The triceps muscle is spared but there is paralysis of all wrist extensors, loss of finger extension at the metacarpophalangeal (MCP) joints, and an inability to extend and radially abduct the thumb. The wrist presents in a flexed position and this deformity is called wrist drop.
- *Radial Tunnel Syndrome*: This occurs when the radial nerve dives beneath the supinator muscle and is compressed at the radial tunnel. Symptoms of pain occur in the dorsal forearm approximately 3–4 cm distal to the lateral epicondyle, and worsen with wrist extension, supination, and resisted gripping with extended

upper extremity. The location of the symptoms serves to differentiate radial tunnel syndrome from lateral epicondylitis.

- *Ulnar Tunnel Syndrome*: A less common ulnar nerve entrapment syndrome, ulnar tunnel syndrome typically occurs with direct pressure to the ulnar aspect of the palm such as weight bearing on an extended upper extremity and is a compression of the distal ulnar nerve as it enters the hand through a space called the ulnar tunnel or Guyon canal. It is also known as Handlebar Palsy as it is more common in cyclists due to the prolonged weight bearing on the bicycle handlebars.

Role of PCP

Typically, the PCP will perform a physical examination, including special tests for specific nerve impingements and sensory threshold testing. Additional tests that the PCP may order to confirm diagnosis include electromyography (EMG) and/or nerve conduction velocity (NCV) or nerve conduction study (NCS) to assess nerve conduction and muscle response to stimulation; imaging studies (X-ray or MRI) to assess for bony or soft tissue abnormalities; and in some cases, nerve ultrasonography to identify sites of nerve compression.

With activity modifications and conservative treatment, most people recover from nerve impingement (neuropraxia and axonotmesis) within several weeks. In severe cases, surgery may be required to restore nerve function and relieve pain.

Patients typically visit their PCP when symptoms last for several days and don't respond to self-care measures. The PCP is usually familiar with the most common nerve impingement syndromes (carpal tunnel, cubital tunnel, thoracic outlet syndrome, radial nerve palsy, and radial tunnel syndromes) and will perform physical assessments and gather subjective information from the patient to diagnose the nerve impingement. The PCP will commonly provide symptomatic relief in the form of acetaminophen and nonsteroidal anti-inflammatory drugs such as ibuprofen and naproxen and prescribe dosage and frequency. Corticosteroids such as cortisone and dexamethasone may be injected directly around the nerve to reduce inflammation and pain. Patients are often referred to OT/PT, or a certified hand therapist (CHT) when available, and if symptoms persist or worsen and dysfunction is more severe than is manageable at the PCP level, patients may be referred for a surgical consult.

Common Comorbidities

Common comorbidities that may increase the risk of, or can occur with nerve impingement include, but are not limited to:

- Diabetes (Chap. 19).
- Autoimmune disorders (e.g., Rheumatoid arthritis) (Chap. 12).

- High blood pressure (Chap. 26).
- Pregnancy or menopause.
- Obesity (Chap. 30).
- Arthritis (Chap. 12).
- Tumors or cysts.
- Edema.
- Thyroid dysfunction.
- Congenital defects.
- Neural disorders.
- Depression (Chap. 18).
- Anxiety (Chap. 11).
- Fractures.

Role of OTP

The OTP in PC can assess for and treat the less severe cases of nerve impingement. This allows the patient to avoid a trip to urgent care, or a referral to specialty OT or PT for more involved treatment than is necessary. The OTP can also address the comorbidities that can be treated with OT interventions, such as depression, anxiety, edema, and arthritis. Addressing the lifestyle choices underlying systemic co-morbid conditions, such as hypertension, thyroid dysfunction, etc., can be helpful. The OTP can also address environmental or worksite concerns that may be contributing to symptoms from the PC setting.

Occupational Impact

Symptoms most commonly reported include:

- Numbness or decreased sensation in the area supplied by the nerve
- Sharp, aching, throbbing, or burning pain which may radiate down the arm
- Tingling and/or pins and needles sensations (paresthesia)
- Muscle weakness or muscle cramping in the area supplied by the nerve

Occupational impact varies from mild impairment to severe disability, depending on type of nerve compression and duration of symptoms. Adults engaged in repetitive occupations are associated with a higher risk for nerve impingement. Repetitive occupations can include work functions, but are also commonly associated with recreational and daily activities.

With prolonged nerve impingement, motor deficits can occur causing difficulty with tasks relying on fine and gross motor coordination. Individuals with nerve impingement syndrome often give up preferred occupations or make significant modifications to daily routines.

Additionally, symptoms tend to intensify when sleeping and may significantly impact sleep participation. Overall, symptoms of nerve impingement impact all aspects of activities of daily living (ADLs) and instrumental activities of daily living (IADLs), which in turn negatively impact mental health and quality of life.

OT Areas of Emphasis

The OTP will perform a comprehensive evaluation to confirm nerve impingement and rule out other pathology, identify patient factors affecting occupational performance, and develop an intervention plan. The OTP will provide patient education regarding identified ergonomic principles, postural changes, activity modifications, body mechanics, and home exercise program adherence. Additionally, the OTP will fabricate prescribed orthoses or recommend appropriate over-the-counter/pre-fabricated orthoses, adaptive equipment and/or durable medical equipment. The OTP can also recommend a referral to a CHT, if the patient requires more involved treatment than can be provided in the PC setting.

Evaluation

Note:
- Videos and images for the assessments mentioned in this chapter can be found online when searching the test name.
- The Shirley Ryan Ability Lab is a good online resource for rehabilitation assessments.

Suggested Areas to Assess:
- Obtain an accurate patient history.

  - Who was involved?
  - What happened?
  - Where did the incident occur?
  - When did the incident occur?
  - What is the injury/issue/chief complaint?
  - To what extent are they injured?
  - What has changed since the incident/injury?

- Patient Specific Functional Scale (PSFS). A self-report outcome measure of function commonly used with musculoskeletal problems; available online and free to use.
- Identify occupational performance barriers. Some possible assessments for upper extremity function and general function include:

- Disabilities of the Arm, Shoulder, and Hand (DASH or QuickDASH). A self-report outcome measure designed to evaluate disorders and measure disability of the upper extremities and monitor change or function over time; available online and free to use.
- Focus on Therapeutic Outcomes (FOTO).

  FOTO requires a subscription/licensing for use. It provides assessment questions relevant to the specific area affected.

- Canadian Occupational Performance Measure (COPM). A client-centered outcome measure for patients to identify and prioritize everyday issues that restrict their participation; available in paper and digital forms and requires a fee to use.

• Perform a proximal screen to rule out cervical involvement (cervical radiculopathy) and thoracic outlet syndrome [1]. If the patient tests positive for TOS, provide postural education and exercises. See the Appendix for Provocative Tests for Proximal Nerve Involvement for instructions and pictures regarding how to do these assessments.

- Spurling's test—to rule out cervical radiculopathy [3, 4]
- Adson, Roos, and Wright's test for TOS [5]

• Inspect skin and upper extremity for changes, deformities, or muscle atrophy and palpate for tenderness and bony/soft tissue abnormalities.
• Perform upper limb tension tests and Provocative Tests for Distal Nerve Compression (Carpal tunnel, cubital tunnel, and radial tunnel syndromes) [1, 2]. See Appendix for *Provocative Tests for Distal Nerve Compression* for instructions.
• Carpal Tunnel Syndrome (Tinel's sign and Phalen's test)

- Cubital Tunnel Syndrome (Tinel's test and elbow flexion test)
- Radial Nerve Palsy (Observe for wrist drop and inability to extend MP joints)
- Radial Tunnel Syndrome (Resisted extension of the long finger with the elbow in full extension, forearm in pronation, and the wrist in neutral)
- Ulnar Tunnel Syndrome (Tinel's test over ulnar tunnel)

Sensory Testing (use what you have available)
• Two-point discrimination
• Light touch/location
• Vibration
• Semmes-Weinstein monofilaments
• Sharp/dull (can use an open paper clip rather than a pin)
• Compare hands/upper extremities to see if there is a difference in acuity of sensation

Range of Motion
• Functional AROM—compare the AROM/PROM and postures during various motions. Have the patient do functional motions:

- Open/close fingers.

- Pinch thumb to each fingertip.
- Touch the back of the head such as when washing hair.
- Touch behind the upper and lower back such as tucking in a shirt and fastening a bra.

Strength
- Manual muscle testing
- Grip/pinch strength

Intervention Strategies

Note
Videos and images for the interventions can be found online when searching the intervention name.

Principles of conservative management include muscle length and myofascial mobility, neural mobilization, orthoses and protection, and activity modification [1, 2]. Patients will require education and training to incorporate these principles into their daily routines.

Muscle Length and Myofascial Mobility

- Often nerve impingement is the product of a cycle of overuse, inflammation, nerve irritation, and muscle guarding, causing hypomobility of the muscles/fascia and increased stress on the nerves during activity.
- Manual techniques such as soft tissue mobilization or massage, low load prolonged stretching and Kinesio® taping can be used to increase muscle length and myofascial mobility. Techniques such as massage, stretching, and simple Kinesio® tape applications can be taught to the patient to perform on their own.
- Thermal modalities (moist hot packs, paraffin, ultrasound, fluidotherapy) may also be beneficial in facilitating blood flow during stretching, if you have these resources available. You can instruct the patient how to safely use heating pad/ moist heat, or paraffin at home.
- Evidence supports the combination of tendon gliding exercises with conventional treatments for nerve distal nerve impingements such as carpal tunnel syndrome [6].

Neural Mobilization

- Evidence suggests neural mobilizations may accelerate recovery of function [7]
- The goal is to improve extraneural and intraneural mobility
- Train patients on appropriate and safe nerve mobilizations or 'nerve gliding/ flossing'. If this is outside of your skill set, you can refer these patients for out-

patient hand therapy. Refer to the *Nerve Glides Handout* in the Appendix for more information.

- Often, therapists make the mistake of doing too much too fast. Use the mnemonic FLOSS to ensure safe and effective neural mobilizations [1].

  - F–Fix the adjacent joint
  - L–Limit the ROM
  - O–Oscillate proximal or distal to the level of compression (progress to both proximal and distal as tolerated)
  - S–Slow, rhythmic motion
  - S–Symptom free

Common Orthoses and Products for Protection

Examples include wrist orthotics, resting night orthotics (custom fabricated or over-the-counter/pre-fabricated), gel pads, elbow flexion block orthotics, counter force straps, yoke orthotics, etc.)

- Orthoses may be necessary to decrease acute symptoms or symptoms that are observed at rest and/or increased with activity
- Custom fabricated orthoses or over-the-counter/pre-fabricated orthoses may be provided
- See the *Common Orthoses in Primary Care* document in the Appendix for patterns and pictures of orthoses that can be fabricated fairly quickly in the PC setting. These include:

  - Wrist cock-up in neutral wrist position (carpal tunnel syndrome, radial tunnel syndrome, ulnar tunnel syndrome)
  - Volar elbow flexion block (cubital tunnel syndrome)

Activity Modifications

Activity modifications and adherence have been shown to positively influence the long-term maintenance of the effects of conservative nerve impingement treatment [8].

- Examples include keyboard ergonomics, reducing gripping/pinching, using headset/keyboard tray vs. holding phone/resting elbows, using a pistol grip, using neutral vs. pronated position, placing a pencil under index finger during typing, etc. The OTP can provide patient-centered education, such as the following:

  - Education on avoiding aggravating motions and techniques to modify identified occupations of concern

- Education on general principles of ergonomics, body mechanics, and activity modifications to decrease stress on the peripheral nerve
- Education to avoid provocative movements such as:

   Wrist flexion/extension with carpal tunnel syndrome
   Extreme elbow flexion with cubital tunnel syndrome (e.g., avoid leaning on ulnar nerve as it runs through the cubital tunnel)
   Avoid activities that cause sensations of vibration (e.g., driving, hair dryer, motor equipment, etc.)

Note: It is important to consider the patient's entire body, especially during activities that provoke symptoms. Poor recruitment of large muscle groups, such as the abdominals and scapular stabilizers, can cause heavy reliance on the small distal musculature of the forearm and wrist. Provide appropriate recommendations to engage core and postural muscles with activity/exercise.

Other Considerations and Resources

(a) Documentation and Billing—Use the *Physical Medicine and Rehabilitation* CPT code that best fits your intervention. If you provide a custom or prefabricated orthotic, use the appropriate L-code or Orthotic Management and Training CPT® code that reflects your intervention. Refer to the *Administrative and Operational Considerations* chapter [9] (Chap. 3).
(b) Suggested referrals if treatment available in the PC office is insufficient:

   • OT/CHT in an outpatient setting for orthosis fabrication, treatment with physical agent modalities, or more intense one-on-one intervention
   • PT for general strengthening exercises
   • Worksite evaluation when posture and work tasks are factors
   • Orthopedic or plastic surgeon for surgery evaluation, if necessary

References

1. Skirven TM, Osterman AL, Fedorczyk JM, Amadia PC. Rehabilitation of the hand and upper extremity. 6th ed. Philadelphia, PA: Elsevier Inc.; 2011.
2. Wietlisbach CM. Cooper's fundamentals of hand therapy: clinical reasoning and treatment guidelines for common diagnoses of the upper extremity. St. Louis, MO: Mosby; 2019.
3. Shabat S, Leitner Y, David R, Folman Y. The correlation between Spurling test and imaging studies in detecting cervical radiculopathy. J Neuroimaging. 2012;22(4):375–8.
4. Thoomes E, Thoomes-de Graaf M, Van Geest S, Vleggeert-Lankamp C, Van der Windt D, Falla D, Verhagen AP, Koes BW, Thoomes-de Graaf M, Kuijper B, Scholten-Peeters W. Value of physical tests in diagnosing cervical radiculopathy: a systematic review. Spine J. 2018;18(1):179–89.

5. Illig K. Thoracic outlet syndrome. Switzerland AG: Springer; 2013.
6. Horng Y, Hsieh S, Tu Y, Lin M, Horng Y, Wang J. The comparative effectiveness of tendon and nerve gliding exercises in patients with carpal tunnel syndrome a randomized trial. Am J Phys Med Rehabil. 2011;90(6):435–42.
7. Ballestero-Pérez R, Plaza-Manzano G, Urraca-Gesto A, Romo-Romo F, Atín-Arratibel M, Pecos-Martín D, Gallego-Izquierdo T, Romero-Franco N. Effectiveness of nerve gliding exercises on carpal tunnel syndrome: a systematic review. J Manip Physiol Ther. 2017;40(1):50–9.
8. Zwolińska J, Kwolek A. Factors determining the effectiveness of conservative treatment in patients with carpal tunnel syndrome. Int J Occup Med Environ Health. 2019;32(2):197–215.
9. American Medical Association. CPT 2020 Professional Edition. Chicago: American Medical Association; 2020.

Chapter 30
Overweight and Obesity

Jill Hurley and Mackenzie Day

Introduction

Overweight and obesity are characterized by an overaccumulation of adipose (fatty) tissue that can lead to biomechanical, psychosocial, and metabolic dysfunction. Like many chronic diseases, obesity is influenced by multiple factors, including environment, behavior, and genetics. Obesity is a prevalent condition, impacting over 40% of American adults, and has widespread and severe impacts on health [1].

Overweight and obesity can be diagnosed and measured in a number of ways, the most common and clinically relevant methods are Body Mass Index (BMI) and Waist Circumference:

- *Body Mass Index (BMI)* is a method for classifying weight along a normed scale, and was issued by the National Institute of Health. BMI is calculated by dividing weight by height squared, the resulting value can place an individual in the following categories; Underweight (<18.5), Normal (18.5–24.9), Overweight (25.0–29.9), Class I Obesity (30.0–34.9), Class II Obesity (35.0–39.9) or Class III Obesity (>40). BMI calculators are available online.

$$\text{Weight} \div \text{Height}^2 = \text{Body Mass Index}\,(\text{BMI})$$

- *Waist Circumference* is a measure that has been found to predict the level of risk an individual is at for developing secondary conditions, such as coronary artery disease or type 2 diabetes. Waist circumference is measured in a stand-

J. Hurley (✉)
Healthe Habits for Living, Lafayette, LA, USA
e-mail: jill@healthehabitsforliving.com

M. Day
Corte Madera, CA, USA

© Springer Nature Switzerland AG 2023   309
S. Dahl-Popolizio et al. (eds.), *Primary Care Occupational Therapy*,
https://doi.org/10.1007/978-3-031-20882-9_30

ing position by placing a measuring tape around one's abdomen just above the hip bones. Greater risk is indicated for men with a waist circumference greater than 40 in and for non-pregnant women with a waist circumference greater than 35 in.

Role of PCP

The PCP tracks weight and BMI, and identifies individuals who are overweight or obese. The provider is likely to discuss health risks associated with overweight and obesity, and suggest strategies for weight loss such as increased activity and improved nutrition. They may refer clients to programs that support weight loss, such as community exercise and nutrition classes. While PCPs are aware of the health implications of being overweight, this condition typically is not effectively managed in the PC setting [2].

Common Comorbidities

- Obesity is related to nearly all chronic conditions. A primary goal in the treatment of obesity is the prevention of chronic complications. Common chronic complications and comorbidities of obesity include arthritis (Chap. 12)
- Obstructive sleep apnea (Chap. 27)
- Hypertension (Chap. 26)
- Diabetes (Chap. 19)
- Fibromyalgia (Chap. 34)
- Peripheral neuropathy
- Skin problems
- Pain, including joint pain, back pain (Chap. 34)
- Cancer (breast, bladder, liver, pancreas, colon)
- Depression (Chap. 18)
- Osteoporosis
- Coronary artery disease
- Chronic obstructive pulmonary disease (COPD) (Chap. 13)

Obesity's link to chronic inflammation plays an important role in potential complications and comorbidities. Inflammation is the body's normal protective response to injury, irritation, disease, or surgery. This inflammation becomes chronic when there is an ongoing stimulus resulting in a complicated interaction occurring between inflammatory messengers. This repetitive cycle is shown in Fig. 30.1: Obesity Cycle is believed to increase chronic disease. For more information on this cycle, see Jill Hurley's Healthe Habits for Living (https://healthehabitsforliving.com).

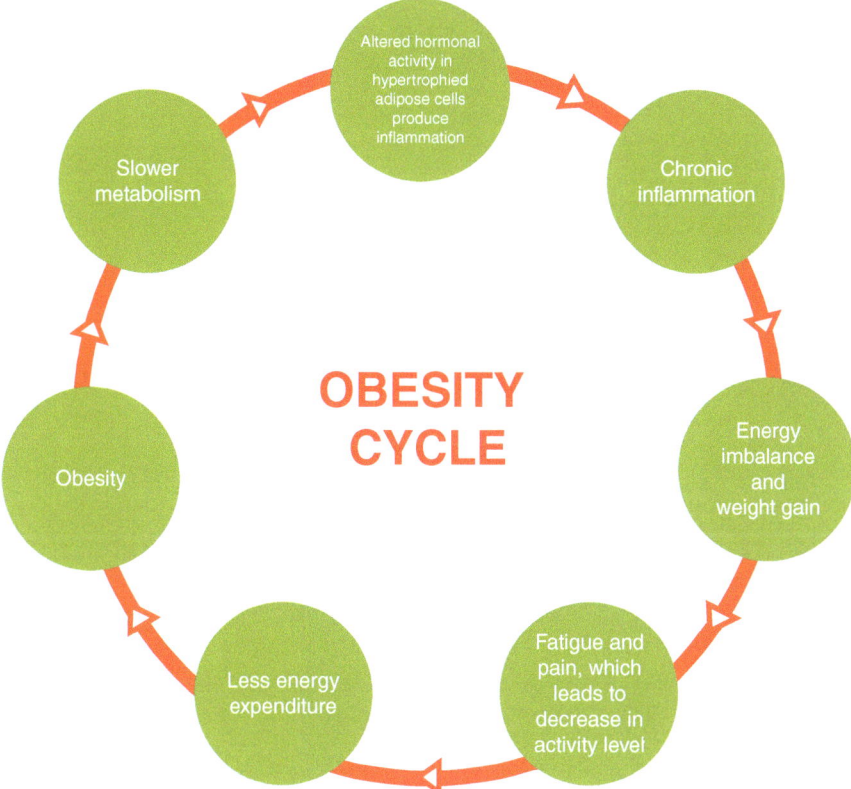

Fig. 30.1 Obesity cycle created by Jill Hurley, OTR, CHT

Role of OTP

Evaluate root causes for this condition, identify barriers to lifestyle modification and condition self-management, and provide realistic strategies the patient can employ to reduce their weight and the related negative effects on their lives. Work with each patient to achieve a healthy lifestyle, improve self-esteem, and achieve an optimal quality of life.

Occupational Impact

Obesity can impact people in a variety of ways, including musculoskeletal, psychological, and social impacts.

- Musculoskeletal consequences include:

- – Poor posture
- – Joint alignment such as "knock knees" or flat arches
- – Modified gait: wider stance, slower stride
- – Increased joint compression
- – Impaired balance

- Psychological impacts include:

  - – Increased depression and anxiety
  - – Reduced quality of life
  - – Poor self-esteem or body satisfaction

- Social impacts include:

  - – Social stigma, resulting in reduced social engagement

Obesity can impact all areas of occupational performance (ADL, IADL, Sleep and rest, work, education, play, leisure, and social participation), depending on the severity of obesity and comorbid conditions. Occupational impacts include:

- Decreased range of motion (ROM) may result in limitations in toilet hygiene, showering, tying shoes, dressing, and functional mobility.
- Low endurance decreases participation. For example, limiting community mobility and ability to participate in tasks like grocery shopping.
- Joint pain can impact sleep, walking, leisure activities such as gardening, sports, or exercise, and may impact work, as standing or sitting for prolonged periods is likely to become uncomfortable.
- Decreased strength may cause difficulty completing household chores and other daily activities.
- Stigma of obesity may discourage participation. For example, not wanting to wear a swimsuit at the beach, or not wanting to try gym class.
- Physical size and weight can also be limiting factors. For example, not fitting on a ride at the fair, booth in a restaurant, seat on an airplane, or exceeding the weight limit on activities like horseback riding or skydiving.

OT Areas of Emphasis

OT intervention should focus on lifestyle changes such as helping people with obesity to engage in meaningful activities, improve nutrition and physical activity, and manage their weight [3, 4]. Lifestyle changes must be sustainable in order to be successful. OTPs help clients to set realistic goals, maintain motivation, and track their progress in order to create a long-term change in habits and routines [5].

Evaluation

Evaluation will include an assessment of the person's medical history and functional abilities, as well as their eating patterns, musculoskeletal status, cardiovascular health, and the person's readiness for behavior change. Assessing a person's attitude and readiness for behavior change is valuable in determining the potential for success with the treatment plan. Many people do not feel it is possible to meet the recommended physical activity guidelines for good health. Because of the relationship between obesity and other chronic conditions, this evaluation is appropriate for nearly all chronic diseases. Evaluation should include the following:

- Personal history, including:
  - Health history: medications, current diagnoses, and past surgeries/procedures, recent lab work, if available
  - Occupations, home environment, social environment
  - History of falls: when, where, and how often and any injuries

- Physical factors including age, weight, body fat%, height, blood pressure, BMI
- Nutritional history
  - Food log

    Available online from the CDC

  - Practices including diets used in the past: successes or failures

- Health literacy
- Standardized functional questionnaire
  - 36-item Short Form Health Survey (SF-36)

    Free, available online

  - Canadian Occupational Performance Measure (COPM)

    Interview-based assessment helps clients to identify and prioritize everyday occupations in which they feel their performance is impaired

- Assessment of musculoskeletal function
  - Standardized balance tests

    Berg Balance Scale

    - 14-item performance-based scale to assess balance.
    - Free, available online

    Balance Evaluation System Test (BESTest)

    - 27-item performance-based scale to assess balance
    - Free, available online

- – Range of Motion (ROM) screening
- – Manual Muscle Testing (MMT)
- Standardized cardiovascular or endurance test
  - – Rockport Walk Test

    Measure based on heart rate, pulse, and walking pace
    Free, available online
- Readiness for behavior change
  - – Physical Activity Readiness Questionnaire (PAR-Q)

    7-item questionnaire
    Free, available online

Intervention Strategies

Ideal intervention for weight loss addresses diet, physical activity, and behavior strategies [2]. OT intervention can target all three of these areas.

Nutrition

- Promote healthy food choices and eating patterns. Provide patient education on nutrition and portion sizing, following standard guidelines such as those published by the United States Department of Agriculture (USDA). Address individual nutritional needs, taking into account any precautions with certain chronic diseases. Take into consideration the person's health literacy, access to healthy food choices, cultural preferences and personal preferences.
- Assist clients in overcoming barriers to healthy eating, including limited time, knowledge, or skills. Help them to create realistic goals around preparing and eating meals. For example, by using a template to plan meals and develop a grocery list. Introduce mindfulness practices, such as avoiding multitasking during eating, to bring awareness to eating habits and reduce caloric intake [6].
- Resources for Nutrition:
  - – USDA ChooseMyPlate
  - – Mindfulness-based Eating Awareness Training (MB-EAT).

Physical Activity

- Physical activity is a key component to weight management [2]. Being active is the best predictor of maintaining success in long-term weight management as well as managing all other chronic diseases. The National Institute of Health suggests 150 min of physical activity per week for health maintenance, and 300 min per week for weight loss [7]. Physical activity should be performed at a moderate level of intensity.
- Assist the individual in identifying and selecting enjoyable physical activities, and developing a realistic plan to incorporate physical activity into their daily routine. Collaborate to create a plan to increase physical activity slowly over time to limit pain and fatigue (for example, see the *Walk to Run Program* in the Appendix. Evaluate and address musculoskeletal and psychological barriers to participation in a fitness plan prior to implementation. Take into consideration the person's health literacy, access to exercise equipment, cultural components, and personal preferences.

Behavioral Strategies

- Set goals. You can use the *SMART Goals & Monthly Tracker* in the Appendix.
  - Set short- and long-term goals. Help clients to make realistic goals, and progress them appropriately. Goals should be individually meaningful and motivating.
- Track progress
  - Monitor daily nutrition and activity, such as by using a log. Monitor weight at regular intervals.
- Establish a support system
- Use mindfulness
  - Interventions such as yoga and meditation can help to reduce the impacts of stigma associated with weight [8, 9].
  - Increasing mindfulness during eating can help to reduce overall consumption [6].
- Readiness for change
  - Evaluate readiness for change, and provide education on the stages of change and the process of developing habits.
  - Provide education on realistic expectations, such as by explaining that results may not be immediately visible upon starting a new program of diet and exercise.

- Address the environment

  - Environmental modifications can help to increase participation and energy expenditure.
  - Durable medical equipment, such as bariatric chairs or reachers, may be appropriate to reduce barriers to participation.
  - Environmental modifications can promote physical activity. For example, placing exercise equipment such as resistance bands on the coffee table to promote use while watching TV.

Other Considerations and Resources

Documentation and Billing

- Most insurances will not reimburse for OT services under a diagnosis of overweight or obesity. However, many will reimburse for services for the comorbid or resultant conditions (such as knee osteoporosis, falls, or limitations in skills like self-care) that an OTP is likely to address. Always be honest and ethical in your billing practices.
- An OTP cannot bill insurance for nutrition counseling or nutrition therapy.

  - Some states have very strict practice guidelines and other states have no guidelines. It would be prudent to find and familiarize yourself with the dietetics practice act typically found through your state government website. (38 states have one at this printing).
  - Disclose you are not a licensed dietician nor a licensed nutritionist unless you have attended an accredited program and are a holder of a valid license for this practice.
  - Do not give a diet plan or calorie count.

Suggested Referrals

- *Registered Dietician:* can provide nutrition therapy, and more detailed guidance on healthy eating habits. Also appropriate for people who need nutrition guidelines for a medical condition, like diabetes or kidney disease.
- *Psychologist/Psychiatrist:* If there are signs of mental illness that are not being addressed. That is, severe anxiety, signs of depression.
- *Bariatric surgeon or Bariatric medicine*: If a client is interested in weight loss surgery or in weight loss medication.
- *Community resources*: such as walking or exercise groups, community centers.

References

1. Centers for Disease Control and Prevention. Overweight and obesity. 2020. https://www.cdc.gov/obesity/index.html.
2. Jensen MD, Ryan DH, Apovian CM Millen BE, Ard JD, Nonas C, Lavelle, ME. Managing overweight and obesity in adults: systematic evidence review from the obesity expert panel, 2014. 2013. https://www.nhlbi.nih.gov/health-pro/guidelines/in-develop/obesity-evidence-review
3. American Occupational Therapy Association. Obesity and occupational therapy (position paper). Am J Occup Ther. 2007;61:701–3. https://doi.org/10.5014/ajot.61.6.701.
4. Dieterly C. Managing obesity in adults: a role for occupational therapy. American Occupational Therapy Association. 2018. https://www.aota.org/~/media/Corporate/Files/Publications/CE-Articles/CE-Article-November-2018.pdf.
5. Smith K, Gamble M, Boggis T. Addressing weight in primary care to help prevent chronic conditions. Administration and Management Special Interest Section Quarterly. 2017;2(4):13–5.
6. Robinson E, Kersbergen I, Higgs S. Eating 'attentively' reduces later energy consumption in overweight and obese females. Br J Nutr. 2014;112(4):657–61. https://doi.org/10.1017/S000711451400141X.
7. National Institute of Health. How much activity do you need? 2019. https://newsinhealth.nih.gov/2019/01/how-much-activity-do-you-need
8. Godsey J. The role of mindfulness based interventions in the treatment of obesity and eating disorders: an integrative review. Complement Ther Med. 2013;21:430–9. https://doi.org/10.1016/j.ctim.2013.06.003.
9. Lillis J, Hayes SC, Bunting K, Masuda A. Teaching acceptance and mindfulness to improve the lives of the obese: a preliminary test of a theoretical model. Ann Behav Med. 2009;37:58–69. https://doi.org/10.1007/s12160-009-9083-x.

Chapter 31
Parkinson's Disease

Gillian Porter and Jyothi Gupta

Introduction

Parkinson's Disease (PD) is a neurodegenerative disease involving the loss of dopaminergic neurons within the basal ganglia [1]. At the time when initial symptoms are observed, it is estimated 30% of cellular death has already occurred [2]. This loss of neurons results in less Dopamine being released into the striatum of the basal ganglia, which is responsible for motor planning [3]. The decreased release of dopamine to the basal ganglia impacts motor and non-motor behavior; the latter includes prefrontal loop and the limbic loop. The symptoms include starting and stopping of cognitive processes, such as planning, short-term memory and attention; emotional processes such as motivation and transitioning from one mood to another are slowed [4].

- *Risk Factors.* Exact causes of cellular death are unknown, though genetic predisposition, environmental factors, and lifestyle influences increase risk [5]. Risk factors include [6, 7]:
- Age: PD occurs in 1% of people over the age of 60 and 5% of people over the age of 85. Approximately 5% of people with PD are diagnosed before the age of 60.
- Family history: Increases risk by 2–5%.
- Types of employment: Farming, factory, and shift work can increase exposure to chemicals and/or conditions linked to Parkinson's.
- Race: More common in White people than other groups.

G. Porter (✉)
Carefree Physical Therapy, Carefree, AZ, USA

Northern Arizona University, Flagstaff, AZ, USA
e-mail: gp288@nau.edu

J. Gupta
University of Texas Medical Branch, Galveston, TX, USA
e-mail: jygupta@UTMB.EDU

© Springer Nature Switzerland AG 2023   319
S. Dahl-Popolizio et al. (eds.), *Primary Care Occupational Therapy*,
https://doi.org/10.1007/978-3-031-20882-9_31

- Serious head injury: A history of head injury can increase risk.
- Gender: Men more than women.
- Where you live: Industrialized and urban areas have higher prevalence and incidence of PD.
- *Types of Parkinsonisms* [8]:
- Primary Idiopathic PD (IPD)

    – 75% of Parkinsonisms

        15% Familial
        85% Sporadic

    – Types of IPD [9]:

        Tremor Dominant 26–40%
        Akinetic Rigid 38–49%
        Mixed Type 12–36%

- Secondary Parkinsonisms

    – 10–12% of Parkinsonisms

        Drug-induced
        Trauma
        Toxin exposure
        Metabolic
        Viral
        Brain tumor
        Vascular

- Atypical

    – 3–5% of Parkinsonisms

        Multiple System Atrophy (MSA)
        Parkinsonism Dementia
        Progressive Supranuclear Palsy (PSP)

- *Factors relating to poor prognosis* [9]
- Older age
- Early cognitive problems
- Associated co-morbidities
- Decreased dopaminergic responsiveness
- Greater baseline impairment
- Combination rigidity and bradykinesia
- *Death* [10]
- Most people die with PD and not from PD.

- PD's potential contribution to death:

  - Falls
  - Pneumonia

Signs and Symptoms

Not every individual with PD has the same symptoms nor severity of symptoms, and disease progression can vary greatly between individuals with PD [11]. Symptoms may also differ due to the asymmetric dopaminergic degeneration in the brain with PD. For example, individuals with left-sided motor symptom dominance (R basal ganglia affected >L) may have greater difficulty with spatial attention, visuospatial orienting, memory, and mental imagery. Individuals with right-sided motor symptom dominance (L basal ganglia affected >R) have greater difficulties with language and verbal memory [12].

- Common pre-diagnosis signs of PD that may remain post-diagnosis [13]:

  - Micrographia
  - Anosmia
  - Abnormal restlessness during sleep
  - Constipation
  - Hypophonia
  - Masked face
  - Dizziness/fainting from hypotension

- Motor Symptoms [3, 14]

  - Bradykinesia*
  - Rigidity*
  - Resting tremor*
  - Postural instability*
  - Gait difficulties (shuffling, decreased arm swing, freezing)
  - Dystonia

- Non-Motor Symptoms [15]

  - Cognitive issues

       Executive function—dual-tasking, reasoning, problem-solving, concentration, complex planning
       Language—word finding
       Memory—difficulty retrieving encoded memories

  - Fatigue
  - Sleep problems

- Anxiety
- Depression
- Apathy
- Pain
- Frequency in urination
- Sexual dysfunction
- Excess saliva or perspiration
- Visual impairments
- Hallucinations

*Primary signs of PD

Disease Stages [16]

PD can follow a typical pattern of progression:

- *Stage One*—mild symptoms with tremor and other movement signs occurring on one side of the body; posture and gait changes as well as changes in facial expressions can occur. Individuals are living independently.
- *Stage Two*—symptoms worsening with tremor, rigidity, and other movement signs affecting both sides of the body; gait and posture appear different. Individuals are living independently.
- *Stage Three*—'mid-stage', loss of balance and bradykinesia occurring with falls being more common. Individuals may still be living independently; however, impairment prompts modification of tasks.
- *Stage Four*—symptoms are more severe, mobility may be occurring with an Assistive Device (AD). Individuals are unable to live independently and require assistance for Activities of Daily Living (ADL's).
- *Stage Five*—most advanced stage with severe disability, likely bedridden, and individuals in this stage require 24 h care.

PCPs and other physicians may refer to rating scales such as the Hoehn and Yahr Stages, that rates symptoms on a scale of 1–5 (essentially matching the five Stages above), or the Unified Parkinson's Disease Rating Scale (UPDRS), which is a more comprehensive tool that also covers non-motor symptoms.

Role of PCP [17–19]

Patients will be seen by a PCP for their general health issues, as well as a general neurologist or neurologist who specializes in movement disorders. These physicians may follow the Movement Disorder Society Clinical Diagnostic Criteria for Parkinson's Disease to guide the initial clinical diagnosis of PD. After taking a medical history, verifying the patient's signs and symptoms are not the result of medication, the physician performs a neurological exam to test balance and muscle tone. A DaTscan may be ordered, and while not a definitive test for PD, can show loss of dopaminergic neurons [14]. Early intervention is desired for symptom management based on functional impairment and to decrease motor and non-motor complications. Consistent follow-up is required throughout the disease progression.

- Medications

  - *To address mild symptoms:* Monoamine oxidase-B (MAO-B) inhibitors, COMT inhibitors, Amantadine, or Anticholinergics.
  - *Improve motor disability* (typically initiated in older patients with more severe motor symptoms): Levodopa, Carbidopa/Levodopa.
  - *Decrease motor complications* (initiated in more mild cases in younger patients): Dopamine agonists.
  - Address Non-motor Symptoms
  - *Depression*—selective serotonin reuptake inhibitors and caution when prescribing tricyclic antidepressants (can exacerbate orthostatic hypotension) (Chap. 18).
  - *Cognitive impairment*—adjust, decrease, or discontinue antiparkinsonian medications and consider a cholinesterase inhibitor.
  - *Constipation*—address with diet and physical activity, discontinue anticholinergics, and add stool softeners/laxatives.
  - *Orthostatic hypotension*—consider medication adjustment, positioning recommendations, and/or prescribing fludrocortisone or midodrine.
  - *Psychosis*—decrease or discontinue antiparkinsonian medications and consider clozapine or quetiapine.
  - *Sleep disturbance*—discontinue dopamine agonists for daytime somnolence and sleep attacks; nighttime awakenings due to bradykinesia consider long-acting Sinemet, adjuvant entacapone, or dopamine agonist (Chap. 27).
  - *Rapid Eye Movement sleep behavior disorder*—decrease or discontinue antiparkinsonian medications and consider clonazepam.
  - *Urinary urgency*—recommendations on adjusting fluid intake and consider tolterodine or oxybutynin; may refer for urology evaluation (Chap. 33).

- Swallowing evaluation for dysphagia.
- Surgical options for symptom management.

  - Deep Brain Stimulation.
  - Duopa™—surgical implantation of a tube in the small intestine to deliver a gel version of carbidopa/levodopa.

- Nonpharmacologic Treatment.

  - Referral to OT, Physical, and Speech Therapy upon initial diagnosis and throughout disease progression, twice annually preferred to monitor and address the impact of disease progression on functional performance.
  - Dietary education to assist with symptom management and promote neuroprotection to slow disease progression.

Role of OTP

The OTP will focus on enhancing client participation in occupations and activities that are of priority to the client.

Occupational Impact

With this progressive condition, patients gradually lose function and the ability to complete ADLs and IADLs. Behavior can become socially inappropriate, which can cause stress to the caregivers. Due to this progressive loss of function, the change in behaviors and overall awareness, there is an increased reliance on family members for all aspects of care. The need for caregiver education and respite must be considered as the OTP creates and modifies the treatment plan.

OT Areas of Emphasis

OTP treatment techniques will focus on large amplitude/high velocity movements that optimize motor control and cognitive attention during functional mobility:

- Encourage participation in occupations and activities that are meaningful to the client.
- Focus on enhancing mobility, while reducing fall risk in the home and community.
- Address upper extremity function/coordination.
- Consider vision and cognitive performance and train, modify, and/or adapt accordingly.
- Maintain a strong relationship with the client's Movement Disorder Specialist.
- Respect medication dosage times and how they may impact quality of movement and cognition.
- Address durable medical equipment, adaptive equipment, or assistive devices needs.
- Provide care-partner/caregiver training.
- Educate on community resources for exercise, support groups, PD-specific community events, PD educational resources, and research initiatives.
- Optimize socialization.
- Encourage neuroprotective habits such as participation in PD-specific exercise and healthy diet.

Note: For information on specialized training programs for this population, see the 'Other Considerations and Resources' section at the end of the chapter.

Evaluation

Common evaluation tools and techniques used in the clinical setting are based on level of impairment impact on performance in daily activities:

- Gait and balance

  - BESTest and Mini-BESTest
  - Timed Up and Go (TUG)

    Can be combined with another task (cognitive, functional, or motor) to test dual-task conditions.

  - Push/Pull Test
  - 3M Backward Walk Test
  - Modified Clinical Test of Sensory Interaction on Balance (CTSIB-M) testing.

- Endurance

  - 6 Minute Walk Test (6MWT)
  - 5× Sit to Stand

- Cognition.

  - Mini Mental State Exam (MMSE), Montreal Cognitive Assessment (MoCA), Trail Making Tests

- Fine Motor Coordination

  - 9-Hole Peg Test
  - Timed tasks

    Buttoning
    Handwriting

- Quality-of-Life scales

  - Parkinson's Disease Questionnaire (PDQ-39)
  - Parkinson's Disease Quality of Life Questionnaire (PDQL)

- ADL performance

  - UPDRS-ADL section
  - Modified Parkinson's Activity Scale

- Subjective movement assessment
  - Time and/or provide subjective description of performance during a reportedly difficult activity such as: getting up from the floor, completing a vehicle transfer, managing a heavy door, transitioning from supine to sitting, etc.

Intervention Strategies

- *Early-Stage*

  Tremor, rigidity, postural changes, and mild gait impairment mark this stage, as well as potential non-motor symptoms such as difficulty with sleeping and hypophonia. People with PD in this stage are still independent with ADLs, though extra time and/or modification of tasks (e.g., modifications to shirt buttoning due to tremor) may be required. Performance in IADLs may be changing or declining such as hiking, playing golf or tennis, or even going out to dinner or the movies. Issues with executive function may be noticeable in this stage, such as planning, maintaining a schedule, and performance in employment.

  - Address occupational performance in IADLs with modification/adaptation techniques to allow for continued participation.
  - Complete home evaluation to assess safety concerns that could increase fall risk.
  - Use movement training techniques such as Lee Silverman Voice Treatment (LSVT) BIG® and Parkinson Wellness Recovery (PWR!)® to promote strategies that counter rigidity, bradykinesia, and issues with initiation and planning of movement.
  - LSVT LOUD® to address voice changes.
  - Encourage exercise as medication for people with PD to optimize neuroprotection and the dopaminergic system; improve motor performance, cognition, and sleep; and decrease fatigue and constipation [20].
  - Encourage socialization to counter the apathy and depression that can occur with PD [21].

- *Mid-Stage*

  Bradykinesia and stiffness are more evident with increased balance impairment, including the potential onset of falling. ADL performance may still be independent with modification, but assistance with IADLs is likely required. Non-motor symptoms are more apparent and likely to interfere with occupational performance.

  - Implement the same interventions listed in the 'early stage', but with increased focus on ADL performance.
  - Driving assessment may be required.

  – Care-partner/caregiver training will be necessary.
  – Encourage use of assistive devices such as canes, walking sticks/hiking poles, and or walkers may be necessary to decrease fall risk.
  – Consider introducing adaptive equipment to assist with feeding.
  – Implement a schedule to assist with time management, reduce anxiety, and ensure consistent participation in exercise, hobbies, IADLs, etc. (external cues can motivate participation).
  – Positioning techniques may be required for comfort due to stiffness, as well as to decrease aspiration.
  – Swallowing may be compromised.
  – Implement diaphragmatic breathing techniques to reduce anxiety and decrease risk of aspiration.
  – When completing a home evaluation or training functional mobility, consider common visual impairments that accompany PD:

  > Decreased contrast sensitivity, color discrimination, depth perception, and visual processing speed [22].

- *Advanced-Stage*
  Severe disability marks this stage of PD with rigidity, bradykinesia, and poor motor initiation/planning interfering with mobility to the degree that ambulation is no longer possible. ADL participation is limited and 24 h care is likely required.
  – Interventions focus on care partner/caregiver training to promote safety in transfers and patient care.
  – Education on positioning, swallowing, and breathing techniques may be required.

Other Considerations and Resources

A Note about Exercise, Mobility, and Home Exercise Programs

Although treating this population in PC requires general OT skills, given the nature of PD being a movement impairment, it is recommended therapists who are working extensively with this population refer to specialty OT, or seek specialized training through LSVT BIG® and/or PWR!® to promote high velocity, high amplitude movement not in exercise training and when addressing functional mobility. A recent study revealed high intensity exercise training decreases worsening of motor symptoms in people with PD [23]. In addition, research has shown that because of PD's pathology impairing the basal ganglia's ability to detect proper movement cues, people with PD have poor movement selection, resulting in impaired gait and postural control. When external cueing techniques, visual or auditory, are applied when training mobility in people with PD, gait dynamics and postural alignment improve [24]. These are important considerations when establishing home exercise programs.

References

1. Mayo Clinic. Parkinson's disease symptoms and causes. 2020. https://www.mayoclinic.org/diseases-conditions/parkinsons-disease/symptoms-causes/syc-20376055.
2. Cheng HC, Ulane CM, Burke RE. Clinical progression in Parkinson disease and the neurobiology of axons. Ann Neurol. 2010;67(6):715–25. https://doi.org/10.1002/ana.21995.
3. Cachope R, Cheer JF. Local control of striatal dopamine release. Front Behav Neurosci. 2014;8:188. https://doi.org/10.3389/fnbeh.2014.00188.
4. Dale Purves et al. Modulation of movement by the basal ganglia. In: Neuroscience, 6th edn. New York: Sinauer Associates, 2001.
5. Barmore R. Parkinson's foundation. Understanding Parkinson's disease: causes. 2021. https://www.parkinson.org/Understanding-Parkinsons/Causes.
6. Melinosky C. WebMD. What causes Parkinson's disease? 2019. https://www.webmd.com/parkinsons-disease/guide/parkinsons-causes#2.
7. Downward E, and Pool J. Parkinson's disease. How common is Parkinson's Disease. 2019. https://parkinsonsdisease.net/basics/statistics/.
8. Jankovic J. The relationship between Parkinson's disease and other movement disorders. In: Calne DB, editor. Handbook of experimental pharmacology. Berlin: Springer; 1989. p. 227–70.
9. Grosset D, Fernandez H, Grosset K, Okun M, editors. Parkinson's disease–Clinician's desk reference. CRC Press; 2009.
10. American Parkinson Disease Association. Death in Parkinson's disease. 2021. https://www.apdaparkinson.org/article/death-parkinsons-disease/.
11. American Parkinson Disease Association. Common symptoms in Parkinson's disease. 2021. https://www.apdaparkinson.org/what-is-parkinsons/symptoms/#motor.
12. Verreyt N, Nys GMS, Santens P, Vingerhoets G. Cognitive differences between patients with left-sided and right-sided Parkinson's disease. Neuropsychol Rev. 2011;21(4):405–24.
13. Barmore R. Parkinson's foundation. Understanding Parkinson's disease: diagnosis. 2021. https://www.parkinson.org/Understanding-Parkinsons/Diagnosis.
14. Johns Hopkins Medical. How Parkinson's disease is diagnosed. 2021. https://www.hopkinsmedicine.org/health/treatment-tests-and-therapies/how-parkinson-disease-is-diagnosed.
15. Davis Phinney Foundation. What are the non-motor symptoms of Parkinson's Disease? 2020. https://davisphinneyfoundation.org/what-are-the-non-motor-symptoms-of-parkinsons/.
16. Barmore R. Parkinson's foundation. Understanding Parekinson's. 2020. https://www.parkinson.org/Understanding-Parkinsons/What-is-Parkinsons/Stages-of-Parkinsons.
17. Postuma RB, Berg D, Stern M, Poewe W, Olanow CW, Oertel W, et al. MDS clinical diagnostic criteria for Parkinson's disease. Mov Disord. 2015;30(12):1591–9. https://www.med.upenn.edu/digitalneuropathologylab/assets/user-content/documents/educational-resources/mds-clinical-diagnostic-criteria-for-parkinson%27s-disease.pdf.
18. Rao S, Hoffmann L, Shakil A. Parkinson's disease: diagnosis and treatment. Am Fam Physician. 2006;74(12):2046–54. https://www.aafp.org/afp/2006/1215/p2046.html.
19. Spears C. Surgical treatment options. Parkinson's foundation. 2020. https://www.parkinson.org/Understanding-Parkinsons/Treatment/Surgical-Treatment-Options.
20. Speelman AD, et al. How might physical activity benefit patients with Parkinson disease? Nat Rev Neurol. 2011;7:528–34.
21. American Parkinson Disease Association. How Parkinson's might affect your friends. 2021. https://www.apdaparkinson.org/article/how-parkinsons-might-affect-your-friends/.

22. Armstrong RA. Visual symptoms in Parkinson's disease. Parkinsons Dis. 2011, 2011:908306.
23. Schenkman M, Moore CG, Kohrt WM, Hall DA, Delitto A, Comella CL, Josbeno DA, Christiansen CL, Berman BD, Kluger BM, Melanson EL, Jain S, Robichaud JA, Poon C, Corcos DM. Effect of high-intensity treadmill exercise on motor symptoms in patients with De novo Parkinson disease. JAMA Neurol. 2017;75:219. https://doi.org/10.1001/jamaneurol.2017.3517.
24. Muthukrishnan N, Abbas JJ, Shill HA, Krishnamurthi N. Cueing paradigms to improve gait and posture in Parkinson's disease: a narrative review. Sensors (Basel). 2019;19(24):5468. https://doi.org/10.3390/s19245468.

Chapter 32
Pediatric Primary Care

Jessica Wood and Katie Serfas

Introduction

This chapter includes common issues that occur which an OTP can address in the PC clinic. These may include education or solutions to remediate small delay or dysfunction to keep the child from further dysfunction, or to prevent further decline and potential health problems while they await a more in-depth evaluation. This chapter includes the commonly used Frames of Reference in pediatric PC and is divided into age groups guided by the American Academy of Pediatrics' guidelines for health supervision of infants, children, and adolescents. The OTP in a pediatric PC setting can assist pediatricians in early identification and treatment of pediatric conditions. This PCP–OTP collaboration can assist in early intervention, early identification or remediation of chronic conditions, and reduced emergency room visits. There are several resources available in the Appendix as well.

J. Wood (✉)
Occupational Therapy, University of Southern Indiana, Evansville, IN, USA
e-mail: jkwood@usi.edu

K. Serfas
Occupational Science and Occupational Therapy, Saint Louis University,
St. Louis, MO, USA
e-mail: kathleen.serfas@health.slu.edu

© Springer Nature Switzerland AG 2023
S. Dahl-Popolizio et al. (eds.), *Primary Care Occupational Therapy*,
https://doi.org/10.1007/978-3-031-20882-9_32

Newborn (0–4 Weeks of Age)

Overview

Infants and their families are often seen in a PC clinic for well-baby checkups, acute illnesses, or development delay concerns. Common concerns in which an OTP may provide insight and direction include strategies for safe and efficient feeding, activities and exercises to increase cardiopulmonary endurance, and activities and exercises to promote development.

Corrected age: If an infant is born preterm (before 36 weeks gestation), you are to correct their age when completing any developmental screening or assessments until the child turns two years of age. To find the corrected age, take the 40 weeks (full term infant) and subtract the amount of weeks a child was born early. For example, a one-year-old who was born at 34 weeks gestation would be 10 months 2 weeks corrected age when completing a standardized assessment or screening. Refer to Table 32.1: *Frames of Reference most commonly used in Pediatric* PC and Table 32.2: *Zero to one month frame of references guide* for the Frame of References that guide PC pediatric OT for this age group.

Table 32.1 Frames of reference most commonly used in pediatric PC

Frame of Reference	Description	Strategies
Developmental	Identify level of skills (motor, social, emotional, cognition) and advance development	Use activities that match the child's abilities and then grade them to the next level
Biomechanical	Based on physics and kinesiology, specifically looking at ROM, strength, and endurance	Positioning, exercises, orthoses
Motor control/motor learning	How children learn movements through direction and regulation	Engage in whole, meaningful tasks, using feedback, practice, demonstration, and/or mental imagery
Sensory integration	Organizing sensory input to produce an adaptive response	Use multi-sensory activities, incorporating vestibular, proprioceptive, and/or tactile input to make an adaptive response
Behavioral/Cognitive Behavioral	One's thoughts and feelings influence behavior within an environment	Positive reinforcement encourages positive behavior. Changing one's thoughts and beliefs can influence behavior
Cognitive (5 and older)	Help child identify, develop, and use cognitive strategies to improve performance	Help child develop strategies and self-evaluate

Source: O'Brien, J.C., & Kuhaneck, H. (2019) *Case-smith's occupational therapy for children and adolescents* (8th ed.). St Louis, MO: Elsevier, Inc.[1]

Table 32.2 Zero to one month frame of references guide

Sensory Integration Frame of Reference	
Developmental Milestone/Norm (0–1 month)	• Begins development of vestibular-proprioceptive-visual connections • Begins the basis of postural control • Development of head control provides a strong base for sensory experiences
Recommended assessment	• Sensory profile, infant/toddler • Observation
Recommended intervention/Parent education	• Swaddling an infant provides proprioceptive input to infant's joints and facilitates autonomic stability and neurological development – Attend to infant as soon as possible when infant is crying • To soothe infant, gently rock, bounce, or sway with infant in caregiver's arms
Motor Learning and Motor Control Frame of reference	
Developmental milestone/Norm (0–1 month)	• Reflexively moves arms and legs • Keeps fingers closed/fisted • Symmetrical in movements
Recommended assessment	• Clinical observation of antigravity movement and repertoire of movements • Assess reflexes
Recommended intervention/Parent education	• Encourage supervised "tummy-time" • Encourage "floor time," in which the infant lies on the floor and moves about [a]If notable asymmetries observed, consult with physician and recommend further OT
Biomechanical frame of reference	
Developmental milestone/Norm (0–1 month)	• Symmetrical in passive range of motion (ROM) • Symmetrical in active ROM, or antigravity movement
Recommended assessment	• Assess movement • Assess caregiver's positioning while holding and feeding infant
Recommended intervention/Parent education	• Encourage caregiver to feed and hold infant in both arms to allow infant room for full cervical rotation
Developmental frame of reference	
Developmental milestone/Norm (0–1 month)	• Makes brief eye contact with the caregiver when held. • Cries with discomfort • Calms or moves to caregiver's voice • Has periods of wakefulness – sleeps between 12–18 h • Reliant on caregiver during ADL tasks
Recommended assessment	• Ages and stages questionnaire • Peabody motor development chart
Recommended intervention/Parent education	• No TV or digital media until 18 months of age. 18 months–4 years should watch no more than 1 h of high-quality programming/day • Read, sing, and talk to the child

[a]Table 32.2 references: Web Resources—Centers for Disease Control and Prevention (CDC). Milestones Checklist: bddd/actearly/pdf/checklists/Checklists-with-Tips_Reader_508.pdf. [3]

Developmental Milestones/Norms

- Makes brief eye contact with the caregiver when held.
- Cries with discomfort.
- Calms or moves to caregiver's voice.
- Reflexively moves arms and legs.
- Keeps fingers closed/fisted.
- Grasps reflexively.
- Has periods of wakefulness, sleeps between 12–18 h.

Caregiver Education

Please see Caregiver Education Handout for Newborns in the appendix.

Recommended Assessments

The following are recommended assessments used to screen infants in a pediatric PC setting. In a fast-paced PC setting, time may be limited. Each assessment has the age range for the given assessment and the time it may take to administer.

- Peabody Motor Development Chart (0–5 years) (Observational chart).
- Ages and Stages Questionnaires, 3rd Edition (0–5 years) (10–15 min).
- Ages and Stages Social-emotional, 2nd Edition (1–72 months) (10–15 min).
- Occupational Profile –Short Child Occupational Profile (SCOPE) (0–21 years) (10–20 min).
- Short Sensory Profile 2, Infant/Toddler (0–36 months) (10–20 min).
- Survey of Well-being of Young Children (SWYC) (2–60 months) (15 min).

Recommended Intervention

Sensory Integration

Sensory integration plays a part in a child's development from the moment of conception, and one's vestibular system is fully integrated at 40 weeks gestation. The child is receiving proprioceptive input when pushing against the walls of the mother's uterus and vestibular input through flipping in the uterus and then spending weeks upside down in preparation for birth. A child's auditory system receives muffled sound and visual system shadows from the outside of its mother body. An infant's taste begins around 12 weeks gestation. In the newborn phase, development of the vestibular-proprioceptive-visual connections begin. During this time, development of head control provides a strong base for sensory experiences.

Motor Learning and Motor Control

A newborn infant's motor learning and motor control can be evaluated through clinical observation. With the infant lying supine and preferably in only a clean diaper, the OTP can observe upper and lower extremity antigravity movements. A variety of movements are observed and will become increasingly smooth and controlled. The movements observed should be symmetrical. In a newborn, extremity flexor tone will be present. If an infant is demonstrating a notable decrease in antigravity movement on one side of the body as compared to the other, their physician should be notified as this could be indicative of a neurological insult or injury.

Biomechanical

Common biomechanical conditions include decreased passive range of motion and/ or decreased active range of motion, or antigravity movements, in extremities. If cervical muscular tightness associated with decreased full range of motion in an infant's cervical spine is observed, remind the caregivers to feed the child holding them in both their left and right arms. Rotating arms allows the child full cervical rotation to the right and the left. If the back of the child's head appears "flat" or "slanted to one side," encourage the caregiver to supervise the child in a variety of lying positions: side lying, prone for "tummy time," prone on the caregiver's chest or inclined on a wedge.

Developmental

Motor movement, arousal states, attention-interaction, and self-regulation are the focus for newborn neurobehavioral development. Full term newborn infants (36–40 weeks gestation) will demonstrate well-defined ranges of arousal states with smooth transitions. The newborn infant begins to develop consistent responses to auditory stimuli, including human voice. An infant begins to visually attend and track objects. Self-regulation, including bringing hands to mouth and face, is also noted.

A newborn's activities of daily living (ADL) and instrumental activities of daily living (IADL) involve the caregiver in every element. The ADL where dysfunction is common is feeding/eating. It is important that any issues or dysfunction in infant feeding is addressed as early as possible to circumvent any future dysfunction and eliminate the formation of bad habits. A newborn feeds on command, in which they nurse, or bottle feed every 2–4 h. Every infant is different; however, it is recommended by the Hagan et al. [2] that if breastfeeding, the caregiver should provide 8–12 feedings in a 24 h frame.

Commonly, issues arise when transitioning an infant from breastfeeding to bottle feeding. In this situation, a PC OTP may observe the mother and infant during feeding. Observe positioning of the infant and mother and the infant's latch. Observe the infant's root and suck reflexes as well as overall oral motor tone and organization. For example, the infant may be latching down onto the nipple using the nipple to evoke a suck reflex. If this is the case, the caregiver would use the nipple of the bottle to evoke this reflex when first giving the bottle to begin the sucking. The OTP would educate the caregiver on weaning off this strategy, as it is important to integrate this reflex. Adaptive bottles may be suggested, if appropriate. The following website is a good resource for appropriate steps to assist with this transition https://www.uhhospitals.org/services/obgyn-womens-health/patient-resources/pregnancy-resources/Breastfeeding-Guide/suck-training

When to Refer for Further Evaluation

If an infant was born prematurely or spent time in the Neonatal Intensive Care Unit (NICU), it is recommended to refer for an early intervention evaluation. If an infant is displaying developmental delay or dysfunction, a referral to early intervention therapy is necessary.

Infants (1–12 Months of Age)

Overview

Infants develop rapidly in the first year of life. They begin to feed more efficiently, recognize faces, roll over, bat at objects, prop in prone, reach for objects, prop in sitting, to eventually sitting upright independently, crawling, and taking their first steps. Infants are often seen in a PC clinic for a well-baby visit, an acute health concern, or a developmental concern. It is important to note that not all children have skills at the same time. While a developmental chart will give developmental norms, the OTP should consider variables, including context, cultural considerations, and pre-existing conditions. These developmental norms are taken from a group of children without developmental delay or conditions. All conditions should be taken into consideration when comparing performance to developmental norms.

Common biomechanical and motor learning/motor planning concerns seen at this age in a PC clinic include decreased passive ROM in cervical spine secondary to muscular tightness (torticollis), unilateral (plagiocephaly) or bilateral (brachycephaly) occipital flattening of the head. Common developmental concerns include hypotonia, hypertonia, or delayed integration of reflexes. Concerns with age-appropriate activities of daily living (ADLs) include feeding issues or sleeping concerns. Refer to Table 32.3 for the Frame of References that guide PC pediatric OT for this age group.

Table 32.3 One to twelve month frame of references guide

Sensory Integration Frame of Reference (FOR)	
Developmental Milestone/Norm (1–12 months)	• Begins development of vestibular-proprioceptive-visual connections • Begins the basis of postural control • Development of head control provides a strong base for sensory experiences
Recommended assessments	• Sensory profile, infant/toddler • Observation
Recommended intervention/Parent education	• Swaddling an infant provides proprioceptive input to infant's joints and facilitates autonomic stability and neurological development (swaddling ceases between 2–3 months, or when an infant is unswaddling self or attempting to roll over.) • Attend to infant as soon as possible when infant is crying • To soothe infant, gently rock, bounce, or sway with infant in caregiver's arms
Motor Learning and Motor Control Frame of reference	
Developmental milestone/ Norm(1–12 months)	• Reflexively moves arms and legs • Reflexes begin to integrate • Symmetrical in movements
Recommended assessments	• Peabody motor development chart • Clinical observation of antigravity movement and repertoire of movements • Assess reflexes. If appropriate reflexes have yet to integrate, consult physician
Recommended intervention/Parent education	• Encourage supervised "tummy-time" • Encourage "floor time," in which the infant lies on the floor and moves about • Congenital clasped thumb (or tightly flexed and adducted) is common, in which a splint may be fabricated to wear while asleep [a]If notable asymmetries observed, consult with physician and recommend further OT
Biomechanical frame of reference	
Developmental milestone/ Norm(1–12 months)	• Symmetrical in passive range of motion (ROM) • Symmetrical in active ROM, or antigravity movement
Recommended assessments	• Assess movement • Assess caregiver's positioning while holding and feeding infant
Recommended intervention/Parent education	• Encourage caregiver to hold and feed infant with both arms, allowing infant room for full cervical ROM

(continued)

Table 32.3 (continued)

Sensory Integration Frame of Reference (FOR)

Developmental frame of reference

Developmental milestone/ Norm(1–12 months)	One month • Calms when picked up or spoken to • Looks at caregiver and follows with eyes • Looks briefly at objects • Alerts to unexpected sound • Makes brief short vowel sounds • Has different types of cries for hunger, tiredness • Moves both arms and legs together • Holds chin up when prone • Opens fingers slightly when at rest • Sleeps between 12–18 h per day Two months • Smiles responsively • Vocalizes with short cooing sounds • Lifts head and chest when prone • Opens and shuts hand *Age-appropriate ADLs* • Moves hand up to the bottle/breast while feeding • Sleeps between 12–18 h per day Four months • Laughs aloud • Looks for the caregiver when upset • Turns to voices • Vocalizes with extended cooing • Supports self on elbows and wrist when in prone • Rolls over prone to supine • Keeps hands unfisted • Plays with fingers at the midline • Grasps objects *Age-appropriate ADL* • Moves hand up to the bottle/breast while feeding • Sleeps between 12–15 h per day Six months • Smiles at own reflection • Looks when name is called • Babbles; makes sounds like "ga," "ma," or "ba" • Rolls over supine to prone • Sits briefly without support • Reaches for objects and transfers toy from one hand to another • Rakes small object with 4 fingers • Bangs small objects on the surface

Table 32.3 (continued)

Sensory Integration Frame of Reference (FOR)

Age-appropriate ADL
- Holds a bottle with both hands
- Uses a cup with help
- Starts holding and mouthing large crackers
- Plays with a spoon; grabs/bangs; puts both ends in mouth
- Sleeps between 12–15 h per day

Nine months
- Uses basic gestures (holding arms out to be picked up, waving bye-bye)
- Looks for dropped objects
- Plays games like peekaboo and pat-a-cake
- Turns when name is called
- Says "Dada" or "Mama" nonspecifically
- Looks around when hearing things like "Where's your blanket?"
- Copies sound that others make
- Sits well without support
- Pulls to stand
- Transitions well between sitting and lying
- Balances on hands and knees
- Crawls
- Picks up a small object with three fingers and thumb
- Releases objects intentionally
- Bangs objects together

Age-appropriate ADL
- Holds a bottle with both hands
- Uses a cup with help
- Picks up food with fingers and eats it
- Sleeps between 10–14 h per day

Twelve months
- Looks for hidden objects
- Imitates new gestures
- Uses "Dada" or "Mama" specifically
- Uses one word other than "Mama" "Dada," or personal names
- Follows a verbal command that includes a gesture "Give me the ball"
- Takes the first independent steps
- Stands without support
- Drops object in a cup
- Picks up a small object with 2-finger pincer grasp, including food

Age-appropriate ADL
- Holds a cup with both hands
- Takes a few sips without help
- Picks up food with 2-finger pincer grasp
- Moves spoon to mouth, but is messy and spills
- Removes socks
- Helps with dressing by pushing arms through sleeves and legs through pant opening
- Sleeps between 10–14 h per day

(continued)

Table 32.3 (continued)

Sensory Integration Frame of Reference (FOR)	
Recommended assessments	• Peabody motor development chart
Recommended intervention/Parent education	• No TV or digital media until 18 months of age. 18 months–4 years should watch no more than 1 h of high-quality programming/day • Read, sing, and talk to the child
Cognitive frame of reference	
Developmental milestone/ Norm(1–12 months)	One month • Calms when picked up or spoken to • Looks at caregiver and follows with eyes • Looks briefly at objects • Alerts to unexpected sound Two months • Smiles responsively Four months • Laughs aloud • Looks for the caregiver when upset • Turns to voices Six months • Smiles at own reflection • Looks when name is called Nine months • Uses basic gestures (holding arms out to be picked up, waving bye-bye) • Looks for dropped objects • Plays games like peekaboo and pat-a-cake • Turns when name is called Twelve months • Looks for hidden objects • Imitates new gestures
Recommended assessments	• Bayley scales of infant and toddler development, third ed. cognitive scales • Bayley scales of infant and toddler development, third ed. cognitive checklist
Recommended intervention/Parent education	• Read, sing, and talk to child • Provide child with a variety of sensory stimuli in environment • Include movement with cognitive approaches • Floor time play

[a]Table 32.3 References: [1, 2, 4–6]

Caregiver Education

Please see *PEDIATRIC. Caregiver Education for Pediatrics and Adolescence* section on Infants in the Appendix.

Recommended Assessments

The following are recommended assessments used to screen infants in a pediatric PC setting. In a fast-paced PC setting, time may be limited. Each assessment has the age range for the given assessment and the time it may take to administer.

- Peabody Motor Development Chart (0–5 years) (Observational chart).
- Ages and Stages Questionnaires, 3rd Edition (0–5 years) (10–15 min).
- Ages and Stages Social-emotional, 2nd Edition (1–72 months) (10–15 min).
- Occupational Profile—Short Child Occupational Profile (SCOPE) (0–21 years) (10–20 min).
- Short Sensory Profile 2 (0–14:11 years) (5–20 min).
- Parenting Stress Index, Fourth Edition Short Form (1 month–12 years) (20 min).
- Bayley Scales of Infant and Toddler Development, 3rd ed. Cognitive Scales (1–42 months) (30–60 min).
- Bayley Scales of Infant and Toddler Development Observation Checklist (1–42 months) (5–10 min). https://www.pearsonassessments.com/content/dam/school/global/clinical/us/assets/bayley-iii/bayley-iii-observational-checklist.pdf
- Bayley Infant Neurodevelopmental Screener (3–24 months) (5–10 min).
- Survey of Well-being of Young Children (SWYC) (2–60 months) (15 min).

Developmental Milestones/Norms

One Month

Developmental Milestones/Norms
- Calms when picked up or spoken to.
- Looks at caregiver and follows with eyes.
- Looks briefly at objects.
- Alerts to unexpected sound.
- Makes brief short vowel sounds.
- Has different types of cries for hunger, tiredness.
- Moves both arms and legs together.
- Holds chin up when prone.
- Opens fingers slightly when at rest.
- Sleeps between 12–18 h per day.

Two Months

Developmental Milestones/Norms
- Smiles responsively.
- Vocalizes with short cooing sounds.
- Lifts head and chest when prone.
- Opens and shuts hands.

Age-Appropriate Activities of Daily Living
- Moves hand up to the bottle/breast while feeding.
- Sleeps between 12–18 h per day.

Four Months

Developmental Milestones/Norms
- Laughs aloud.
- Looks for the caregiver when upset.
- Turns to voices.
- Vocalizes with extended cooing.
- Supports self on elbows and wrist when in prone.
- Rolls over prone to supine.
- Keeps hands unfisted.
- Plays with fingers at the midline.
- Grasps objects.

Age-Appropriate Activities of Daily Living
- Moves hand up to the bottle/breast while feeding.
- Sleeps between 12–15 h per day.

Six Months

Developmental Milestones/Norms
- Smiles at own reflection.
- Looks when name is called.
- Babbles; makes sounds like "ga," "ma," or "ba."
- Rolls over supine to prone.
- Sits briefly without support.
- Reaches for objects and transfers toy from one hand to another.
- Rakes small object with four fingers.
- Bangs small objects on the surface.

Age-Appropriate Activities of Daily Living
- Holds a bottle with both hands.
- Uses a cup with help.
- Starts holding and mouthing large crackers.
- Plays with a spoon; grabs/bangs; puts both ends in mouth.
- Sleeps between 12–15 h per day.

Nine Months

Developmental Milestones/Norms
- Uses basic gestures (holding arms out to be picked up, waving bye-bye).
- Looks for dropped objects.
- Plays games like peekaboo and pat-a-cake.
- Turns when name is called.
- Say "Dada" or "Mama" nonspecifically.
- Looks around when hearing things like "Where's your blanket?"

- Copies sound that others make.
- Sits well without support.
- Pulls to stand.
- Transitions well between sitting and lying.
- Balances on hands and knees.
- Crawls.
- Picks up a small object with three fingers and thumb.
- Releases objects intentionally.
- Bangs objects together.

Age-Appropriate Activities of Daily Living
- Holds a bottle with both hands.
- Uses a cup with help.
- Picks up food with fingers and eats it.
- Sleeps between 10–14 h per day.

Twelve Months

Developmental Milestones/Norms
- Looks for hidden objects.
- Imitates new gestures.
- Uses "Dada" or "Mama" specifically.
- Uses one word other than "Mama" "Dada," or personal names.
- Follows a verbal command that includes a gesture "Give me the ball."
- Takes the first independent steps.
- Stands without support.
- Drops object in a cup.
- Picks up a small object with 2-finger pincer grasp, including food.

Age-Appropriate Activities of Daily Living
- Holds a cup with both hands.
- Takes a few sips without help.
- Picks up food with 2-finger pincer grasp.
- Moves spoon to mouth, but is messy and spills.
- Removes socks.
- Helps with dressing by pushing arms through sleeves and legs through pant opening.
- Sleeps between 10–14 h per day.

Recommended Intervention

Sensory Integration

During the infant phase, a child's sensory system continues to integrate. A child starts to have increased mobility, developing body scheme and spatial perception. Early sensorimotor experiences help a child understand the effect of their actions on themselves and others, learning cause and effect. By the end of a child's first year, they are experiencing many new sensory experiences during self-feeding.

Feeding: Oftentimes, infants with sensory processing dysfunction have difficulty with latching during breastfeeding. They may not tolerate being talked to or rocked during feeding. The PC OTP may educate the caregiver on swaddling the infant while breast- or bottle-feeding and give the caregiver education on sensory-friendly environments (quiet room, dim lighting, decreased noise).

While transitioning to textured feeding, a child may demonstrate aversion to foods. Recommend the caregiver include a variety of sensory play in which the child experiences a variety of textures in their hands that are also common in foods, including smooth and crunchy, and a variety of temperatures.

Sleeping: Children with sensory processing issues have increased sleep problems. Help the caregivers establish appropriate bedtime and sleep routines, as well as a sensory-friendly environment. Increased full-body proprioceptive input prior to bedtime may help the child with sleep issues. Oftentimes, children with sensory issues have nutrient deficiencies that may impact their ability to fall and remain asleep. The PC OTP may consult the physician if this is suspected [4].

Motor Learning and Motor Control

An infant's motor learning and motor control are evaluated through clinical observation. With the infant lying supine and preferably in only a clean diaper, the OTP can observe upper and lower extremity antigravity movements. A variety of movements are observed and will become increasingly smooth and controlled. The movements observed should be symmetrical. In a newborn, extremity flexor tone will be present. If an infant is demonstrating a notable decrease in antigravity movement on one side of the body as compared to the other, their physician should be notified as this could be indicative of a neurological insult or injury.

Biomechanical

Upper limb formation is complete by 8 weeks gestation. Therefore, any abnormalities observed should be communicated to the physician and intervention should begin immediately. One of the most common congenital upper limb issues is congenital clasped thumb. This condition is treated conservatively, if found early. The PC OTP would educate the caregiver on PROM and stretching intervention. Depending on the severity, or if this family will receive continued OT services within the next week or two, a splint may be fabricated to keep the MCP joint in a functional position. This splint is to be worn while the infant is asleep. Skin checks for redness or breakdown should be completed every 2–3 h, or before/after feedings and diaper changes.

Developmental

An infant's activities of daily living (ADL) and instrumental activities of daily living (IADL) involve the caregiver in every element. Refer to each age in months above for age appropriate ADLs. Two common areas of dysfunction in infants include feeding/eating and sleeping.

Feeding: Feeding disorders are relatively common. It is important that any issues or dysfunction in infant feeding is addressed as early as possible to circumvent any future dysfunction and eliminate the formation of bad habits. Feeding issues can be related to things, including gastroesophageal reflux, food allergies, oral motor function, sensory issues, and behavioral issues, or a combination of these.

Infants receive breast or formula milk until around 6 months of age when pureed vegetables, fruits, and meats are introduced. Commonly, issues arise when transitioning an infant from breastfeeding to bottle feeding. In this situation, observe the mother and infant during feeding (refer to feeding section). When transitioning to food, a child may demonstrate oral motor dysfunction. The OTP would observe then palpate the child's oral musculature for difference in tone. If a neurological condition is suspected, a simple lateralization screen may be beneficial. To check for lateralization, the OTP would place a small probe in the child's mouth and move the probe to the right and left sides of the mouth. The child's tongue should follow the probe instinctually. If unable to lateralize to one side, a neurological condition may be present, and it would be important to inform the physician.

Sleep: Infants between the ages of 1–11 months sleep approximately 12–18 h per night. Between 1–2 months, infants nap throughout the day, and between 3–11 months an infant takes 3–4 naps (30 min–2 h) daily. OTPs may play a key role in helping caregivers establish good bedtime and sleep habits.

Cognitive

Infants utilize cognition through attention, interaction, and self-regulation. It is critically important that caregivers interact directly and intentionally with the child in ways that encourage a response. For example, making eye contact and talking to the child, pausing to allow the infant to respond, then smiling and using a positive, encouraging tone of voice once he/she does.

- If delays are suspected, screen an infant's cognitive abilities using cognitive screeners such as Bayley Infant Neurodevelopmental Screener (3–24 months) (5–10 min to administer).

When to Refer for Further Evaluation

If an infant was born prematurely or spent time in the Neonatal Intensive Care Unit (NICU), it is recommended to refer for an early intervention evaluation.

When to Refer for Further Evaluation (1–6 Months)
- Child has difficulty lifting head in prone, sitting.
- Arches back and stiff legs.
- No anti-gravity movements in supine or anti-gravity alignment in prone during horizontal suspension.
- Difficulty reaching in supine, prone, sitting.
- Unable to visually track 180° in supine.

When to refer for swallowing evaluation:
- Increased congestion, wet vocal quality, or coughing/choking during or after eating.
- Oral motor dysfunction.
- Frequent respiratory illnesses.

When to Refer for Further Evaluation (9–12 Months) Because the Following Are Red Flags for Autism Spectrum Disorder (ASD)
- The child fails to orient to name.
- The child does not point at objects.
- The child does not play with a variety of toys.
- The child lacks appropriate eye gaze.
- The child lacks sharing interest or enjoyment.
- The child lacks warm, joyful expressions.
- The child lacks coordination of nonverbal communication.
- The child has delayed speech and language skills.
- The child demonstrates repetitive movements or posturing of body.
- The child demonstrates repetitive movements with objects.

Toddler (1–2 Years of Age)

Overview

Toddlers learn while actively exploring their environment. Lots of changes occur between 1 and 2 years of age, and children progress at different rates. They are starting to communicate through words, follow simple commands, point to ask for something, or point to objects they know. Toddlers walk, squat, and start to climb stairs. They can throw a small ball and will scribble if given a crayon. Toddlers can feed themselves with a 2-finger pincer grasp, scoop food with a spoon, and drink from a cup. They can help dress and undress simple clothes without buttons or zippers. Toddlers may begin to say "no" more frequently and have temper tantrums.

By 24 months of age, speech is becoming clearer as toddlers begin to form simple sentences and understand two-step questions or commands such as "Go to your room and get a book." They can name pictures and point to body parts when asked. Gross motor skills continue to develop as children demonstrate more coordination with running, jumping, kicking, and catching larger balls. They have good thumb and finger control and can turn doorknobs and lids, build a tower, and turn pages in a book, one at a time. Toddlers can spear food with a fork, unbutton larger buttons, and help with hand washing. Toilet training can be initiated as children gain bladder control and urinate in the toilet. Toddlers imitate adults and peers and play alongside other children (parallel play), while also engaging in pretend or make-believe play (i.e., imitate housework or feed a doll).

Toddlers are often seen in a PC clinic for a well-check visit, an acute health concern, or a developmental concern. Common biomechanical and developmental concerns seen at this age include decreased strength and endurance, hypotonia, hypertonia, delayed integration of reflexes, or overall delay of skill development. Common behavioral/sensory concerns include increased or decreased activity level, sensitivity or reactivity to the environment, adaptability to changes in routine, intensity of responses, and engagement with others. Concerns with age-appropriate occupations include feeding and sleeping issues, dressing, toileting readiness, and play exploration, along with decreased motor performance skills. Refer to Table 32.4 for the Frame of References that guide PC pediatric OT for this age group.

Caregiver Education

Please see *PEDIATRIC. Caregiver Education for Pediatrics and Adolescence* section on Toddlers in the Appendix.

Recommended Assessments

The following are recommended assessments used to screen infants in a pediatric PC setting. In a fast-paced PC setting, time may be limited. Each assessment has the age range for the given assessment and time it may take to administer.

- Peabody Motor Development Chart (0–5 years) (Observational chart).
- Ages and Stages Questionnaires, 3rd Edition (0–5 years) (10–15 min).
- Ages and Stages Social-emotional, 2nd Edition (1–72 months) (10–15 min).
- Occupational Profile—Short Child Occupational Profile (SCOPE) (0–21 years) (10–20 min).
- Short Sensory Profile 2, Infant/Toddler (0–36 months) (10–20 min).
- Survey of Well-being of Young Children (SWYC) (2–60 months) (15 min).
- Modified Checklist for Autism in Toddlers (M-Chat)(16 and 30 months) (15 min).
- Parenting Stress Index, Fourth Edition Short Form (1 month–12 years) (20 min).
- Survey of Well-being of Young Children (SWYC) (2–60 months) (15 min).

Table 32.4 One to two year frame of reference guide

Sensory Integration Frame of Reference	
Developmental Milestone/ Norm(1–2 years)	• Sensory input affects development, learning, and behavior which impacts childhood engagement and participation in occupations • Differences in sensory functions can create challenges in daily life • Specific sensory strategies can be offered to help the child feel more comfortable
Recommended assessment	• Short sensory profile • Observation • Parent report
Recommended intervention/Parent education	• Create a sensory diet to embed sensory experiences throughout the day to support an optimal level of alertness or calming • Proprioceptive or heavy muscle activities and linear movement are good activities to incorporate. Examples of regulating activities can be found in regulating activities handout in the appendix • The environment or the activity itself can be modified to avoid unpleasant sensation • Provide textured objects, teethers, vibrating toys, and playfully encourage exploration with hands, face, and mouth
Behavioral frame of reference	
Developmental milestone/ Norm(1–2 years)	15 months • Points to ask for something or to get help 18 months • Engages with others for play • Points to object of interest to draw attention to it • Turns and looks at adult if something new happens • Uses words to ask for help 24 months • Plays alongside other children (parallel play) • Uses 50 words • Combines two words into short phrase or sentence • Follows 2-step command 30 months • Engages in pretend or imaginary play • Tries to get a caregiver to watch by saying, "Look at me!"
Recommended assessment	• Ages and stages • Parent report
Recommended intervention/Parent education	• Provide simple rules with clear and reasonable expectations that should be communicated in a developmentally appropriate manner • Use firm, consistent, and appropriate discipline without shaking, yelling, or hitting • Behavior may be a result of sensory dysregulation. Have parents consider the environment the child is in when the behavior begins. What led up to the behavior?

Table 32.4 (continued)

Sensory Integration Frame of Reference
Developmental and Biomechanical Frames of reference

| Developmental milestone/ Norm(1–2 years) | 15 months
• Looks around after hearing "Where's your blanket?"
• Uses three words other than names
• Speaks in jargon
• Follows a verbal command without a gesture
• Squats to pick up objects
• Climbs onto furniture
• Crawls up a few steps
• Begins to run
• Imitates scribbling with a crayon
• Drops object in and takes the object out of a container
Age-appropriate ADL
• Drinks from a cup with minimal spilling
• Picks up food with 2-finger pincer grasp
• Scoops food with a spoon and feeds self
• Uses a straw
• Removes socks
• Helps with dressing by pushing arms through sleeves and legs through pant opening
• Sleeps between 12–14 h per day
18 months
• Identifies at least two body parts
• Points to pictures in a book
• Names at least five familiar objects
• Walks up steps with two feet per step with hand held
• Sits in a small chair
• Carries a toy while walking
• Scribbles spontaneously
• Throws small ball a few feet while standing
Age-appropriate ADL
• Uses a straw
• Scoops food with a spoon and feeds self
• Removes socks
• Helps with dressing by pushing arms through sleeves and legs through pant opening
• Sleeps between 12–14 h per day
24 month
• Names at least five body parts
• Uses words that are 50% intelligible to strangers
• Kicks a ball
• Jumps off the ground with two feet
• Runs with coordination
• Stacks objects
• Turns pages in a book
• Uses hands to turn objects like lids, toys, knobs
• Draws lines
Age-appropriate ADL
• Drinks from a cup (no lid) without spilling
• Scoops well with a spoon |

(continued)

Table 32.4 (continued)

Sensory Integration Frame of Reference	
	• Takes off simple clothing such as pushing pants or pulling off socks • Removes shoes • Once the shirt is over their head, they can find and push arms through shirt opening • Sleeps between 12–14 h per day 30 months • Engages in pretend or imaginary play • Tries to get a caregiver to watch by saying, "Look at me!" • Uses pronouns correctly • Begins to walk upstairs alternating feet • Runs well without falling • Grasps crayon with thumb and fingers instead of fist • Copies a vertical line • Catches large balls Age-appropriate ADL • Urinates in a potty or toilet • Spears food with a fork • Washes and dries hands • Attempts to don socks • Unbuttons a large button • Dons easy clothing such as jackets or open-front shirts without zipping or buttoning them • Sleeps between 12–14 h per day
Recommended assessment	• Ages and stages • Observation • Parent report • Peabody motor development chart
Recommended intervention/Parent education	• Allow plenty of time to practice dressing. See getting dressed handout in the appendix • Select clothes with minimal fasteners • Elastic waist pants and pull-on shirts are easiest to manage • Use self-help toys, books, or adult clothes for dress-up • Pop-apart beads, playdoh, and simple construction toys can help improve hand coordination and strength • Provide handouts with developmentally appropriate activities for fine motor development, hand strengthening, and simple self-care skills. See the fine motor development, bilateral coordination, and hand strengthening handout and the self-care skills handout in the appendix • Consider toilet readiness

References: Web Resources:https://www.aap.org/en-us/Documents/ttb_bring_out_best.pdf

Fifteen Months

Developmental Milestones/Norms

• Points to ask for something or to get help.
• Looks around after hearing "Where's your blanket?"
• Uses three words other than names.
• Speaks in jargon.

- Follows a verbal command without a gesture.
- Squats to pick up objects.
- Climbs onto furniture.
- Crawls up a few steps.
- Begins to run.
- Imitates scribbling with a crayon.
- Drops object in and takes the object out of a container.

Age-appropriate Activities of Daily Living

- Drinks from a cup with minimal spilling.
- Picks up food with 2-finger pincer grasp.
- Scoops food with a spoon and feeds self.
- Uses a straw.
- Removes socks.
- Helps with dressing by pushing arms through sleeves and legs through pant opening.
- Sleeps between 12–14 h per day.

18 Months

Developmental Milestones/Norms

- Engages with others for play.
- Points to pictures in a book.
- Points to object of interest to draw attention to it.
- Turns and looks at adult if something new happens.
- Uses words to ask for help.
- Identifies at least two body parts.
- Names at least five familiar objects.
- Walks up steps with 2 feet per step with hand held.
- Sits in a small chair.
- Carries a toy while walking.
- Scribbles spontaneously.
- Throws small ball a few feet while standing.

Age-appropriate Activities of Daily Living

- Uses a straw.
- Scoops food with a spoon and feeds self.
- Removes socks.
- Helps with dressing by pushing arms through sleeves and legs through pant opening.
- Sleeps between 12–14 h per day.

24 Months

Developmental Milestones/Norms

- Plays alongside other children (parallel play).
- Uses 50 words.
- Combines two words into short phrase or sentence.
- Follows 2-step command.
- Names at least five body parts.
- Uses words that are 50% intelligible to strangers.
- Kicks a ball.
- Jumps off the ground with two feet.
- Runs with coordination.
- Stacks objects.
- Turns pages in a book.
- Uses hands to turn objects like lids, toys, knobs.
- Draws lines.

Age-appropriate Activities of Daily Living

- Drinks from a cup (no lid) without spilling.
- Scoops well with a spoon.
- Takes off simple clothing such as pushing pants or pulling off socks.
- Removes shoes.
- Once the shirt is over their head, they can find and push arms through shirt opening.
- Sleeps between 12–14 h per day.

30 Months

Developmental Milestones/Norms

- Engages in pretend or imaginary play.
- Tries to get a caregiver to watch by saying, "Look at me!"
- Uses pronouns correctly.
- Begins to walk upstairs alternating feet.
- Runs well without falling.
- Grasps crayon with thumb and fingers instead of fist.
- Copies a vertical line.
- Catches large balls.

Age-appropriate Activities of Daily Living

- Urinates in a potty or toilet.
- Spears food with a fork.
- Washes and dries hands.
- Attempts to don socks.

- Unbuttons a large button.
- Dons easy clothing such as jackets or open-front shirts without zipping or buttoning them.
- Sleeps between 12–14 h per day.

Recommended Intervention

Sensory Integration

Sensory input affects development, learning, and behavior which impacts childhood engagement and participation in occupations. Differences in sensory functions can create challenges in daily life with feeding, dressing, grooming, bathing, sleeping, social participation, movement, and play. Some children with sensory difficulties may avoid or reject engaging in such activities and often become anxious, fearful, frustrated, or aggressive if forced to participate. Other children seem oblivious to touch, pain, movement, taste, smells, sights, or sounds. While others seek intense sensory stimulation. Some children may need a referral for a sensory integration evaluation and regular therapy to change the neuroplasticity in the brain.

Specific sensory strategies, however, can be offered to help the child feel more comfortable, manage his/her behavior, and increase attention. A *sensory diet* can be created to embed sensory experiences throughout the day to support an optimal level of alertness or calming in the child's environment. A sensory diet is an activity plan specifically tailored to an individual's sensory needs in order to assist in self-regulation [7]. This tool is based on the framework developed by Wilbarger [8]. Proprioceptive or heavy muscle activities (chair push-ups or animal walks) and linear movement (jumping on a trampoline) are typically regulating activities and good to incorporate every 90 min–2 h. Environmental modifications can be provided as well to help manage sensory input or the activity itself can be modified to avoid the unpleasant sensation. Examples of regulating activities can be found in the Regulating Activities Handout in the appendix.

Feeding: Deep pressure can be applied to the child's gums or palate to help reduce oral hypersensitivity. Provide textured objects, teethers, vibrating toys, and playfully encourage exploration with hands, face, and mouth. Introduce new flavors and textures gradually while also changing food temperatures. A spoon, toy, or teething ring can be dipped into new food items.

Dressing: Tags or seams in clothes can be unbearable. They can be cut out or seamless clothes can be purchased. Soft cotton tends to be most tolerated and compression garments like compression tees and biking shorts can be helpful to provide uniform pressure. The smell of clothing may contribute to sensitivities, so no-scent laundry detergent should be used. Allow the child to pick his/her own clothes.

Bathing: Let the child perform touching on him/herself to wash face and body parts. Encourage water play with a variety of toys, use deep or firm pressure and rhythmic touch with a washcloth. Deep pressure to the head can be helpful before shampooing. A hand-held shower allows the child to operate direction of water pressure on the body. Wrap the child tightly in a towel while applying pressure after the bath.

Sleep: Children this age should sleep 12–14 h a day and have at least one nap during the day. Regular naptime and bedtime routines are essential. Lack of sleep may compromise physical growth, health, cognition, attention, and behavior. Encourage sleep-promoting activities. Put the child in the crib drowsy but awake so he/she can learn to self-regulate and fall asleep independently. Establish quiet time before bedtime and read a book, rock in a rocking chair, sing quiet songs, take a warm bath, give a back rub, or hold a favorite stuffed animal. Consider the sensory qualities of the sleep environment such as light, sounds, odors, and bedding. Children do best in a dark, quiet room. Use soft, rhythmic music with natural sounds. Vanilla, lavender, or rose scents are calming. Cotton, flannel, or other smooth textures are best for clothes and bedding. Weighted blankets may help facilitate calmness to fall asleep; however, it should be removed once the child falls asleep or after approximately 30 min. Weighted blankets should be no more than 10% of the child's body weight, per weighted blanket protocol [9]. Minimize screen time (turn off at least 1 h before bed). Social stories or video modeling can be used to help establish a healthy bedtime routine. Social stories use words and pictures to explain a specific occurrence. Incorporate actual pictures of the child in the story and use first person language (In the evening, I get ready to go to sleep. I take a warm bath, read a book, and cuddle with my teddy bear…) Video modeling involves recording an individual completing a desired behavior and then watching the video for reinforcement. Parents, siblings, or the child can be videotaped.

Behavioral: Children at this age start showing frustration and getting upset when unable to accomplish a task, communicate needs, or get what they want. It is important to provide simple rules with clear and reasonable expectations that should be communicated in a developmentally appropriate manner. Use firm, consistent, and appropriate discipline without shaking, yelling, or hitting. Positive reinforcement can be used to increase desired behaviors (playing a game sets the stage to reward and reinforce good behaviors with time together in enjoyable activities.)

An effective tool for discipline is positive attention. Pay attention and praise good or desired behaviors while ignoring undesired ones, as long as they do not put the child or others in danger. Model and role-play desired behaviors. Prepare the child for changes in routine in advance. Use a time-out to deal with undesirable behaviors. Time-out at this age should be brief 60–90 s. Use a calm voice and few words. If a negative problem behavior persists, try to identify the purpose of it – escape, avoid, attention, obtain, or transition. Children may also be acting out if their sensory system is dysregulated. Consider all possibilities for undesirable behavior before reacting. For more information on how to shape a child's behavior, please refer to the following website from the American Academy of Pediatrics: https://www.aap.org/en-us/Documents/ttb_bring_out_best.pdf

Developmental and Biomechanical

Children may demonstrate decreased range of motion, strength, endurance, coordination, low tone, delayed integration of reflexes, and an overall delay in skill development. These deficits can impact the participation in age-appropriate activities of daily living and motor skills.

Dressing is a slow process for young children, so allow plenty of time to practice and select clothing that will present a minimum of frustration. Use pull-on shirts, elastic waist pants, and clothing with minimal closures (buttons, zippers, snaps). Self-help toys, books, or adult clothes for dress-up may aid in teaching some basic dressing skills. A handout for age-appropriate self-care skills (Self-Care Skills Handout) is available in the appendix as well as a handout on getting dressed (Getting Dressed Handout).

Fine motor coordination and hand strength are required for children to engage in the childhood occupations of play, activities of daily living, and preschool. A child with decreased skills in these areas will have difficulty with eating utensils, writing utensils, and basic object manipulation. They can engage in a variety of activities to improve these skills such as playing with pop-apart beads, squeeze playdoh, make a snake or other shapes, dig in dirt or sand, pop packaging bubbles, squeeze hand rockets, and build with Duplos or any simple construction toy. Caregivers can be provided handouts with developmentally appropriate activities for fine motor development and hand strengthening (see Fine Motor, Bilateral Coordination, and Hand Strengthening Activities Handout in the appendix). Refer to specific age-appropriate skills on preceding pages.

When to Refer for Further Evaluation

If a child is displaying developmental delay or dysfunction, a referral to early intervention or school-based therapy is recommended. If sensory concerns are significantly impacting the quality of life for the child and family, refer for sensory integration evaluation.

The following are red flags for Autism Spectrum Disorder (ASD) and the child should be further evaluated:

- The child fails to orient to name.
- The child does not point at objects.
- The child does not play with a variety of toys.
- The child lacks appropriate eye gaze.
- The child lacks sharing interest or enjoyment.
- The child lacks warm, joyful expressions.
- The child lacks coordination of nonverbal communication.
- The child has delayed speech and language skills.
- The child demonstrates repetitive movements or posturing of body.
- The child demonstrates repetitive movements with objects.

Additional Recommendations

No TV or digital media until 18 months of age. 18 months–4 years should watch no more than 1 h of high-quality programming/day.
   Read, sing, and talk to the child.
   Promote physically active family time.

Preschool (3–4 years of Age)

Overview

The ages between 3 and 4 are often called the preschool years and full of curiosity and a growing sense of independence. Increasing motor skills provide opportunities for a variety of physical activities and group games. Ball skills continue to develop, and a child can copy shapes while drawing and use scissors. He/she can dress and undress, but may need help with fasteners, maintain bladder and bowel control with occasional accidents, manage utensils well to feed self, wash and dry hands, and brush teeth. The child can carry on conversations and tell stories. He/she is learning how to manage feelings in socially acceptable ways and attempt to solve problems. Cooperative and well-developed imaginative play are reflective of this period. Argumentative behavior can be frustrating and challenging at times as the child is attempting to understand how and why things happen. Media use has a strong appeal during this period and should be limited to 1–2 h of high-quality programming/day.

   Preschool children are often seen in a PC clinic for a physical or well-check visit, an acute health concern, or a developmental concern. Common biomechanical and developmental concerns seen at this age in a PC clinic include decreased strength, endurance, coordination, postural control, hypotonia, and overall delay of skill development. Common behavioral/sensory concerns include increased or decreased activity level, sensitivity or reactivity to the environment, adaptability to changes in routine, intensity of responses, and engagement with others. Concerns with age-appropriate occupations include picky eating, sleeping, dressing, toileting, play, and social participation, along with decreased motor and process performance skills. Refer to Table 32.5 for the Frame of References that guide PC pediatric OT for this age group.

Caregiver Education

Please see *PEDIATRIC. Caregiver Education for Pediatrics and Adolescence* section on 2–5 Years of Age in the appendix.

Recommended Assessments

The following are recommended assessments used to screen Preschool-age children in a pediatric PC setting. In a fast-paced PC setting, time may be limited. Each assessment has the age range for the given assessment and the time it may take to administer.

- Peabody Motor Development Chart (0–5 years) (Observational chart).
- Ages and Stages Questionnaires, 3rd Edition (0–5 years) (10–15 min).
- Ages and Stages Social-emotional, 2nd Edition (1–72 months) (10–15 min).

Table 32.5 Preschool (3–4 Year) frame of reference guide

Sensory Integration Frame of Reference	
Developmental Milestone/ Norm(3–4 year)	• Sensory input affects development, learning, and behavior which impacts childhood engagement and participation in occupations • Differences in sensory functions can create challenges in daily life • Specific sensory strategies can be offered to help the child feel more comfortable during dressing and sleeping
Recommended assessment	• Short sensory profile • Observation • Parent report
Recommended intervention/ Parent education	• For dyspraxia, provide opportunities for active participation in safe environments to help increase self-esteem and confidence. Sports, swimming, gymnastics, obstacle courses, running, jumping, and climbing on playground equipment are all great activities
Behavioral frame of reference	
Developmental milestone/ Norm(3–4 year)	• Preschoolers are notorious picky eaters, often limiting foods to just a couple favorite items. It's a common concern that many children will eventually outgrow • Children this age show frustration when attempting to understand how and why things happen
Recommended assessment	• Ages and stages • Parental report
Recommended intervention/ Parent education	• Prepare one meal with a couple of approved foods your child will eat • Offer incentives such as stickers or special toys to try new foods • Offer regular mealtimes and snack times • Serve food family style and allow the child to put food on their own plates • Allow child to play with food • Be patient. Some kids must be exposed to new foods at least ten times before they will try it • For behavior, it is important to provide rules with clear and reasonable expectations that should be communicated in a developmentally appropriate manner • Children may also be acting out if their sensory system is dysregulated. Consider all possibilities for undesirable behavior before reacting

(continued)

Table 32.5 (continued)

Sensory Integration Frame of Reference	
Developmental and Biomechanical Frames of reference	
Developmental milestone/ Norm(3–4 year)	3 years • Engages in imaginative play • Plays in cooperation and shares • Uses 3-word sentences • Uses words that are 75% intelligible to strangers • Tells you a story from a book or TV • Compares things using words like *shorter* or *bigger* • Understands simple prepositions, such as *under* or *on* • Pedals a tricycle • Climbs on and off chair or couch • Jumps forward • Draws a single circle • Draws a person with a head and one other part • Cuts with child scissors Age-appropriate ADL • Enters bathroom and urinates independently • Dons coat, jacket, or shirt with little help • Dons shoes, although right and left orientation may be incorrect • Dons socks with little help for heel orientation • Pulls down simple clothing (elastic waist pants) independently • Buttons large front buttons • Zips/unzips if the shank is connected • Eats independently • Sleeps between 12–14 h per day 4 years • Engages in well-developed imaginative play • Uses 4-word sentences • Uses words that are 100% intelligible to strangers • Follows simple rules when playing games • Answers questions like "What do you do when you are sleepy?" • Tells caregiver a story from a book • Skips on one foot • Climbs stairs alternating feet without support • Draws a person with at least three body parts • Draws a simple cross • Grasps pencil with thumb and fingers instead of fist Age-appropriate ADL • Enters bathroom and has a bowel movement independently • Brushes teeth • Inserts shank and zips/unzips a jacket with practice • Buttons 3 or 4 buttons • Finds front side of clothing and dresses self with supervision • Laces shoes • Dons socks with the correct orientation • Sleeps between 11–13 h per day • A handout for age-appropriate self-care skills (see the self-care skills handout in the appendix)

Table 32.5 (continued)

Sensory Integration Frame of Reference	
Recommended assessment	• Ages and stages • Parent report observation • Peabody motor development chart
Recommended intervention/ Parent education	• Catch and throw games, obstacle courses, rhythm pattern hand games, squirt (water) bottle games, paper punch around a picture, build with Legos, pick up items with tweezers, textured rubbings, climbing, swinging, swimming, gymnastics, scooter board activities, card games, hopscotch, and tug-of-war can be used to improve fine motor coordination, bilateral hand skills, hand strength, and postural control. Schedules, checklists, social stories, and video modelling can be used for any ADL • Caregivers can be provided handouts with developmentally appropriate activities for fine motor and bilateral hand skill development, and hand strengthening (see the fine motor, bilateral coordination, and hand strengthening handout in the appendix)

References: Web Resources:https://www.aap.org/en-us/Documents/ttb_bring_out_best.pdf

- Occupational Profile—Short Child Occupational Profile (SCOPE) (0–21 years) (10–20 min).
- Parenting Stress Index, Fourth Edition Short Form (1 month–12 years) (20 min).
- Survey of Well-being of Young Children (SWYC) (2–60 months) (15 min).
- Short Sensory Profile 2 (0–14:11 years) (5–20 min).
- Bruininks-Oseretsky Test of Motor Proficiency (BOT-2) Brief Form (4–21:11 years) (15–30 min).

Three Years

Developmental Milestones/Norms

- Engages in imaginative play.
- Plays in cooperation and shares.
- Uses 3-word sentences.
- Uses words that are 75% intelligible to strangers.
- Tells you a story from a book or TV.
- Compares things using words like *shorter* or *bigger.*
- Understands simple prepositions, such as *under* or *on.*
- Pedals a tricycle.
- Climbs on and off chair or couch.
- Jumps forward.
- Draws a single circle.
- Draws a person with a head and one other part.
- Cuts with child scissors.

Age-appropriate Activities of Daily Living

- Enters bathroom and urinates independently.
- Dons coat, jacket, or shirt with little help.
- Dons shoes, although right and left orientation may be incorrect.
- Dons socks with little help for heel orientation.
- Pulls down simple clothing (elastic waist pants) independently.
- Buttons large front buttons.
- Zips/unzips if the shank is connected.
- Eats independently.
- Sleeps between 12–14 h per day.

Four Years

Developmental Milestones/Norms

- Engages in well-developed imaginative play.
- Uses 4-word sentences.
- Uses words that are 100% intelligible to strangers.
- Follows simple rules when playing games.
- Answers questions like "What do you do when you are sleepy?"
- Tells caregiver a story from a book.
- Skips on one foot.
- Climbs stairs alternating feet without support.
- Draws a person with at least three body parts.
- Draws a simple cross.
- Unbuttons and buttons medium-sized buttons.
- Grasps pencil with thumb and fingers instead of fist.

Age-appropriate Activities of Daily Living

- Enters bathroom and has a bowel movement independently.
- Brushes teeth.
- Inserts shank and zips/unzips a jacket with practice.
- Buttons 3 or 4 buttons.
- Finds front side of clothing and dresses self with supervision.
- Laces shoes.
- Dons socks with the correct orientation.
- Sleeps between 11–13 h per day.

Recommended Intervention

Sensory Integration

The Alert Program for Self-Regulation: How Does Your Engine Run? By Williams and Shellenberger [10] can be introduced to help children identify and manage their level of alertness for optimal function at home and school. Please see Toddler (1–2 year) sensory integration intervention.

Dressing: Same as for Toddler (1–2 year).

Sleep: Children this age should sleep 11–14 h a day, with possibly one nap during the day. Regular bedtime routines are essential. Lack of sleep may compromise physical growth, health, cognition, attention, and behavior. Encourage sleep-promoting activities by establishing quiet time before bedtime and read a book, play calming music, take a warm bath, give a back rub, or hold a favorite toy or blanket. Consider the sensory qualities of the sleep environment such as light, sounds, odors, and bedding. Children do best in a dark, quiet room. Use soft, rhythmic music with natural sounds. Vanilla, lavender, or rose scents are calming. Cotton, flannel, or other smooth textures are best for clothes and bedding. Weighted blankets may help facilitate calmness to fall asleep; however, it should be removed once the child falls asleep or approximately after 30 minutes. Weighted blankets should be no more than 10% of the child's body weight, per weighted blanket protocol [9]. Minimize screen time (turn off at least 1 h before bed). Social stories or video modeling can be used to help establish a healthy bedtime routine. Social stories use words and pictures to explain a specific occurrence. Incorporate actual pictures of the child in the story and use first person language (In the evening, I get ready to go to sleep. I take a warm bath, read a book, and cuddle with my teddy bear…) Video modeling involves recording an individual completing a desired behavior and then watching the video for reinforcement. Parents, siblings, or the child can be videotaped.

Praxis: Children with dyspraxia have difficulty planning and executing novel tasks and appear awkward and clumsy. They often have difficulty with dressing, object manipulation, drawing, and play as well. Active participation in safe environments is essential to help increase self-esteem and confidence. Encourage sports participation, swimming, and gymnastics through the local community center where the child is welcomed and supported. The focus is less on competition and more on participation. Provide opportunities to create and navigate obstacle courses, run, jump, and climb on playground equipment. Break down activities into smaller steps and then practice doing a small part of a task at a time. Have the child observe others performing everyday activities.

Behavioral

Picky Eaters-Preschoolers are notorious picky eaters, often limiting foods to just a couple favorite items. It's a common concern that many children will eventually outgrow. Here are several tips to help picky eaters:

- Prepare one meal with a couple of approved foods your child will eat. Limit processed food and sugary drinks. Sugary drinks include soda, fruit juice, lemonade, and sports drinks. Sugary drinks can lead to cavities and unhealthy weight gain. Water and milk are best to build strong bones.
- Offer incentives such as stickers or special toys to try new foods.
- Offer regular mealtimes and snack times. Limit foods between these times because children who graze throughout the day will not be hungry at mealtimes. Sit together at the table and turn off the TV.
- Serve food family style and allow the child to put food on their own plates. It helps them get used to sights and smells of different food items. Use smaller plates, bowls, cups, and utensils.
- Allow child to play with food.
- Be patient. Some kids must be exposed to new foods at least ten times before they will try it. Encourage, but do not pressure kids to eat.

Behavior: Children this age show frustration when attempting to understand how and why things happen. It is important to provide rules with clear and reasonable expectations that should be communicated in a developmentally appropriate manner. Use firm, consistent, and appropriate discipline without yelling or hitting. Positive reinforcement can be used to increase desired behaviors (playing a game sets the stage to reward and reinforce good behaviors with time together in enjoyable activities.) An effective tool for discipline is attention. Pay attention and praise good or desired behaviors, while ignoring undesired ones, as long as they do not put the child or others in danger. Model and role-play desired behaviors. Prepare the child for changes in routine or schedule in advance. Use a time-out to deal with undesirable behaviors. Time-out should be 1 min of time-out for every year of age. For example, for a 3-year-old, the time-out would be 3 min. If a negative problem behavior persists, try and identify the purpose of it (escape, avoid, attention, obtain, or transition). Children may also be acting out if their sensory system is dysregulated. Consider all possibilities for undesirable behavior before reacting. For more information on how to shape a child's behavior, please refer to the following website from the American Academy of Pediatrics: https://www.aap.org/en-us/Documents/ttb_bring_out_best.pdf

Developmental and Biomechanical

Children seen in a PC setting may demonstrate decreased strength, endurance, coordination, postural control, hypotonia, and overall delay of skill development. These delays or deficits can impact the participation in age-appropriate activities of daily living, motor skills, and process skills.

Toilet training: most children this age are ready to toilet train if he/she can remain dry for 2 h at a time, recognizes the need to use the toilet (sensation), can get on/off toilet, manage clothing, clean self after toileting, and wash/dry hands. Schedules, checklists, social stories, and video modelling can be used.

Fine motor coordination, bilateral hand skills, and hand strength are all required for children to engage in the childhood occupations of play, activities of daily living, and preschool. A child with decreased skills in these areas will have difficulty with eating utensils, writing utensils, and basic object manipulation. They can engage in a variety of activities to improve these skills such as playing catch/throw games, completing obstacle courses, rhythm pattern hand games, squirt water from a water bottle, use a paper punch around a picture, build with Legos, pick up items with tweezers, and make rubbings of textured surfaces. Caregivers can be provided handouts with developmentally appropriate activities for fine motor and bilateral hand skill development and hand strengthening (see the Fine Motor, Bilateral Coordination, and Hand Strengthening Handout in Appendix).

Postural control is the ability to maintain the center of mass over the base of support. It is required for refined movement and mobility and is an interplay between the sensory, motor, and musculoskeletal systems. It can be observed while a child is standing, sitting, and or during movement tasks. To improve postural control, the child can be encouraged to climb, swing, use pull-up bars on a playground, swim, participate in gymnastics, complete scooter board activities while prone, play board or card games in prone, hopscotch, jumping jacks, jump on a trampoline, pull/push a wagon with someone inside, wheelbarrow walks, and play tug-of-war.

When to Refer for Further Evaluation

If a child is displaying developmental delay or dysfunction, a referral to early intervention or school-based therapy is recommended.

If sensory concerns are significantly impacting the quality of life for the child and family, refer for sensory integration evaluation.

If food preferences and limitations persist and start to affect growth, weight gain, sleep, and bowels, a referral for intervention should be made.

Additional Recommendations
No TV or digital media until 18 months of age. 18 months–4 years should watch no more than 1 h of high-quality programming/day.

Read, sing, and talk to the child.

Promote physically active family time.

School-Aged Children (5–14 Years of Age)

Overview

Children grow and develop greatly in the "school-age" years. They enter school around 5 or 6 years of age, learning to print their name and complete all ADLs independently, to leaving school around 14 years of age having complex problem solving skills and resiliency with life's stressors. When a child reaches school-age years, they are seen by their PCP once a year for a well-visit and as needed for acute illness visits. Commonly seen issues in PC to which an OTP would be beneficial include behavioral issues, such as attention and hyperactivity, sensory processing issues, psychosocial concerns, including bullying and conflict-resolution, issues with independently completing age-appropriate ADLs, as well as sexuality. The OTP is prepared to help an adolescent and their caregiver navigate the complexities of sexuality, especially those with developmental delays. Refer to Table 32.6 for the Frame of References that guide PC pediatric OT for this age group.

Table 32.6 School age (5–14 years) frame of reference guide

Sensory Integration Frame of Reference	
Developmental Milestone/Norm(5–14 Years)	• Exploratory in self-feeding • Becomes increasingly more independent in ADLs • Explores new foods
Recommended assessment	• Short sensory profile 2 • Observation
Recommended intervention/Parent education	• Provide a variety of sensory stimuli during play • Encourage outdoor and "rough and tumble" play
Motor Learning and Motor Control Frame of reference	
Developmental milestone/Norm(5–14 years)	• Child develops more complex motor movements: jumping → hopping on one leg → skipping
Recommended assessment	• BOT-2
Recommended intervention/Parent education	• Encourage activities that cross midline • Encourage activities in prone
Biomechanical frame of reference	
Developmental milestone/Norm(5–14 years)	• Symmetric strength in extremities • Functional ROM in joints
Recommended assessment	• ROM testing • MMT
Recommended intervention/Parent education	• Encourage outdoor play • Provide appropriate home exercises and activities, as necessary

Table 32.6 (continued)

Sensory Integration Frame of Reference

Developmental frame of reference	
Developmental milestone/ Norm(5–14 years)	5 and 6 years • Balances on one foot; hops; skips • Can draw a person with at least six body parts • Prints some letters/numbers • Can copy squares and triangles • Has good articulation/language skills • Can count to 10 • Names four or more colors • Follows simple directions Age-appropriate ADL • Is able to tie a knot • Dresses with minimal assistance • Sleeps between 10–11 h per day 7 and 8 years • Demonstrates social and emotional competence (including self-regulation) • Forms caring, supportive relationships with family members, other adults, and peers Age-appropriate ADL • Engages in healthy nutrition and physical activity behaviors • Sleeps between 10–11 h per day 9 and 10 years • Demonstrates social and emotional competence (including self-regulation) • Forms caring, supportive relationships with family members, other adults, and peers • Uses independent decision-making skills (including problem-solving) • Displays a sense of self-confidence and hopefulness Age-appropriate ADL • Engages in healthy nutrition and physical activity behaviors • Sleeps between 10–11 h per day 11–14 years • Forms caring, supportive relationships with family members, other adults, and peers • Engages in a positive way with the life of the community • Demonstrates physical, cognitive, emotional, social, and moral competencies (including self-regulation) • Exhibits compassion and empathy • Exhibits resiliency when confronted with life stressors • Uses independent decision-making skills (including problem-solving) • Displays a sense of self-confidence, hopefulness, and well-being Age-appropriate ADL • Engages in behaviors that optimize wellness and contribute to a healthy lifestyle • Sleeps between 8–9 h per day

(continued)

Table 32.6 (continued)

Sensory Integration Frame of Reference	
Recommended assessment	• BOT-2 • Skilled observation
Recommended intervention/Parent education	• Create a family plan around the quantity, quality, and location of media use • Promote physical activity (>60 min/day)
Cognitive/Psychosocial frame of reference	
Developmental milestone/ Norm(5–14 years)	• Self-esteem and self-identity development • Incidence of symptoms related to depression are much higher around puberty • Anxiety disorder is the most common childhood mental health issue
Recommended assessment	• Child depression inventory • Beck depression inventory • COPM
Recommended intervention/Parent education	• Encourage environmental modifications (communication on routines, daily schedule, daily planner) • Self-regulation strategies • Build self-efficacy with "just-right" challenges

Caregiver Education

Please see *PEDIATRIC. Caregiver Education for Pediatrics and Adolescence* section for School-Aged Children in the Appendix.

Recommended Assessments

The following are recommended assessments used to screen school-age children in a pediatric PC setting. In a fast-paced PC setting, time may be limited. Each assessment has the age range for the given assessment and the time it may take to administer.

- Occupational Profile—Short Child Occupational Profile (SCOPE) (0–21 years) (10–20 min).
- Short Sensory Profile 2 (0–14:11 years) (5–20 min).
- Bruininks-Oseretsky Test of Motor Proficiency (BOT-2) Brief Form (4–21:11 years) (15–30 min).
- BRIEF2 Screening (5–18 years) (10 min).
- Parenting Stress Index, Fourth Edition Short Form (1 month–12 years) (20 min).
- Child Depression Inventory (7–17 years) (10 min).
- Beck Depression Inventory (13–80 years) (10 min). https://www.ismanet.org/doctoryourspirit/pdfs/Beck-Depression-Inventory-BDI.pdf
- Canadian Occupational Performance Measure (COPM) (6–100 years) (10–45 min).

Developmental Milestones/Norms

5 and 6 Years

Developmental Milestones/Norms

- Balances on one foot; hops; skips.
- Can draw a person with at least six body parts.
- Prints some letters/numbers.
- Can copy squares and triangles.
- Has good articulation/language skills.
- Can count to 10.
- Names four or more colors.
- Follows simple directions.

  Age-appropriate Activities of Daily Living

- Is able to tie a knot.
- Dresses with minimal assistance.
- Sleeps between 10–11 h per day.

Seven and Eight Years

Developmental Milestones/Norms

- Demonstrates social and emotional competence (including self-regulation).
- Forms caring, supportive relationships with family members, other adults, and peers.

  Age-appropriate Activities of Daily Living

- Engages in healthy nutrition and physical activity behaviors.
- Sleeps between 10–11 h per day.

Nine and Ten Years

- Demonstrates social and emotional competence (including self-regulation).
- Forms caring, supportive relationships with family members, other adults, and peers.
- Uses independent decision-making skills (including problem-solving).
- Displays a sense of self-confidence and hopefulness.

  Age-appropriate Activities of Daily Living

- Engages in healthy nutrition and physical activity behaviors.
- Sleeps between 10–11 h per day.

Eleven and Twelve Years

- Forms caring, supportive relationships with family members, other adults, and peers.
- Engages in a positive way with the life of the community.
- Demonstrates physical, cognitive, emotional, social, and moral competencies (including self-regulation).
- Exhibits compassion and empathy.
- Exhibits resiliency when confronted with life stressors.
- Uses independent decision-making skills (including problem-solving).
- Displays a sense of self-confidence, hopefulness, and well-being.

    Age-appropriate Activities of Daily Living

- Engages in behaviors that optimize wellness and contribute to a healthy lifestyle.
- Sleeps between 8–9 h per day.

Recommended Intervention

Sensory Integration

Ayres hypothesized that between 3–7 years of age is a crucial period for sensory integration because of the brain's receptiveness to sensation and its capacity for organizing sensory stimuli. A child's sensorimotor skills continue to mature. At this time, children develop strong inner drives to produce more complicated sensorimotor skills and meet the sensorimotor demands of peers. In this time frame, a child goes from learning to jump to learning to jump rope, from learning to catch a ball to learning to play a motor-complex game of basketball. During this time, children also become more autonomous in completing daily tasks and routines. Parents of school-age children with sensory processing issues often present to a PCP with concerns related to sensory integration. Sensory processing dysfunction may make morning routine hectic (getting dressed, eating breakfast, and getting out the door) and eating at school and home difficult. However, sensory processing dysfunction also impacts other areas of a child's life. These include behavioral (difficulty disciplining child), cognitive (problems paying attention in class, executive functioning), fine/visual motor (difficulty with self-dressing, including learning to tie shoes).

Motor Learning and Motor Control

Coordination and motor control can be assessed through quick screening tools, including the BOT-2 short form. If a child is demonstrating motor concerns such as clumsiness, difficulty coordinating the two sides of the body, or difficulty crossing midline, a referral should be made for further evaluation.

Biomechanical

A quick biomechanical screen would be advantageous in school-aged children. If deficits are noted in active range of motion or strength is significantly different in one side of the body compared to the other, this should be communicated to the PCP. While growing pains are common in this age group, if pain is consistent and/or lasts for longer than 3 months, a referral to a chronic pain OTP or physical therapist may be appropriate. For children with orthotics, the pediatric PC OTP may complete an orthotic fit check and skin check, in which he/she ensures the orthotic is still a good fit and the skin that comes in contact with the orthotic for any redness, rubbing, or skin breakdown. The OTP may also assess a child's wheelchair for fit and appropriateness, as well as a skin assessment for any redness, rubbing, or skin breakdown.

Developmental

Children develop rapidly during their school-age years. Their ability to participate in and complete age appropriate ADLs evolve from learning to tie one's shoe to being responsible for babysitting another child. If a child is demonstrating delay in development, they may require further OT services or suggestions to modify the environment for continued growth and development.

Cognitive/Psychosocial

As children develop in their gross, fine and visual motor skills, it is important that a PC OTP considers social emotional development and executive functioning as well. Anxiety Disorder is the most common childhood mental health issue. While symptoms of anxiety and depression can appear at any stage in childhood, the highest prevalence of depression is during the puberty years. It is important for the pediatric PC OTP to screen for anxiety and depression and refer to the appropriate provider. Attention Deficit Hyperactive Disorder (ADHD) is a condition widely seen in the pediatric population. Behavioral issues seen in ADHD are also widely seen in children with sensory processing differences [11], therefore it may be beneficial to screen for sensory dysfunction as well.

When to Refer for Further Evaluation

If a child is displaying concerns in developmental progress, including independence in ADLs, IADLs, a referral to continued OT services is recommended. It may also be appropriate to recommend the child receives evaluation by a physical therapist (PT), speech therapist, and/or psychotherapist or social worker.

If a child is displaying developmental delay or dysfunction, a referral to school-based therapy is recommended.

If sensory concerns are significantly impacting the quality of life for the child and family, refer for sensory integration evaluation.

If food preferences and limitations persist and start to affect growth, weight gain, sleep, and bowels, a referral for intervention should be made.

Adolescence (15–21 Years of Age)

Overview

Adolescence marks the time of transition from childhood to adulthood. Children and parents begin to prepare for the future. This is often a time to transition into paid employment, post-secondary education, and establishing healthy and meaningful relationships. The pediatric PC OTP addresses pediatric concerns of development while also considering what supports the child and caregiver may need in relation to psychosocial issues. See Table 32.7 for the Frame of References that guide PC pediatric OT for this age group.

Developmental Milestones/Norms

Adolescence (15–21 Years)

- Forms caring, supportive relationships with family members, other adults, and peers.
- Engages in a positive way with the life of the community.
- Demonstrates physical, cognitive, emotional, social, and moral competencies (including self-regulation).
- Exhibits compassion and empathy.
- Exhibits resiliency when confronted with life stressors.
- Uses independent decision-making skills (including problem-solving).
- Displays a sense of self-confidence, hopefulness, and well-being.

  Age-appropriate Activities of Daily Living

- Engages in behaviors that optimize wellness and contribute to a healthy lifestyle.

Table 32.7 Overview of adolescence (15–21 years) frame of reference guide

Sensory Integration Frame of Reference	
Developmental Milestone/Norm(15–21 years)	• Sensory integration is building foundation for executive functioning
Recommended assessment	• Adolescent/adult sensory profile
Recommended intervention/Parent education	• Daily planner • Heavy proprioceptive input prior to task requiring attention
Motor Learning and Motor Control Frame of reference	
Developmental milestone/Norm(15–21 years)	• Motor learning and motor control foundation is now being tested in higher level academic contexts
Recommended assessment	• BOT-2
Recommended intervention/Parent education	• Accommodations including: Typing instead of handwriting for school assignments; Reading strategies
Biomechanical frame of reference	
Developmental milestone/Norm(15–21 years)	• Functional ROM and strength
Recommended assessment	• ROM • MMT
Recommended intervention/Parent education	• Orthotic checks • Skin checks • Wheelchair fitting
Developmental and Cognitive/psychosocial frame of reference	
Developmental milestone/Norm(15–21 years)	• Forms caring, supportive relationships with family members, other adults, and peers • Engages in a positive way with the life of the community • Demonstrates physical, cognitive, emotional, social, and moral competencies (including self-regulation) • Exhibits compassion and empathy • Exhibits resiliency when confronted with life stressors • Uses independent decision-making skills (including problem-solving) • Displays a sense of self-confidence, hopefulness, and well-being *Age-appropriate ADL* • Engages in behaviors that optimize wellness and contribute to a healthy lifestyle • Sleeps between 8–9 h per day
Recommended assessment	• BRIEF2 screening • Child depression inventory • Beck depression inventory • COPM
Recommended intervention/Parent education	• Create a family plan around the quantity, quality, and location of media use • Promote physical activity (>60 min/day) • Daily planner • Accommodations and modifications to environment to support executive functioning

References: [1, 2]

Caregiver Education

Please see *PEDIATRIC. Caregiver Education for Pediatrics and Adolescence* in the Appendix.

Recommended Assessments

The following are recommended assessments used to screen school-age children in a pediatric PC setting. In a fast-paced PC setting, time may be limited. Each assessment has the age range for the given assessment and the time it may take to administer.

- Occupational Profile—Short Child Occupational Profile (SCOPE) (0–21 years) (10–20 min).
- Adolescent/Adult Sensory Profile (11+ years) (5–20 min).
- Bruininks-Oseretsky Test of Motor Proficiency (BOT-2) Brief Form (4–21:11 years) (15–30 min).
- BRIEF2 Screening (5–18 years) (10 min).
- Child Depression Inventory (7–17 years) (10 min).
- Beck Depression Inventory (13–80 years) (10 min). https://www.ismanet.org/doctoryourspirit/pdfs/Beck-Depression-Inventory-BDI.pdf
- Canadian Occupational Performance Measure (COPM) (6–100 years) (10–45 min).

Recommended Intervention

Sensory Integration

Sensory processing dysfunction in adolescence can cause difficulty in executive functioning, including attention and organization. The PC OTP would help the patient and caregiver/parent with environmental modification and accommodations. A daily planner is one accommodation. Another intervention recommendation would be to encourage the patient to participate in heavy proprioceptive input (running, lifting weights, jumping rope, push-ups) prior to any activity that requires sustained attention.

Motor Planning/Motor Control

Coordination and motor control can be assessed through quick screening tools including the BOT-2 short form. Motor concerns typical to be seen in a PC setting may include visual motor integration deficits and/or dyslexia that would impact the child's ability to fully participate in the academic setting. Fine motor deficits may elicit accommodations from the OTP, such as a child who is inefficient with hand-writing may be recommended typing for school assignments. If a child is demon-strating these motor concerns, a referral should be made for further evaluation.

Biomechanical

A quick biomechanical screen would be advantageous in adolescents. If deficits are noted in active range of motion, or strength is significantly different on one side of the body compared to the other, this should be communicated to the PCP. While growing pains are common in this age group, if pain is consistent and/or lasts for longer than three months, a referral to a chronic pain OTP or physical therapist may be appropriate. For children with orthotics, the pediatric PC OTP may com-plete an orthotic fit and skin check, in which he/she ensures the orthotic is still a good fit and the skin that comes in contact with the orthotic for any redness, rub-bing, or skin breakdown. The OTP may also assess a child's wheelchair for fit and appropriateness, as well as a skin assessment for any redness, rubbing, or skin breakdown.

Developmental and Cognitive/Psychosocial

Development in adolescence centers around the teenager's social/emotional and cognitive development. As a child develops, it is important that a PC OTP considers social emotional development and executive functioning as well. Anxiety Disorder is the most common childhood mental health issue. While symptoms of anxiety and depression can appear at any stage in childhood, the highest prevalence of depres-sion is during the puberty years. It is important for the pediatric PC OTP to screen for anxiety and depression and refer to the appropriate provider. Attention Deficit Hyperactive Disorder (ADHD) is a condition widely seen in the pediatric popula-tion. Behavioral issues seen in ADHD are also widely seen in people with sensory processing differences [11], therefore it may be beneficial to screen for sensory dysfunction as well.

When to Refer for Further Evaluation

If an adolescent is displaying concerns in any of the aforementioned areas that are impeding independence in ADLs, IADLs, a referral to continued OT services is recommended. It may also be appropriate to recommend the child receives evalua-tion by a physical therapist (PT), speech therapist, and/or psychotherapist or social worker (Table 32.7).

References

1. O'Brien JC, Kuhaneck H. Case-smith's occupational therapy for children and adolescents. 8th ed. St Louis, MO: Elsevier, Inc.; 2019.
2. Hagan JF, Shaw JS, Duncan PM, editors. Bright futures: Guidelines for health supervision of infants, children, and adolescents. 4th ed. Elk Grove Village, IL: American Academy of Pediatrics; 2017.
3. Centers for Disease Control and Prevention. Learn the signs. Act Early. 2019. https://www.cdc.gov/ncbddd/actearly/index.html.
4. Johnson CR, Turner K, Stewart PA, Schmidt B, Shui A, Macklin E, Reynolds A, James J, Johnson SL, Courtney PM, Hyman SL. Relationships between feeding problems, behavioral characteristics and nutritional quality in children with ASD. J Autism Dev Disord. 2014;44(9):2175–84.
5. Shreve M, Chu A. Pediatric Thumb Deformities. Bull Hosp Jt Dis. 2016;74(1):98–108.
6. Pathway Awareness Foundation. Early Infant Assessment Redefined. n.d.
7. Pingale V, Fletcher T, Candler C. The effects of sensory diets on children's classroom behaviors. J Occup Ther Sch Early Interv. 2019;12(2):225–38.
8. Wilbarger P, Wilbarger JL. Sensory defensiveness in children aged 2–12: an intervention guide for parents and other caretakers. Framingham, MA: Therapro; 1991.
9. Gee BM, Peterson TG, Buck A, Lloyd K. Improving sleep quality using weighted blankets among young children with an autism spectrum disorder. Int J Ther Rehabil. 2016;23(4):173–81.
10. Williams MS, Shellenberger S. "How does your engine run?" In: A leader's guide to the Alert Program for Self-regulation. Albuquerque: Therapy Works; 1994.
11. Ghanizadeh A. Sensory processing problems in children with ADHD, a systematic review. Psychiatry Investig. 2011;8:89–94. https://doi.org/10.4306/pi.2011.8.2.89.

Chapter 33
Pelvic Floor Dysfunction

Claire Giuliano, Laura M. Milligan, and Cindy C. Ivy

Introduction

Pelvic floor dysfunction refers to impaired function in the bladder, bowel, sexual organs, and/or surrounding tissue structures. Treatment varies based on the type of dysfunction or condition, and seeks to address the accompanying symptoms of pain, tension, weakness, and limitations in ADL performance. The Centers for Medicare and Medicaid Service (CMS) recognizes the pelvic floor diagnoses below as treatable and reimbursable by rehabilitation professionals. This list of conditions represents the most commonly treated diagnoses and are not a full representation of pelvic floor dysfunction treated by OTPs.

- Urinary Incontinence
- Fecal Incontinence
- Pelvic Organ Prolapse
- Constipation
- Dyspareunia

Common Pelvic Floor Dysfunction

Urinary incontinence (UI) is the involuntary loss of bladder control, and can range from occasional urinary leaking to complete voiding of the bladder. Studies show

C. Giuliano
Department of Health Sciences, Northern Arizona University, Flagstaff, AZ, USA

L. M. Milligan (✉)
Department of Health Sciences, Northern Arizona University, Phoenix, AZ, USA

C. C. Ivy
Northern Arizona University, Phoenix Biomedical Campus, Phoenix, AZ, USA
e-mail: Cynthia.ivy@nau.edu

© Springer Nature Switzerland AG 2023
S. Dahl-Popolizio et al. (eds.), *Primary Care Occupational Therapy*,
https://doi.org/10.1007/978-3-031-20882-9_33

that about 50% of women and 25% of men report suffering from bladder incontinence [1]. The American College of Obstetricians and Gynecologists recognizes
three main types of UI: stress UI, urge UI, and mixed incontinence.

- *Stress Urinary Incontinence*

  - Stress UI is characterized by leaking urine when coughing, laughing, or
    sneezing, or engaging in high impact activities such as running or jumping.

- *Urge Urinary Incontinence*

  - Urge UI is characterized when an individual experiences a strong and sudden
    urge that is difficult to control. Urge UI may also be referred to as detrusor
    instability or spastic bladder.

- *Mixed Incontinence*

  - Mixed UI combines the symptoms of Urge and Stress UI.

Fecal Incontinence is the unexpected leakage of feces in the form of solid, liquid,
or gas. This can range from occasional leaking of stool or gas, to complete emptying
of the bowel.

Constipation describes the difficulty of passing feces through bowel movements,
usually due to hardened stool and/or pain. This occurs when the colon absorbs too
much water, or the contraction of the colon is slow or delayed in transit time. This
can be due to diet, physical inactivity, dysfunction of gastrointestinal mobility, medication side effects, or dehydration. Constipation is the most common gastrointestinal complaint [2].

Pelvic Organ Prolapse is the descent of one or more of the following: Anterior
vaginal wall, posterior vaginal wall, uterus, or the vaginal vault [3].

Dyspareunia is pain with sexual intercourse, which can occur before, after, or
during intercourse. Pain can occur on external genitals, deep pelvic layers, or the
lower abdomen. Pain can be due to a medical condition or psychological cause such
as trauma or negative feelings toward a partner. Common causes of dyspareunia
include childbirth, imperforate hymen, coarse pubic hair, small introitus, endome-
triosis, diabetes (due to fragile mucosa), vaginismus, vulvodynia, chronic gastrointestinal disorders, fibroids, and urinary tract infection [4]. Dyspareunia exists in the
absence of organic disease.

Role of PCP

The PCP will often diagnose these conditions and refer to a specialist such as a uro-
gynecologist, urologist, gastroenterologist, obstetrics and gynecologist (OBGYN),
pain specialist, psychologist, physical therapist and/or OTP, as deemed warranted.
The PCP may also order special tests and prescribe medications or durable medical
equipment (DME) for symptom management. If the PCP is trained in pessary insertion for prolapsed pelvic organs, the PCP will fit and insert this device for structural
support and symptom management.

Common Comorbidities

There are many conditions potentially causing or co-existing with pelvic dysfunction. These include, but are not limited to, malignancies, pelvic congestion syndrome, pelvic inflammatory disease, radiation lesions, interstitial cystitis, urinary tract infections, abdominal or pelvic trigger points, lower back pain, nerve entrapment, depression, anxiety, obesity, urinary tract infections, irritable bowel syndrome, and peripartum pelvic syndrome [5]. Individuals may also experience sleep deficiency related to pelvic dysfunction, which may in turn create additional health concerns, including hypertension, dyslipidemia, cardiovascular disease, weight-related issues, metabolic syndrome, Type 2 Diabetes, and even colorectal cancer [6]. A short pelvic floor may also contribute to pelvic pain and dysfunction [7].

Role of OTP

Identify factors that affect function and quality of life; provide actionable interventions and recommendations.

Occupational Impact

Any of the diagnoses associated with pelvic floor dysfunction may have a profound occupational impact by way of disruption, deprivation, or imbalance in a person's daily occupations.

Self-care is impacted through difficulty with keeping clothes clean, mobility, home management, and community activities. One patient stated that she bought two pairs of every type of jeans and slacks that she wore and carried large handbags so that she would always have a change of clothing with her. She went on to say that she sometimes carried two extra sets.

Productivity is similarly impacted. One teacher left her job due to urge incontinence. She was unable to leave the students unattended in the classroom for her frequent bathroom needs. People may be hesitant to participate in both paid and unpaid work due to distractions from, and preoccupation with, the symptoms associated with pelvic floor dysfunction.

Enjoyment of leisure, social, and sexual activities is disrupted. Smells created from incontinence may be embarrassing and shameful to the individual experiencing pelvic floor dysfunction, rendering the individual to avoid leisure or social activities. If restrooms are unavailable in public areas, this may create further isolation. Pain and fear of accidents may interrupt enjoyment of sexual intercourse.

Rest and sleep can be disrupted by nocturia, urinary frequency, and/or pelvic pain.

Individuals may face financial burden, especially with urinary and fecal incontinence management. The average annual cost of urinary incontinence alone is over
$25 billion in the United States, which averages over $3500 in bladder management
costs for each individual [8].

OT Areas of Emphasis

The OTP will provide intervention by way of both remediation and compensation.
The therapy for remediation includes strengthening and mobility, life management,
bladder retraining, biofeedback, electrical stimulation, relaxation and breathing
techniques, and activity modification. Compensation techniques will also include
life management and activity modification, along with environmental modifications,
training in adaptive equipment, schedule planning and coordinating with other team
members. The OTP should also assess for common behavioral health comorbidities
such as depression and anxiety with this population.

Evaluation

Occupational profile should be obtained with identification from patients regarding
impact of condition or dysfunction on I/ADLs, work, sleep, social participation,
leisure activities, education, and play. Assessment tools should be used for thorough
patient feedback. Biomechanics of the pelvis should be assessed externally, including the surrounding structures of hips, back, and lower extremities. If indicated, an
internal exam should be conducted after informed consent is given by the patient.
Internal exams should be used to identify muscle strength, endurance, coordination,
reflex function, and stability of all three layers of the pelvic floor. Prolapse stage
and scar integrity can also be assessed with an internal exam. *Internal exam requires
advanced clinical training or certification and should not be performed otherwise.*

Suggested Assessment Tools

- Occupational profile should be obtained with the use of open-ended questions
  and keen listening and communication techniques due to sensitivity of discuss-
  ing this topic. Eye contact, affirmation and clarifying questions help to move this
  portion of the evaluation forward. Use a private room with soft lighting and free
  from distractions. Table lamp, comfortable chair, and commode chair (in case of
  emergency) should be in the room to put the patient at ease. During the occupational profile, ask the patient if they are having intercourse without consent. This
  can cause dyspareunia.

- General health and comorbidities status can be gleaned from the medical record; it is also reassuring to the patient to have them repeat some of this information as it is often relevant to the pelvic floor diagnosis.
- Determine history of past therapies (PT, OT, Psychology, Nutrition, other). What has worked? This section of the evaluation may lead to a solution-oriented approach to therapy. At times, focusing on what worked in the past will lead to an excellent OT plan for intervention in the present.
- Evaluate mobility, sensation, posture, upper and lower extremity active range of motion: this is important to understand patient factors that may be contributing to problems (slowness, lack of coordination with clothing, general deconditioning leading to pelvic floor weakness or prolapse, additive effects of pain concerns).
- General profile of urination and defecation schedules. Typical bladder health consists of urination every 3–4 hours, and every 1–3 days for defecation [3]. Dietary profile, including fluid and fiber intake.
- Pain scale.
- Pelvic Floor Impact Questionnaire-Short Form (PFIQ-7).
- Pelvic Floor Disability Index (PFDI-20).
- Pelvic Organ Prolapse Questionnaire (POP-Q).
- Urogenital Distress Inventory Short Form (UDI-6).
- Incontinence Impact Questionnaire-Short Form (IIQ-7).
- Incontinence Quality of life Questionnaire (I-QOL).
- Bristol Stool Chart.
- Bowel or Bladder Diary.
- Vulvar Pain Functional Questionnaire (V-Q).
- Manual Muscle Testing of pelvic floor: *this requires advanced training and should not be performed without proper training or certification.* This involves testing of muscle strength, endurance, coordination, and stability of the three layers of the pelvic floor starting from the superficial perineum to the deep layer of the pelvic floor.
- If pelvic floor biofeedback equipment is available, baseline measurement can be obtained of the pelvic floor muscle contraction and relaxation responses. It is recommended to use this tool during intervention if it is used as part of the evaluation.

Intervention Strategies

Urinary Incontinence

- *Stress:*
  - Instruction in finding and contracting the pelvic floor muscles is the first and most important evidence-based intervention, which should be done through external observation of perineal reflexes, muscle contraction and control, as

well as internal exam [9, 10]. *Internal exam requires advanced clinical training or certification and should not be performed otherwise.*

- The patient can use a hand mirror or their own hand as feedback by placing near the anus or vagina so they can practice contracting. If biofeedback equipment is available, this is also a helpful tool in identifying the pelvic floor muscles which must be performed by the therapist. Biofeedback can be used to guide with down-training of spastic or high tone pelvic floor muscles, or aid in contraction of weak pelvic floor muscles.
- Electrical stimulation using a probe intended to insert in the vagina can also stimulate a muscle contraction and may be used as a teaching tool to identify and self-contract if stress incontinence is due to weak pelvic floor muscles.
- Setting a smart phone or other device to provide reminders to contract can be helpful, or link the contractions with an activity that is done frequently throughout the day such as turning a door knob or answering a phone.

- *Urge:*

  - Detrusor instability or urge incontinence may be successfully treated through a combination of bladder retraining and dietary modification such as:
  - Bladder diaries.
  - Track exactly when one urinates. One can estimate the volume by counting seconds while urinating. Each second is about 15 ml. Normal urination is about 250–400 mL each urination. Have the patient bring the diary with them to therapy.
  - Timed/scheduled voiding.

    The goal of timed voiding is to gradually increase the time between voids while keeping it at regular intervals. Thus, if a person can only wait 40 min between voids, they are to void every 40 min, then gradually increase to every 45 min, then every 50 min, etc. until they are about 2 hour or greater increments. Use of the diary is helpful in the training. A wearable device reminder may also be useful.

  - Relaxation strategies.

    Any number of relaxation strategies may be helpful with detrusor instability. One effective technique is to take a deep breath in, and then let it out very slowly through pursed lips over a count of 4 s.
    Guided visual imagery and progressive relaxation techniques may also help to relax the detrusor muscle.
    Simple diaphragmatic breathing may also be helpful in relaxing the detrusor.

  - Contraction of the Pelvic floor muscles/ "Kegel" exercises.
  - Contraction of the pelvic floor muscles produces a reflex relaxation of the detrusor muscle. This technique may be used while undergoing timed voiding schedule to control accidents during a detrusor spasm. The patient should be taught to contract the pelvic floor muscles when they have the urge to void.

– Diet modification.

> Teach the patient to avoid citrus, highly acidic foods, caffeine, spicy foods, and carbonated drinks. These can be irritating and simulating to the detrusor muscle.
> A column of food and drink could be added to the bladder diary to assist in changing eating and drinking behavior.

– Myofascial release around the urethra, bladder, and/or ureters may relieve symptoms if muscles are spastic or tight.

• *Mixed*

– This type of incontinence should be treated with both intervention methods from stress and urge incontinence methods. If one type of incontinence is more prominent in an individual, then interventions for that type of incontinence should have more of a focus.
– Urinary incontinence

> May also be a cause of a neurogenic bladder. Neurogenic bladder is caused by neurological damage from a disease process, acquired injury, or congenital condition. Neurogenic bladder is not curable, but can usually be managed through medication or intermittent catheterization.

Fecal Incontinence

– Strong rapport should first be established with the patient due to the nature of this condition causing embarrassment and shame. Give the patient hope to aid in feelings of isolation.

> Skin care should be addressed with patient. Feces can significantly compromise skin integrity and cause infection. Hand mirror can be recommended for skin checks. Barrier creams can be suggested for skin protection.
> Digital exam should be used to assess the external anal sphincter (EAS) and internal anal sphincter (IAS) for reflex function, sensory awareness, pain assessment, and muscle tone.
> Strengthening exercises may be indicated for patients with low tone, and may include the surrounding pelvic structures of the abdominal muscles and lower back with functional coordination between both. E-stim should be considered if muscles are very weak.
> Balloon techniques can be used for sensory awareness and retraining of stretch receptors in anus and rectum, and retraining of recto-sphincteric striated reflex. This method is performed by insertion of a pressure-controlled balloon into the rectum. This technique can increase rectal sensitivity to improve bowel control.

Diet should be reviewed with patients through a bowel diary or during evaluation intake. Foods that trigger diarrhea and gas should be considered, as well as consistency in meal times, and appropriate fiber intake for bulking stool. Well documented research exists for the use of biofeedback for fecal incontinence, which can be used to monitor contractions, coordination, overuse of muscles, over overdistention [11].

Pelvic Organ Prolapse

- The prolapse stage should be assessed through an internal exam prior to the design of the treatment plan.
- Breathing pattern should be assessed for epigastric rise during inhale; if breathing pattern is maladaptive, diaphragmatic breathing should be a primary component of treatment plan. Education regarding avoidance of breath holding or straining during toileting, high pressure activities, or ADL tasks in order to prevent further descent of organs should be provided to the patient.
- Proper lifting techniques should be taught to the patient in order to protect prolapse. Digital splinting should be taught to the patient with the use of a single digit inserted into the vaginal canal (by patient) during toileting in order to push out pocketed urine or feces for complete emptying.
- Strengthening exercises of the pelvic floor are helpful for support of prolapse since prolapse is frequently associated with tissue laxity and weakness, and/or loss of nerve, muscle, or ligament integrity. Patients generally do better with strengthening exercises in gravity-reduced or gravity-eliminated positions such as quadruped.

    - Hip elevated exercises such as bridges or clams can be used for pelvic floor strengthening with cued pelvic and abdominal bracing. Use of pillows, wedges, or large balls can be used for up- or downgrading activities. Dosage should be based on the patient's strength, endurance, coordination, and stability of pelvic floor muscles and surrounding musculature, which is gathered during the evaluation.

- A pessary prosthetic may be helpful to a patient for reduced protrusion of prolapse, or to provide slow and controlled release of medication. A physician should fit a patient for this device.
- Individuals may be asymptomatic and still have evidence of prolapse. Additionally, if the prolapse stage is at III or IV, surgical intervention may be required for management of symptoms.

Constipation

- Successful rehabilitation of constipation helps the patient achieve optimal stool consistency and correct maladaptive defecation patterns. Eating and toileting habits should be assessed, as well as posture, muscle tone of the pelvic floor, abdomen, hips, and reflex function.
- Ergonomic assessment with instruction to sit down on the toilet (no crouching) with posterior pelvic tilt to manage intra-abdominal pressure appropriately. Feet should be on a flat surface or stool to assist in hip flexion. A Squatty Potty®, small step stool, or stacked books can aid the patient in body mechanics. Patients should never strain or hold breath during a bowel movement.
- Reflexes should be observed by asking the patient to squeeze, relax, and bear down. The patient should be educated on breathing patterns to ensure there is no straining during bowel movements.
- Manual techniques, including visceral mobilization or abdominal wall massage, can be used to help relax the abdominal wall and increase circulation in the intestinal tract. Abdominal wall massage can be taught to the patient by instructing them to use light strokes in a clockwise direction starting by ascending on the right side, moving across the upper abdomen, and descending on the left side of the abdomen.
- Meditation, visualization, and/or biofeedback can be used for relaxation techniques and can be practiced with the patient sitting on the toilet.
- Strengthening exercises may be indicated if a patient has a weak trunk or hips. Abdominal activation should be taught during exhalation for proper management of intra-abdominal pressure.
  - A bowel diary can be used to help the patient establish a bowel routine, and can include exercise and diet.

Dyspareunia

- Pelvic floor muscles should be assessed for trigger points and hypersensitivity. Trigger points can be found on any number of trigger point charts. Pastore and Katzman provide an overview of assessing trigger points [12].
- Biomechanics should be assessed for areas of stiffness or dysfunction, including spinal mobility and hip range of motion, in order to treat underlying issues of structures connected to the pelvis.
- Lubricant education should be provided to the patient with attention to use of brands that are in range of vaginal pH (3.5–5.5), and are free of scents, parabens, phthalates, or heating gels. Attention to menstrual cycles should be tracked by the patient to rule out hormonal issues related to lubrication or pain (handout in appendix).

- DME can be largely helpful to patients, including dilators for stretching, vibrators for nerve habituation, and/or *Ohnuts* for relief with deep thrusting.
- Relaxation training is helpful for patients with spastic pelvic floor during intercourse. This can include visualization, meditation, positive affirmations, and diaphragmatic breathing. See *Progressive Muscle Relaxation* handout in the Appendix.
- Patient education regarding consent to sexual intercourse is important with dyspareunia. One 22-year-old female told the OTP that it wasn't until an aunt told her that rape could occur with a married partner that she understood that she was being raped by her boyfriend. The conversation with the aunt led her to seek medical advice and counseling. She did not realize that was the cause of her pain.
- Education with a partner may be helpful, if applicable.

Other Considerations and Resources

- Documentation and Billing

  - Herman & Wallace list of most common ICD-10 codes for pelvic floor dysfunction. (https://hermanwallace.com/common-ICD-10-codes).
  - It should be noted that most insurance does not cover Dyspareunia, and some do not cover pelvic floor rehabilitation at all.
  - Many pelvic floor treatments and goals fall under the umbrella of activities of daily living (ADLs).

- Suggested referrals or DME

  - CMT Medical for DME equipment and therapist tools
  - The Ohnut (https://ohnut.co/)
  - Bedside commodes
  - Squatty Potty®
  - Pessaries for organ prolapse

      Impressa-disposable one-time use pessary (These can be found on Amazon.com and in many grocery and drug stores)

  - Dilators
  - Vaginal weights
  - Lubricants and moisturizers
  - Wands
  - Suppositories for pain relief
  - Desert Harvest Oil "Releveum" for pelvic pain relief (https://www.desertharvest.com/)

Additional Resources for Provider and Patient
- Useful tools, videos, and articles can be found through the Mayo Clinic at the following link: https://www.mayoclinic.org/departments-centers/physical-medicine-rehabilitation/minnesota/services/pelvic-floor-dysfunction-program
- Urinary Incontinence Toolkit provides tools for initial evaluation of a patient, along with free education handouts for patients addressing the following: urinary incontinence and treatment approaches; simple cystometrics; daily habits; bladder training; pelvic muscle exercise; urge incontinence; drug treatment for urge incontinence; urodynamics; biofeedback; surgical treatments; radical prostatectomy [13]. http://www.gericareonline.net/tools/eng/urinary/index.html

References

1. Rubilotta E, Balzarro M, Bassi S, Corsi P, Pirozzi M, Nicolò T, Benito Porcaro A, D'Amico A, Artibani W. Pure stress urinary incontinence: analysis of the prevalence, estimation of costs and financial impact. J Urol. 2017;197(4):E836.
2. National Institute of Diabetes and Digestive and Kidney Diseases. Constipation. 2019. https://www.niddk.nih.gov/health-information/digestive-diseases/constipation
3. Haylen BT, de Ridder D, Freeman RM, Swift SR, Berghmans B, Lee J, Schaer GN. An international Urogynecological association (IUGA)/international continence society (ICS) joint report on the terminology for female pelvic floor dysfunction. Int Urogynecol J. 2010;21(1):5–26.
4. Jones KD, Lehr ST, Hewell SW. Principles & practice: dyspareunia: three case reports. J Obstet Gynecol Neonatal Nurs. 1997;26(1):19–23.
5. Bordman R, Jackson B. Below the belt: approach to chronic pelvic pain. Can Fam Physician. 2006;52(12):1556–62.
6. Medic G, Wille M, Hemels ME. Short- and long-term health consequences of sleep disruption. Nat Sci Sleep. 2017;9:151–61. https://doi.org/10.2147/NSS.S134864.
7. Fitzgerald MP, Kotarinos R. Rehabilitation of the short pelvic floor. II: treatment of the patient with the short pelvic floor. Int Urogynecol J Pelvic Floor Dysfunct. 2003;14(4):269–75.
8. Hunjan R, Twiss KL. Urgent interventions: promoting occupational engagement for clients with urinary incontinence. OT Pract. 2013;18(21):8–12.
9. Miller JM. Criteria for therapeutic use of pelvic floor muscle training in women. J Wound Ostomy Cont Nurs. 2002;29(6):301–11.
10. Dougherty MC. Current state of research on pelvic muscle strengthening techniques. J Wound Ostomy Cont Nurs. 1998;25(2):75–83.
11. Shafik A, El Sibai O, Shafik IA, Shafik AA. Stress, urge, and mixed types of fecal incontinence: pathogenesis, clinical presentation, and treatment. Am Surg. 2007;73(1):6–9.
12. Pastore EA, Katzman WB. Recognizing myofascial pelvic pain in the female patient with chronic pelvic pain. J Obstet Gynecol Neonatal Nurs. 2012;41(5):680–91. https://doi.org/10.1111/j.1552-6909.2012.01404.x.
13. American Geriatrics Society, John A. Hartford Foundation, & Practicing Physician Education in Geriatrics. Urinary Incontinence Toolkit. 2006. http://www.gericareonline.net/tools/eng/urinary/index.html

Chapter 34
Persistent Pain

John V. Rider and Katie Smith

Introduction

Persistent pain, historically known as chronic pain, is not consistently defined but is typically categorized as pain that persists for more than 3 months beyond the expected time period for healing or pain that does not serve an evolutionary adaptive function. The International Association for the Study of Pain defines pain as "an unpleasant sensory and emotional experience associated with, or resembling that associated with, actual or potential tissue damage [1]." It is important to note that the definition includes both an unpleasant *sensory* and *emotional* experience, indicating the importance of addressing both the physical and psychological experience of pain. Persistent pain is the most common reason for adults seeking medical care in the United States. Estimates range from 11 to 40% of the population reporting persistent pain [2], and costs are estimated at $560 billion each year [3]. Pain is always a personal experience that is influenced to varying degrees by biological, psychological, and social factors, indicating the complexity of the pain experience [1]. Although pain usually serves an adaptive role, persistent pain may have adverse effects on function as well as social and psychological well-being [1]. The most current theories related to persistent pain identify the contribution of memory, social context, emotional responses, and cognitive perspective as significant to the development and perpetuation of persistent pain [4]. Hence, interventions for persistent pain must be broader than just addressing the physical and sensory responses.

Physical medicine and pain management, until recently, has focused on addressing the physical and sensory responses of pain, believing the pain was related to

J. V. Rider (✉)
School of Occupational Therapy, Touro University Nevada, Henderson, NV, USA
e-mail: jrider@touro.edu

K. Smith
Revolutionary Alignment, LLC, Detroit, MI, USA
www.RevolutionaryAlignment.com

© Springer Nature Switzerland AG 2023
S. Dahl-Popolizio et al. (eds.), *Primary Care Occupational Therapy*,
https://doi.org/10.1007/978-3-031-20882-9_34

structural pathology. Historically, health professionals have been trained to treat pain using a biomedical model. This biomedical model, when applied to pain, supposes a direct relationship between identifiable soft-tissue damage and the experience of pain. This approach does not consider the psychological or social aspects of pain, which recent studies suggest play a large role in the persistent pain experience [5–10]. Many individuals with persistent pain experience minimal relief from a purely biomedical approach and continue to live with a decreased quality of life. These individuals may feel like the healthcare system has "failed them," causing them to lose hope in ever managing their persistent pain. The biopsychosocial model is now widely accepted as the most heuristic evidence-based approach for assessing and treating persistent pain [4, 11–13]. This approach encapsulates the interactions among the biological, psychological, and social components unique to each individual. As the biopsychosocial model acknowledges the interactions of each of these components in the experience of pain, it also supports the interdisciplinary approach to pain management [4]. As a result, this model allows OTPs to maintain their holistic view and use physical, psychological, social, cognitive, affective, and behavioral measures, as well as their interactions, to best assess and treat each patient's unique pain experience. This multimodal and multidimensional approach is key to successfully changing the pain experience and helping patients live well with persistent pain.

Role of PCP

Persistent pain is complex and multifaceted and, therefore, may not be readily identified using common diagnostic tests. Many of the diagnostic tests listed below are performed in the PC setting and others may be ordered by the PCP. However, it is important to remember that there is little correlation between "abnormal" findings on imaging and the pain your patient may be experiencing. Persistent pain cannot be broken down into discrete physical or psychosocial elements. These diagnostic tests can be used as a guide to address physical aspects of pain, but the presence of "abnormal" or "normal" findings should not be cause to exclude further evaluation of psychosocial constructs that can modulate the patient's experience of pain and perception of disability. Having the OTP available on the PC team allows the PCP to refer immediately to the professional who has the skills to assess these more intangible aspects of pain.

Common tests performed in the management of persistent pain:

- *Imaging tests*

  - X-ray—Used to identify bony abnormalities such as osteophyte formation or fractures
  - Computerized Tomography scan (CT)—Used to identify soft tissue abnormalities such as a torn ligament or herniated intervertebral disc

- Magnetic Resonance Imaging (MRI)—Used to identify abnormalities among the relationship between the bones and soft tissue without radiation
- Ultrasound—Uses high-frequency sound waves to produce images of body structures to identify abnormalities
- Myelogram—Used to identify abnormalities of the spinal cord such as compression or tumors
- Bone scan—Used to identify bony abnormalities such as osteoarthritis and fractures

- *Nerve tests*

  - Electromyography test (EMG)—Measures muscle response or electrical activity in response to a nerve's stimulation of the muscle
  - Nerve Conduction Velocity test (NCV)—Measures how fast an electrical impulse moves through your nerve to identify any nerve damage
  - Nerve block—Used to determine if the pain is associated with a specific nerve or joint

- *Blood tests*

  - May be used to rule out diagnoses such as rheumatoid arthritis, and check levels of inflammation and examine metabolic health

- *Quantitative Sensory Testing*

  - Used to examine general sensory perception after application of various mechanical and thermal stimuli to determine absence, presence, and level of detection, pain thresholds, and stimulus-response curves

- *Physical performance tests*

  - General range of motion, muscle testing and palpation of structures for a comprehensive musculoskeletal examination
  A comprehensive PCP assessment may include, but is not limited to

- Review of all pertinent medical records for: medical history, comorbidities, current medications, and psychosocial factors.
- Detailed history of any acute and persistent pain.
- Past trauma history.
- Past medical treatments, consultations, and diagnostic testing.
- Present disabilities, mental health disorders, substance abuse history, prescription, and illicit substance use and nicotine dependence.
- Physical exam including neurological and orthopedic special tests.
- Discussion of expectations and realistic outcomes.
- Development of a management plan, including goals, relevant diagnoses, treatment, appropriate referrals, and re-evaluation.

In general, the PCP emphasizes the pharmacological aspects of pain management and provides referrals to appropriate disciplines to further manage persistent pain.

Common Comorbidities

Persistent pain may increase the likelihood of other health problems, including cardiovascular issues (e.g., hypertension, postural orthostatic tachycardia syndrome), gastrointestinal issues (e.g., opioid-induced constipation, irritable bowel syndrome, canaboid hyperemesis syndrome), substance use disorders, depression, anxiety, stress, sleep disturbances (insomnia), fatigue, headaches, cognitive impairments (e.g., decreased attention span, impaired concentration and executive functioning, etc.), poor appetite, weight gain or obesity, attention deficit hyperactive disorder, fibromyalgia, hyperlipidemia (high cholesterol), diabetes mellitus, osteoporosis, weakened immune system, adverse events related to medications, and suicide.

Role of OTP

People experiencing persistent pain face many obstacles to occupational performance, ranging from a mild to severe impact. Persistent pain has the potential to impair a person's ability to engage in preferred activities of daily living (ADLs) and instrumental activities of daily living (IADLs), ultimately reducing their quality of life. The OTP evaluates the impact of pain and provides pain management strategies the patient is able to effectively employ with the goal of improving quality of life (e.g., supported self-management).

Occupational Impact

Persistent pain may be present both at rest and with activity and can invade all occupations (e.g., rest and sleep, education, work, play, leisure, social participation, sexual activity, mobility, etc.), interfering with physical, emotional, and spiritual functioning. Persistent pain does not respect contexts or environments and can negatively affect a person's ability to function properly in various environments (physical, social, and virtual). Client factors, such as values, beliefs, and spirituality, are impacted by the presence of persistent pain and can further negatively impact performance skills and patterns. Persistent pain can impair cognitive abilities (e.g., executive functioning, attention, and working memory) and motor abilities (e.g., joint stiffness, decreased strength, and endurance), affecting a person's ability to perform work duties, take care of housework, engage in social activities, etc. Often, people experiencing persistent pain are forced to alter chosen habits and routines and are unable to fulfill personal roles, thus negatively affecting their identity and life satisfaction.

OT Areas of Emphasis

The role of OT in supporting patients in addressing and managing persistent pain is multidimensional, much like the experience of pain itself. OTPs first assess how persistent pain has impacted a patient's life, including quality and satisfaction with task performance. This is accomplished by obtaining a comprehensive occupational profile. Once a plan of care is established, several intervention techniques can support an individual with persistent pain's ability to return to function, gain independence, and achieve positive health outcomes. OTPs must promote the distinct value of their services by empowering patients with supported self-management strategies and shifting goals from reducing pain to managing a chronic condition to increase occupational participation and performance.

Evaluation

- *Suggested Areas To Evaluate* (if the assessment is mentioned in multiple domains, link provided, when availableEvaluation, to the first mention of the assessment)
    - *ADLs*—'How does your pain impact your ability to do things such as getting ready for the day and taking care of yourself?'

        Assessments include: Barthel ADL Index or patient-specific assessments, such as the Canadian Occupational Performance Measure (COPM), Occupational Performance History Interview (OPHI-II), or Patient-Specific Functional Scale (PSFS)
    - *IADLs*—'How does your pain impact your ability to do things such as go out into the community, take care of your house, prepare meals, etc.?'

        Assessments include: Lawson IADL Scale or patient-specific assessments, such as the COPM, OPHI-II, PSFS, or PROMIS Profile 29)
    - *Performance patterns, habits, and routines*—'Tell me about your typical daily routine?' 'What changes, if any, have you made to your daily routine because of your pain?' 'Have you given up any important things in your life?' (Occupational Experience Profile (OEP), PROMIS Profile 29)
    - *Sleep behaviors*—'How much sleep are you getting on average each night?' 'How many times are you waking up each night?' 'How are you preparing for sleep each night?' 'Do you feel rested in the morning?' 'How has your sleep been impacted by pain?' (PROMIS Profile 29) (Chap. 27).
    - *Psychosocial responses to pain*—Common emotional responses to pain can include anxiety, depression, anger, feeling misunderstood, and demoralization. 'How would you describe your general mood?' 'Does your mood change throughout the day based on your pain?' 'How do you currently cope with your pain?' (Pain Anxiety Symptoms Scale 20 (PASS-20), Pain Coping Inventory Questionnaire (PCI), PROMIS Profile 29)

  – *Environmental barriers*—Ergonomic considerations for work and home
  – *Support system*—'Do you have support at work or at home?' 'Do you have someone you can call when you need help?'

• *Additional Suggested Assessment Tools*

  – Patient-Specific Functional Scale—Free and available online. A useful questionnaire that can be used to quantify activity limitation and measure functional outcome for patients.
  – Functional Pain Scale—Free and available online. Assists the individual in identifying if persistent pain affects function.
  – The Pain Disability Questionnaire—Free and available online. Assesses perception of disability in relation to pain. Designed for chronic disabling musculoskeletal disorders.
  – Pain Self-Efficacy Questionnaire—Free and available online. 10-item questionnaire developed to assess the confidence of individuals with persistent pain in performing activities while in pain.
  – Motivational interviewing (MI). See Appendix for *Motivational Interviewing Information*. MI is an approach that identifies the individual's priorities, readiness for change, and potential barriers to change and guides them away from ambivalence or uncertainty towards finding the motivation to make positive decisions and accomplishing established goals.
  – Occupational Self-Assessment—Short Form—Measures the individual's perceptions of their occupational competence and valued activities and how illness and disability impact occupational competence.
  – Neurophysiology of Pain Questionnaire—Free and available online. Devised to assess how an individual conceptualizes the biological mechanisms that underpin their pain. Can be used as a baseline to provide client education on pain neuroscience.
  – Pain Catastrophizing Scale—Free and available online. A questionnaire that measures the individual's level of pain catastrophizing and breaks it down into three constructs: magnifying the pain threat, ruminating on the pain, and feelings of helplessness.
  – Chronic Pain Acceptance Questionnaire-Revised (CPAQ-R)—Free and available online. Measures acceptance of pain within activity engagement and pain willingness.
  – Fear-Avoidance Beliefs Questionnaire (FBAQ)—Free and available online. Measures how fear-avoidance beliefs about physical activity and work may affect and contribute to their pain and resulting disability.
  – Pain Anxiety Symptoms Scale 20 (PASS-20)—Free and available online. Measures pain-related anxiety.
  – Pain Coping Inventory Questionnaire (PCI)—Free and available online. Measures cognitive and behavioral strategies for dealing with chronic pain.
  – Brief Pain Inventory (BPI)—Free and available online. Measures the severity of pain, activity interference, and affective interference.

- West Haven-Yale Multidimensional Pain Inventory (WHYMPI)—Free and available online. Assesses pain across the pain experience, responses of others to the client's communicated pain, and participation in daily activities.
- McGill Pain Questionnaire (MPQ)—Free and available online. Assesses the quality and intensity of pain with a drawing of the human body and pain descriptors across sensory, affective, and evaluative dimensions.
- Range of motion and manual muscle testing.
- ADL/IADL Measures:
- Barthel Index (Free and available online) or observed/narrative ADLs.
- Lawton IADL Scale (Free and available online) or observed/narrative IADLs.

Intervention Strategies

The overall aim of all intervention strategies is to re-engage the patient in their preferred occupations. OTPs in PC should focus on helping patients apply evidence-based strategies to improve occupational participation and performance and provide referrals for ongoing specialized persistent pain management services when warranted. Most of the following interventions can be provided or initiated in a single visit and then continued care can be provided via the OTP in PC or through a referral for outside services.

Suggested Intervention Strategies

Education and Training

- *Understanding persistent pain*
  - Pain Neuroscience Education (PNE) is an educational strategy to help patients better understand the neurobiology and neurophysiology of pain and pain processing by the nervous system and has been shown to help change a patient's perception of pain and reduce fear avoidance behaviors, enhance movement and activity participation, and minimize healthcare utilization [14].
  - OTPs in PC can use simplified scientific language with pictures, metaphors, and drawings in one or several visits.
  - Adrian Louw has published booklets for clinicians and patients to aid in pain neuroscience education

    Why Do I Hurt? Workbook.
    Why You Hurt Therapeutic Neuroscience Education System
    Why Do I Hurt? A Patient Book About The Neuroscience of Pain
  - Additional resources for advancing the understanding of Pain Neuroscience:

Explain Pain by Butler & Mosely

Pain *Neuroscience Education: Teaching People About Pain* by Louw & Puentedura.

- *Body mechanics/ergonomics*
  - Patients with persistent pain may exhibit protective behaviors leading to alterations in posture that make it difficult to tolerate certain positions and activities. OTPs in PC can help patients identify more comfortable postures to reduce overall pain with activity to increase occupational participation.
  - OTPs should also encourage movement in preferred activities and throughout the day by helping patients understand that feared and avoided movements will not cause increased damage by using a graded exposure approach coupled with education.
  - Some examples include:

    Education and training on sleeping positions with proper support to decrease low back pain
    Resting one foot on a footstool when standing for a prolonged time to decrease low back pain
    Sitting and standing techniques to decrease excessive spinal flexion
    Adaptive driving positions
    Recommendations for proper ergonomics at home and work

- *Adaptive equipment*
  - Some examples include long-handled reacher to reduce bending, bath bench to avoid fatigue during bathing, long-handled sponge to decrease spinal flexion during bathing, built-up handles or easy grip items to decrease hand and upper extremity pain, etc.

- *Self-management strategies*
  - Activity tolerance/pacing activities can help patients learn to balance time spent on an activity and rest to increase function and participation in meaningful and preferred activities. OTPs in PC can use the following metaphors to help patients begin to utilize activity pacing as a self-management strategy.
  - Spoon Theory of energy management, where spoons are a unit of energy used to estimate the "cost" of daily tasks, and prioritizing "spending" spoons on valued or necessary activities (see *Spoon Tracking* handout in Appendix).
  - Overcoming the 'boom-bust' cycle of overexertion and resulting 'crash;' 'shifting' instead to staying within a moderate and well-paced 'energy budget.'
  - Water Pitcher with 'energy' pouring out during daily activities.

- *Developing a 'flare-up' plan*

  - The goal of a flare-up plan is to maintain control rather than allowing pain to take control.
  - OTPs in PC can help patients develop an individualized written plan on how they will manage a flare-up. (e.g., make a list of potential triggers and include ways to pace or change the triggering activity, include skills to relax or distract from the pain, skills to use modalities to relieve pain, short-term changes to medications to manage pain, and necessary modifications to maintain occupational engagement in preferred activities despite pain).
  - Training patients on safe and appropriate use of physical agent modalities to manage pain and improve occupational performance (e.g., cryotherapy (Cold packs), thermotherapy (Hot packs, heat pads, paraffin baths), and electrotherapy (TENS unit).

- *Lifestyle interventions/modifications*

  - Anti-inflammatory diet for persistent pain
  - Proper hydration
  - Medication adherence and management
  - Sleep hygiene (e.g., helping patients review current sleep hygiene routine and make changes such as maintaining a consistent sleep/wake cycle, getting enough exercise/activity/sun exposure during the day, avoiding stimulating activities and substances, incorporating "wind-down" routines leading up to sleep, modifying sleep environment, etc.) (See Sleep Hygiene handout in Appendix)
  - Increasing physical activity (See Walk to Run handout in Appendix)
  - QUOTA Exercise: aerobic, strengthening, balance, and flexibility for persistent pain
  - Developing a baseline over 3 days/3 repetitions (Baseline is where pain level is exacerbated or triggered.)

    > Calculate 80% of the baseline. This is the starting point for your exercise program. You will do this exercise every day regardless of whether you are feeling better or worse (unless severe acute exacerbation) for the first week. After 1 week, add 5% to the baseline, complete every planned day for the next week.
    > After the second week, add another 5% to this level. Complete for the next 3 sessions/repetitions. If this goes well, add another 5% and repeat.

- *Lifestyle balance*

  - Help patients identify occupations that provide pleasure, productivity, restoration, and social connection, using the Occupational Experience Profile by Karen Atler, to achieve a better lifestyle balance.
  - See Occupational Balance handout in Appendix.

- *Psychological interventions*
  - Cognitive Behavioral Therapy (CBT) and Acceptance and Commitment Therapy (ACT) frameworks can be used to address negative thoughts and pain catastrophizing. OTPs in PC can introduce these approaches and provide simple tools to begin managing persistent pain. If patients are open to taking a cognitive behavioral approach, the appropriate referral can be made to OTPs or mental health professionals specializing in treating persistent pain using these approaches.

    CBT emphasizes changing how the individual thinks, which, in turn, changes how they feel about pain. The OTP can work with the client to *stop* (notice their thoughts), *ask* (ask whether it is helpful or unhelpful), and *choose* (choose a helpful thought to replace the negative one). OTPs in PC can help patients identify unhelpful thoughts such as "should statements," focusing only on the negative, overgeneralizing, or all-or-nothing thinking and choose accurate, flexible, and helpful thoughts as a replacement.

    ACT emphasizes coping with persistent pain by helping the individual accept negative feelings as a normal part of life and learning to base choices and actions on personal values, rather than the negative feelings. ACT helps individuals to accept that while pain may be unpleasant, their lives don't need to be put on hold to manage it. The OTP can help patients work through the following principles. A—accepting experiences as they are instead of rejecting them simply because they may cause pain. Help patients learn to see pain as a normal aspect of life, rather than trying to escape it. C—choosing behaviors mindfully rather than allowing automatic thoughts or conditioned responses to guide choices, which often results in avoidance behavior. Help patients step back and take a mindful approach to selecting meaningful occupations for engagement. T—Taking action and having agency in their life rather than being paralyzed by unpleasant thoughts, memories, emotions, or sensations. Help patients develop self-efficacy, commit to changing their behavior, and taking actions that support their values, despite persistent pain. Using a biopsychosocial approach, OTPs should incorporate psychosocial approaches, such as CBT and ACT, to improve occupational engagement, overall well-being, and support patients in living well with persistent pain [15]. CBT and ACT can be used one-on-one, in group formats, single sessions, or as part of ongoing OT and are easily combined with other evidence-based approaches. Multiple handouts, worksheets, and resources are available online.

– Relaxation training and mindfulness

OTPs in PC can help patients identify relaxation strategies such as dia-phragmatic breathing, progressive muscle relaxation, guided meditation, visualization, light stretching, music therapy, etc., and how to incorporate them into their daily routines to improve persistent pain management and increase occupational engagement *(see Progressive Muscle Relaxation handout in Appendix).*

Biofeedback strategies include helping patients to regulate physiological processes through the use of feedback mechanisms (e.g., visual, auditory, or tactile) and can be incorporated into relaxation training.

Mindfulness training can be used to help patients improve their present-moment awareness and offer practical strategies to act more reflectively rather than impulsively. Mindfulness-based interventions have been shown to improve sleep participation, stress, pain acceptance, pain intensity, and many psychological components of pain, allowing for greater occupational participation [16, 17] *(see Mindfulness handouts in Appendix).*

– Assertiveness and communication training

OTPs in PC can help patients learn effective communication principles to become more assertive, such as being clear about their intentions in state-ments to others, clarifying facts, feelings, and needs, encouraging honest and direct communication instead of maladaptive coping behaviors, actively listening and assuming responsibility for self and consequences of actions.

Help patients develop self-advocacy strategies such as keeping a pain diary, being honest about their pain, educating themselves about pain research and available treatment options, etc.

– Motivational Interviewing

Motivational interviewing is a client-centered counseling method to help elicit behavioral change by helping patients explore and resolve their own ambivalence (see *Motivational Interviewing handout* in Appendix).

Rather than trying to convince the patient how important it is to make life-style changes in order to improve pain, the OTP focuses on understanding and collaborating with the patient. The OTP in PC can use the *OARS* method. O—ask **o**pen-ended questions. A—provide **a**ffirming responses. R—use **r**eflective listening skills. S—**s**ummarize what the patient says, giving special attention to change statements.

- Occupational engagement
  - All intervention strategies should emphasize the power of occupational engagement and assist the client in the resumption of preferred occupations despite persistent pain (e.g., living well with pain).
- Suggested referrals or DME
  - Referrals should be individualized, but some recommendations that are commonly used include:

    Mental health counseling for clients at risk for suicide ideations
    Pain Specialist Physician or Orthopedic Surgeon for surgical options and injections
    Podiatrist for specialized foot or ankle evaluation of pain
    Outpatient OT/PT for continued services
    Adaptive equipment to address pain during ADLs/IADLs (e.g., shower chair, sock aid, jar opener, etc.)
    Raised seating options in the bathroom, home, work to address pain with standing
    Adaptive driving positioning equipment to address pain while driving
    Ergonomic evaluation and ergonomic equipment and recommendations to address pain at home or work
    Multidisciplinary intensive pain program (day treatment or inpatient)

Other Considerations and Resources

Additional resources for provider and patient.

Handouts available:
- Nourishing and depleting activities https://www.getselfhelp.co.uk/docs/NourishingDepleting.pdf
- Anti-inflammatory diet Handout https://www.fammed.wisc.edu/files/webfm-uploads/documents/outreach/im/handout_ai_diet_patient.pdf
- Anti-inflammatory diet Handout 2 https://www.peacehealth.org/sites/default/files/anti-inflammatory_diet.pdf
- Dr. Greg Lehman. (2017) Recovery Strategies: Pain guidebook. www.greglehman.ca Retrieved from: https://static1.squarespace.com/static/57260f1fd51cd4d1168668ab/t/590dca266b8f5b01a7f97ceb/1494075961206/recovery+strategies+pain+guidebook+2017.pdf
- Sleep Hygiene Handouts: https://www.sleepfoundation.org/articles/sleep-hygiene
- Sleep Diary handouts: https://www.sleepfoundation.org/sites/default/files/inline-files/SleepDiaryv6.pdf?ada=1
- https://www.sleepfoundation.org/excessive-sleepiness-osa/living-and-managing/diet-and-exercise-changes-help-excessive-sleepiness

References

1. Raja SN, Carr DB, Cohen M, Finnerup NB, Flor H, Gibson S, Keefe FJ, Mogil JS, Ringkamp M, Sluka KA, Song X, Stevens B, Sullivan MD, Tutelman PR, Ushida T, Vader K. The revised International Association for the Study of Pain definition of pain: concepts, challenges, and compromises. Pain. 2020;161(9):1976–82. https://doi.org/10.1097/j.pain.0000000000001939.
2. Dahlhamer J, Lucas J, Zelaya C, Nahin R, Mackey S, DeBar L, Kerns R, Von Korff M, Porter L, Helmick C. Prevalence of chronic pain and high-impact chronic pain among adults—United States, 2016. MMWR Morb Mortal Wkly Rep. 2018;67:1001–6.
3. Kuehn B. Chronic pain prevalence. JAMA. 2018;320(16):1632. https://doi.org/10.1001/jama.2018.16009.
4. Gatchel RJ, Peng YB, Peters ML, Fuchs PN, Turk DC. The biopsychosocial approach to chronic pain: scientific advances and future directions. Psychol Bull. 2007;133(4):581–624. https://doi.org/10.1037/0033-2909.133.4.581.
5. Fisher GS, Emerson L, Firpo C, Ptak J, Wonn J, Bartolacci G. Chronic pain and occupation: an exploration of the lived experience. Am J Occup Ther. 2007;61:290–302.
6. Linton SJ, Shaw WS. Impact of psychological factors in the experience of pain. Phys Ther. 2011;91(5):700–11. https://doi.org/10.2522/ptj.20100330.
7. Karayannis NV, Baumann I, Sturgeon JA, Melloh M, Mackey SC. The impact of social isolation on pain interference: a longitudinal study. Ann Behav Med. 2018;53(1):65–74. https://doi.org/10.1093/abm/kay017.
8. Ferreira-Valente MA, Pais-Ribeiro JL, Jensen MP. Associations between psychosocial factors and pain intensity, physical functioning, and psychological functioning in patients with chronic pain: a cross-cultural comparison. Clin J Pain. 2014;30(8):713–23. https://doi.org/10.1097/AJP.0000000000000027.
9. Blyth FM, Macfarlane GJ, Nicholas MK. The contribution of psychosocial factors to the development of chronic pain: the key to better outcomes for patients? Pain. 2007;129(1):8–11. https://doi.org/10.1016/j.pain.2007.03.009.
10. Varela AJ, Van Asslet LW. The relationship between psychosocial factors and reported disability: the role of pain self-efficacy. BMC Musculoskelet Disord. 2022;23(21):21. https://doi.org/10.1186/s12891-021-04955-6.
11. American Occupational Therapy Association. Position statement—role of occupational therapy in pain management. Am J Occup Ther. 2021;75(Suppl. 3):7513410010. https://doi.org/10.5014/ajot.2021.75S3001.
12. Bevers K, Watts L, Kishino ND, Gachtel RJ. The biopsychosocial model of the assessment, prevention, and treatment of chronic pain. Neurology. 2016;12:98–104. https://doi.org/10.17925/USN.2016.12.02.98.
13. Gatchel RJ, Howard KJ. The biopsychosocial approach. Practical Pain Management. 2018; 8(4). https://www.practicalpainmanagement.com/treatments/psychological/biopsychosocial-approach.
14. Louw A, Zimney K, Puentedura EJ, Diener I. The efficacy of pain neuroscience education on musculoskeletal pain: a systematic review of the literature. Physiother Theory Pract. 2016;32(5):332–55. https://doi.org/10.1080/09593985.2016.1194646.
15. Rider J, Tay M. Increasing occupational engagement by addressing psychosocial and occupational factors of chronic pain: a case report. Open J. Occup. Ther. 2022; 10(3), 1–12.
16. Chiesa A, Serretti A. Mindfulness-based interventions for chronic pain: a systematic review of the evidence. J Altern Complement Med. 2011;17(1):83–93. https://doi.org/10.1089/acm.2009.0546.
17. Khusid MA, Vythilingam M. The emerging role of mindfulness meditation as effective self-management strategy, part 2: clinical implications for chronic pain, substance misuse, and insomnia. Mil Med. 2016;181:969–75. https://doi.org/10.7205/milmed-d-14-00678.

Further Reading

American Occupational Therapy Association. Role of occupational therapy in pain management. Am J Occup Ther, 2021; 75(Supplement_3), 7513410010.

Antcliff D, Keeley P, Campbell M, Woby S, Keenan AM, McGowan L. Activity pacing: moving beyond taking breaks and slowing down. Qual Life Res Int J Qual Life Asp Treat Care Rehab. 2018;27(7):1933–5. https://doi.org/10.1007/s11136-018-1794-7.

Breeden K, Rowe N. A biopsychosocial approach for addressing chronic pain in everyday occupational therapy practice. OT Pract. 2017;22:CE-1.

Caneiro JP, Bunzli S, O'Sullivan P. Beliefs about the body and pain: the critical role in musculoskeletal pain management. Braz J Phys Ther. 2021;25(1):17–29. https://doi.org/10.1016/j.bjpt.2020.06.003.

Dueñas M, Ojeda B, Salazar A, Mico JA, Failde I. A review of chronic pain impact on patients, their social environment and the health care system. J Pain Res. 2016;9:457–67. https://doi.org/10.2147/JPR.S105892.

Jihad A, Hana K, Emilie R, et al. Nutrition interventions in rheumatoid arthritis: the potential use of plant-based diets. A review. Front Nutr, 2019; 6: 141. https://www.frontiersin.org/article/10.3389/fnut.2019.00141 DOI: https://doi.org/10.3389/fnut.2019.00141.

Kroll HR. Exercise therapy for chronic pain. Phys Med Rehabil Clin N Am. 2015;26:263–81. https://doi.org/10.1016/j.pmr.2014.12.007.

Mittinty M, Vanlint S, Stocks N, et al. Exploring effect of pain education on chronic pain patients' expectation of recovery and pain intensity. Scand J Pain. 2018;18(2):211–9. https://doi.org/10.1515/sjpain-2018-0023.

Moseley GL. Whole of community pain education for back pain. Why does first-line care get almost no attention and what exactly are we waiting for? Br J Sports Med. 2019;53:588–9.

Owen GT, Bruel BM, Schade CM, Eckmann MS, Hustak EC, Engle MP. Evidence-based pain medicine for primary care physicians Proceedings (Baylor University: Medical Center). 2018;31(7):37–47. https://doi.org/10.1080/08998280.2017.1400290.

Thompson BL, Gage J, Kirk R. Living well with chronic pain: a classical grounded theory. Disabil Rehabil. 2020; 42(8);1141–52.

Chapter 35
Tendinopathies

Sue Dahl-Popolizo and Cindy C. Ivy

Introduction

Tendinitis is a term historically used as the diagnosis for pain and swelling of a tendon [1]. Current nomenclature differentiates tendinitis from tendinosis and other terms as follows:

Tendinitis: Acute pain and inflammation in a tendon, absent of microscopic tendon damage.

Tendinosis: Chronic tendon pain due to degenerative damage of tendon tissue. Tendon fibers are disorganized and appear scarred.

Tendinopathy is another term used, indicating a chronic tendon pathology.

Tenosynovitis: Inflammation and swelling of a tendon, typically caused by repetitive activities/movements.

Common tendinopathies seen in PC occur at the lateral epicondyle (lateral epicondylitis/tennis elbow), medial epicondyle (medial epicondylitis/golfer's elbow), rotator cuff tendons, and Achilles tendon [1–3]. DeQuervain's tenosynovitis and stenosing tenosynovitis (STS) or *trigger finger* are also common tendinopathies seen in PC. The descriptions below use the common names you will likely see. Keep in mind, when you see the diagnosis of tendinitis, most of these will be tendinosis.

S. Dahl-Popolizo (✉)
Arizona State University, Phoenix, AZ, USA

AT Still University, Mesa, AZ, USA
e-mail: Sue.Dahlpopolizio@asu.edu; sdahlpopolizio@atsu.edu

C. C. Ivy
Northern Arizona University, Phoenix Biomedical Campus, Phoenix, AZ, USA
e-mail: Cynthia.ivy@nau.edu

© Springer Nature Switzerland AG 2023
S. Dahl-Popolizio et al. (eds.), *Primary Care Occupational Therapy*,
https://doi.org/10.1007/978-3-031-20882-9_35

- *Lateral Epicondylitis/ "tennis elbow":* Pain at the lateral epicondyle region in the origin or anchor site of the wrist extensor tendons. Typically the extensor carpi radialis brevis is the primary muscle that is involved, but the other wrist and finger extensors can be involved as well. The most common cause of this condition is the overuse of these tendons through repetitive gripping tasks, especially with some level of elbow extension (e.g., painting, mechanical work, cutting, etc.). Trauma can cause this condition, as in excessive force applied to the extended wrist, or a direct blow to the tendon. This is less common, but can increase susceptibility to future injury [4].
- *Medial Epicondylitis/"golfer's elbow":* Pain at the medial epicondyle at the origin of the flexor pronator mass which includes pronator teres, flexor carpi radialis (primarily); flexor digitorum superficialis, palmaris longus, flexor carpi ulnaris (possibly). Pain worsens with gripping and forearm motion. Sports involving repetitive wrist flexion and pronation (e.g., golfing, throwing, racquet sports), or repetitive or forceful activities that involve repeated or sustained resistance to flexed wrist/fingers (lifting heavy objects, forceful grip, repetitive or sustained vibration, etc.). It can also occur traumatically [5].
- *Stenosing Tenosynovitis/"trigger finger":* The finger flexor tendons are encased in a tendon sheath, and are kept in place against the volar surface of the bones of the digits via a pulley system. The most proximal pulley, the A-1 pulley, can become inflamed and can thicken over time. The flexor tendon that passes through the pulley can become inflamed, and develop a nodule just distal to the pulley. As the tendon continues to pass through the pulley with finger flexion, the nodule moves proximally through the pulley and may get stuck on the proximal aspect, causing the patient to experience painful locking of the PIP in flexion, or *triggering.* In more severe cases, the patient uses the contralateral hand to unlock or extend the finger [6]. Trigger finger often progresses in stages from pain with palpation just proximal to the metacarpal head to locking in flexion, which is only released by passive extension.
- *DeQuervain's Tenosynovitis:* Tendons, (extensor pollicis brevis and abductor pollicis longus),and the tendon sheath at the lateral aspect of the base of the thumb become irritated and inflamed due to constriction of the tendons in the first dorsal compartment of the extensor retinaculum. This can be caused by overuse, specifically with resisted radial deviation, and is also common with pregnancy or soon after childbirth. It is most common in middle aged women, and can comorbidly occur with rheumatoid conditions [7].

Rotator Cuff Tendinitis: This term technically refers to tendinitis of the rotator cuff tendons including the

Supraspinatus (most commonly injured tendon)—initiates abduction, and tends to become compressed against the acromion process and coracoacromial arch when there is a muscle balance discrepancy (weakness of posterior shoulder girdle).
Infraspinatus—primary function is external rotation
Teres minor—assists with external rotation
Subscapularis—primarily responsible for internal rotation

Additional Issues that Present Pain and Dysfunction in the Shoulder

Long head of the bicep—is another commonly injured tendon. It is part of the shoulder joint capsule, and it can become tethered or impinged from the ligament in the bicipital groove of the humerus. At times a long head of the biceps will rupture without pain and the patient will present with a mass at the mid-anterior aspect of their arm, even months or years after the injury. This is sometimes referred to as *Popeye arm* and does not require treatment from the OTP if the patient is not having pain or other functional deficits as a result.

Impingement—irritation to any of the rotator cuff muscles or the long head of the biceps is sometimes referred to as *impingement* as it is thought that there is compression on the natural gliding action of the tendon in the close space occupied within the scapula and the attachment on the humerus. Impingement is caused by abrasion of the cuff by the acromion, intrasubstance degenerative tearing, tendinosis, aging, overuse, or avascularity.

Bursitis-bursae are fluid filled sacs that help protect the rotator cuff tendons and facilitate normal gliding. Inflammation of the bursae can be quite painful.

Adhesive Capsulitis-rotator cuff pathology is often mistaken for adhesive capsulitis which is a tightening of the joint capsule resulting in reduced range of motion and pain with unknown cause. It is also called *frozen shoulder*. At times, this condition may occur with no known cause.

Role of PCP

For all of these conditions, the PCP typically completes: diagnostic testing, pain management through over-the-counter or prescription medication, referrals to OT or physical therapy (PT), or to an orthopedic surgeon for evaluation for surgery or steroid injections. Some PCPs may do a steroid injection in their office. The PCP may refer chronic or recalcitrant conditions to pain management specialists, usually anesthesiologists.

Diagnostic Tests and Thresholds

Ultrasound of the affected musculoskeletal tissue can be used to detect whether the pain is due to inflammation or degenerative changes. This helps determine the optimal course of treatment.

Other diagnostic techniques used by the PCP include palpation, X-ray to rule out other issues, MRI to determine lesion site, aspiration of fluid, if appropriate, to rule out/in infection, anesthetic injection to determine if pain is alleviated.

Common Comorbidities

Many of these conditions occur as a result of overuse, and they can be very frustrating for the patient, especially when they become chronic. Comorbidities to assess for include:

- Arthritis (Chap. 12)
- Depression (Chap. 18)
- Anxiety (Chap. 11)
- Advanced age (pathogenesis is likely a degenerative process in many cases)

Role of OTP

Assess to ensure you know what you are treating and provide appropriate intervention to minimize pain and maximize function. It is a good idea to complete a quality of life assessment or assess whether the patient is experiencing stress or dissatisfaction at work as this can be a factor in how quickly, or whether, the patient will respond to treatment.

Occupational Impact

Occupational impact varies from mild impairment to severe disability, depending on which tendon is involved, its function, and duration of symptoms. Adults engaged in repetitive occupations tend to be at higher risk for chronic tendinopathy. Repetitive occupations can include work functions but are also commonly associated with recreational and daily activities. With prolonged tendon involvement, patients experience weakness, loss of function in the activities that require use of the involved tendon(s). Patients often employ modified postures to avoid using the injured tendon/extremity and exacerbating the pain. Further weakness and additional tendon and postural problems can occur as a result. Sleep may be affected as well due to pain in the affected area. Symptoms can impact all aspects of ADL/IADLs, which in turn negatively impact mental health and quality of life.

OT Areas of Emphasis

Many of these patients respond well to conservative treatment. They may require only one or a few visits of OT, or they may require two to three visits a week for a few weeks. If your setting is conducive to providing the treatment, these patients respond very well to OT in the PC office, especially if they are referred soon after the symptoms present. If they require more treatment than you can provide in this setting, you can refer them to an outpatient therapy center.

Evaluation

- Occupational profile—special attention to all activities which aggravate the symptoms and activities in which symptoms are not aggravated or are resolved
- Grip and pinch strength
- Place involved tendon in lengthened position to see if pain is provoked
- Resist involved tendon to assess strength (manual muscle testing [MMT]), and for pain with resistance
- Palpation over involved tendon insertion or distal palm in the case of stenosing tenosynovitis/trigger finger
- In case of suspected lateral epicondylitis, resisted middle finger extension and palpation over the supinator can assess for radial nerve impingement
- In case of suspected rotator cuff involvement, there are a number of provocative maneuvers https://www.healthline.com/health/rotator-cuff-tear-test that can be assessed by the OTP-videos and instructions available free online if you search 'provocative tests for rotator cuff'.
- Gross sensory test to rule out co-morbid nerve compression
- Edema (circumferential measurement compared to uninvolved side and ipsilateral side over time)
- Pain scale
- Outcome measure such as QuickDASH

Intervention Strategies

- The most important intervention for the OTP in the case of tendinoses is to assess and modify the aggravating activities. This may involve problem-solving alternative positions and techniques as well as use of tools and adaptive techniques.
- Orthosis used to rest the inflamed area and stop the aggravating function. Patterns and pictures of 'Common Orthoses in Primary Care' can be found in the Appendix. Some examples include:
  - Trial of volar wrist orthosis for medial and lateral epicondylitis-wear during activity and at night, removing for wrist ROM exercises. The wrist should be in about 10–15° of extension in both cases.
  - Trial of custom PIP flexion block or prefabricated Oval 8 (™) orthosis to block PIP flexion for trigger finger—wear 3 weeks day and night, followed by 3 weeks night only for a total of 6 weeks. The Oval 8 (™) should not be restrictive. At times, two are needed as options to change orthosis to accommodate changes in swelling. If the thumb is involved, a custom figure-8 orthotic preventing IP flexion can be very effective.

- For DeQuervains tenosynovitis, use an over-the-counter or custom thumb spica orthosis with the wrist included and the IP joint of the thumb left free to move.
- A "tennis elbow", also called "Nirschl" strap can be helpful in the case of both medial and lateral epicondylitis to redistribute the force at the common flexor and extensor tendon attachment points at the elbow. This should be worn during activity during the day. Make sure that the strap is tight enough to support but not too tight that it is restrictive on the blood vessels. At least one finger should fit beneath the strap when testing. Place the strap approximately two fingers distal to the elbow crease.

- Stretching and range of motion exercises throughout the day.

  - For medial and lateral epicondylitis, it is helpful to do approximately 20–25 repetitions of active range of motion to wrist extension and flexion in a pain free range several times per day. If performing the range of motion is painful, try placing the wrist and forearm in a gravity-reduced plane. Stretching should also not provoke pain, however, the client will feel the stretch. Holding the stretch for a minimum of 30 seconds and repeating throughout the day will give the best results.
  - For trigger finger, it is important to maintain AROM without aggravating the tenosynovitis. Performing isolated DIP, PIP, and MCP AROM is usually effective and non-aggravating. The finger should not be painful or trigger during the AROM. This may be performed 3× per day up to 10 repetitions each time.
  - For DeQuervain's tenosynovitis, the thumb and the wrist should be isolated when performing AROM and stretching. In other words, do not allow the wrist to ulnarly deviate simultaneously with thumb CMC, MCP, or IP flexion until this can be done without causing pain. If the patient continues to have pain that is not resolving after about 2 weeks, it would be appropriate to refer to a therapist who specializes in the hand and upper extremity.
  - For the shoulder, it is often best to begin with Codman's Pendulum exercises. Instruct the client to begin with a wide stance, hips slightly flexed, and hold on to the table or counter surface with the uninvolved side. Gently rock the body forward and backward with the shoulder and arm relaxed (passively swinging gently) until the involved shoulder naturally picks up momentum with the swing of the arm and gravity with no active muscle movement at the glenohumeral joint. Repeat swaying side to side. Repeat with a cone shape movement. This exercise will require practice with the therapist, perhaps mirror feedback, and hip movement to avoid active engagement of the shoulder muscles. After a week or so of doing pendulum exercises several times per day, it would be appropriate to try dowel exercises, wall climbs, and scapular protraction and retraction by gliding arms forward with hands on a large ball on the table.
  - If the patient continues to have pain at this point, it would be appropriate to refer to a physical therapy (PT) or OT shoulder specialist.

- Use of hot and cold modalities for pain and inflammation management.
- If the therapist is skilled in the administration of manual therapy techniques, they can be implemented in this setting.
- If general hand weakness is a concern, theraputty is an excellent strengthening tool to have in the clinic. See the Appendix for *Theraputty Handout* for specific exercises.

Other Considerations and Resources

Many of the references listed provide more extensive information that may be helpful to the OTP working in PC.

References

1. National Institute of Arthritis and Musculoskeletal and Skin Diseases. Sports injuries basics. National Institute of Health. https://www.niams.nih.gov/health-topics/tendinitis#tab-overview.
2. King D and Genin J. Tendinitis or tendinosis? Why the difference is important, what treatments can help. Cleveland Clinic. 2016. https://health.clevelandclinic.org/tendinitis-tendinosis-difference-important-treatments-help/.
3. Wilson JJ, Best TM. Common overuse tendon problems: a review and recommendations for treatment. Am Fam Physician. 2005;72(5):811–8. https://www.aafp.org/afp/2005/0901/p811.html.
4. Hand Care: The Upper Extremity Expert. Tennis elbow–lateral epicondylitis. American Society for Surgery of the Hand. 2017. https://www.assh.org/handcare/hand-arm-conditions/tennis-elbow.
5. Abbasi D and Ahmad CS. Ortho bullets: medial epicondylitis (golfer's elbow). American Shoulder and Elbow Surgeons. 2021. https://www.orthobullets.com/shoulder-and-elbow/3083/medial-epicondylitis-golfers-elbow.
6. OrthoInfo. Trigger finger. https://orthoinfo.aaos.org/en/diseases%2D%2Dconditions/trigger-finger/.
7. OrthoInfo. De Quervain's tenosynovitis. https://orthoinfo.aaos.org/en/diseases%2D%2Dconditions/de-quervains-tendinosis/.

Chapter 36
Visual Impairments

Jason Vice

Introduction

Visual impairment can occur at any point along the visual pathway, including optical irregularities associated with anatomy of the eye, pathology of the retina and optic nerve, or damage to visual processing areas in the brain. Vision screening should begin as early as infancy [1] and continue throughout the lifespan, as prevalence of both natural and pathological changes increase with age [2]. Visual acuity or sharpness of vision is one of the primary measures of visual performance. Additionally, the visual field or area that can be seen while focusing on a single point, eye movements, and pupillary response may be assessed to determine the integrity of the neurological components of the visual system.

Visual perception refers to the ability to interpret and understand what is seen. It plays an important role in childhood development and occupational performance at all ages. Visual perception is dependent upon accurate input from the visual system as well as integration with other sensory inputs and cognitive processes in the brain [3]. Assessments of visual perceptual skills vary in length and time for completion; therefore, they may not routinely be evaluated by a PCP unless otherwise indicated.

- *Visual Acuity*—Measured as a Snellen fraction (testing distance/distance at which normal eye can resolve targets on chart) or equivalent. Typically measured in feet, meters or LogMAR. Typical testing distances are 20 ft. or 6 m (Table 36.1).

  - Notes about Visual Acuity:

    Most children do not achieve adult levels of vision (20/20 using Snellen measures) until at least 5 years of age [5].

J. Vice (✉)
University of Alabama, Birmingham, AL, USA
e-mail: jvice02@uab.edu

Table 36.1 Visual acuity [4]

Ranges	U.S Notation (feet)	Snellen Fraction (meters)	LogMAR
Normal vision	20/12.5–20/25	6/3.8–6/7.5	−0.2–+0.1
Near Normal vision	20/32–20/63	6/9.5–6/19	0.2–0.5
Moderate low vision	20/70–20/160	6/21–6/48	0.54–0.9
Severe low vision	20/200–20/400	6/60–6/120	+1.0–1.3
Profound low vision	20/500–20/1000	6/150–6/300	1.4–1.7
Near blindness	20/1250–20/2000	6/380–6/600	1.8–+2.0
Blindness	No light perception (NLP)	No light perception (NLP)	NLP

Table 36.2 Visual fields [6]

Average Limits of the Visual Field		
Vertical degrees	Superior field	60°
	Inferior field	75°
Horizontal degrees	Temporal field	100°
	Nasal field	60°

Visual acuity measures are typically for distance viewing which does not require accommodation (focusing of the lens) to clearly see targets. Persons with focusing issues or adults over 40 years of age (due to presbyopia) may have reduced visual acuity when viewing at near distances.

A best-corrected visual acuity of 20/200 or worse is often referred to as "Legal Blindness." Legal blindness is merely a definition used to determine eligibility for certain disability benefits and provides little functional information about how well a person can see.

Physicians may denote the progressive terms "counting fingers" (CF), "hand motion" (HM), and "light perception only" (LPO) when unable to quantify visual acuity.

- *Visual Field*—Measured in vertical and horizontal degrees as the total area to which a person can detect a static or moving target in each eye while fixating on a central point. A visual field test can assess both central and peripheral vision integrity (Table 36.2).

  - Notes about Visual Field:

    The visual field of each eye overlaps centrally. Therefore, it is important to test the visual field monocularly (one eye) versus binocularly (both eyes together).

    Degrees of visual field are expected to be slightly different between the left and right eye and from person-to-person, due to facial characteristics.

    The person being tested must keep their gaze steady during visual field assessment. Movement of the head or eye makes test results less reliable.

    The physiological blind spot (where the optic nerve exits each eye) is a normal landmark of visual field testing.

Table 36.3 Cranial nerve palsy [7]

Cranial nerve palsy	Exam findings (in primary gaze)
3rd nerve palsy	Eye turns downward and outward
4th nerve palsy	Eye turns upward and outward
6th nerve palsy	Eye turns medially toward nose

- *Eye Movements and Alignment*—Measured as conjugate movements of both eyes in the same direction at the same time and vergence movements of both eyes in opposite directions at the same time to maintain fixation on an object of interest. Abnormal response or misalignment of one eye may result in loss of visual fusion or the perception of double vision (diplopia). Examination of eye movements tests the integrity of cranial nerves 3, 4, and 6, extraocular eye muscles, and higher-order centers that control eye movements (Table 36.3).

  - Notes about Eye Movements and Alignment:

    Near point of convergence (NPC) tests visual fusion as an object approaches the face. Both eyes should be fixated on the object and the patient should not report seeing the object in double. Normal NPC is 10 cm (4 in.) or less. Eye deviations may interfere with depth perception and coordination. -Tropia (eye misalignment at all times) and -phoria (eye drift only some of the time).

    Esotropia (one or both eyes turned inward, "cross-eyed") and exotropia (one or both eyes turned outward, "lazy-eye") are referred to as strabismus. Uncorrected strabismus in childhood can result in amblyopia, a decrease or loss of vision in one eye. Uncorrected strabismus in adults usually results in double vision.

    Nystagmus is repetitive, involuntary oscillating movement of the eyes. Physiologic nystagmus is a normal response when the eyes are moved to an extreme position or after spinning. Pathologic nystagmus can be present at birth and may be associated with dysfunction of the vestibular system.

- *Pupillary Response*—Measures integrity of the optic nerve and parasympathetic branch of the oculomotor nerve to changes in light levels or accommodation. In typical room light, pupils should be round, symmetrical, and 3–6 mm in diameter.

  - Notes about Pupillary Response:

    In the direct light reflex, the pupil tested constricts to direct light. A normal response includes a consensual reflex by the opposite pupil. Failure of the tested pupil to constrict or failure of the opposite pupil to constrict suggests oculomotor nerve lesion to one of the eyes. Failure of either pupil to constrict suggests a lesion of the optic nerve.

    In some cases, the pupil may intentionally be dilated by the PCP in order to examine the fundus or back of the eye. Some stimulant medications and illicit substances may also cause dilation of the pupils.

Common Conditions Affecting the Eye
- Myopia—"nearsightedness"; a condition in which the eyeball is too long causing close objects to appear clearly, but distant objects to appear blurry.
- Hyperopia—"farsightedness"; a condition in which the eyeball is too short causing close objects to appear blurry, but distant objects to appear clearly.
- Astigmatism—a condition related to irregular curvature of the cornea causing blurry vision.
- Dry Eye—a condition in which there is insufficient or ineffective lubrication of the eye, resulting in reduced visual acuity.
- Ptosis—drooping of the upper eyelid, which decreases the visual field.
- Nystagmus—repetitive, involuntary oscillations of the eye which reduce visual acuity.
- Strabismus—misalignment of the eyes which may cause blurred or double vision.
- Amblyopia—"lazy eye"; reduction or loss of vision associated with misalignment of the eyes in early life.
- Conjunctivitis—redness or inflammation of the transparent layer of tissue which covers the sclera (white of the eye) and lines the inner eyelid.

Common Conditions Affecting the Retina
- Age-Related Macular Degeneration (AMD)—a condition resulting in blurring or loss of central visual acuity as a result of cellular debris or abnormal blood vessel growth in the macula (retina). Can be dry (non-exudative) or wet (exudative) types.
- Diabetic Retinopathy (DR)—a condition related to diabetes in which persistently elevated blood glucose damages small blood vessels and cells in the retina.
- Glaucoma—a group of eye diseases most frequently associated with increased intraocular eye pressure which result in permanent damage to the optic nerve.
- Retinitis Pigmentosa—genetic disorder involving progressive loss of rod photoreceptor cells, resulting in decreased peripheral vision and night blindness.

Common Conditions of Neurologic Processing of Vision
- Homonymous Hemianopia—a visual field loss typically involving either the left or right halves of vision from both eyes.
- Visual Neglect—a neurologic disorder of attention in which a person fails to respond to stimuli in the side of visual space contralateral to the brain lesion, typically the left visual field.
- Cortical Visual Impairment—a bilateral visual impairment due to neurologic injury, such as hypoxia, ischemia, or developmental brain defects often seen in children.

Role of PCP

Vision screening is typically completed by a PCP as part of a regular checkup [8]. The vision screen is not a diagnostic process, but a means to detect disorders of vision that require further comprehensive examination by an eye doctor, such as an ophthalmologist or optometrist. An ophthalmologist is a medical doctor who specializes in the complex medical and surgical management of visual impairment. An optometrist is a health care professional who specializes in refractive errors of the eye, but is also trained to identify and treat other eye disorders. Further examination and treatment for benign conditions may be completed by the PCP depending on signs and symptoms [9].

Vision Screening for Low-Risk Patients

A typical examination by a PCP will include a basic assessment of eye alignment, pupillary response, eye movements, red reflex, and eye examination. A penlight is used to measure eye alignment by assessing for uniform corneal light reflection and also to inspect the shape and response of the pupil to light. The ability to move the eyes in unison through the six cardinal points of gaze may be assessed using a penlight, finger, or other target. An ophthalmoscope may be used to observe reflection of light from the retina and through the intervening structures of the eye. Visual acuity in children may be tested annually with a symbols chart. Visual acuity in persons ages 6–40 should be tested every 3 years with a Snellen chart. All persons over age 40 should have a baseline comprehensive exam.

Current guidelines from the Centers for Disease Control and Prevention (CDC) recommend that persons with diabetes get a dilated eye exam every year. In addition, people at higher risk for glaucoma (African Americans age 40 and older and everyone older than 60 years of age) need a dilated eye exam once every 2 years.

Common Comorbidities

Common comorbidities that may contribute to vision loss
- Chronic health conditions
- Cerebrovascular accident
- Parkinson's disease
- Diabetes
- Hypertension
- Multiple sclerosis (MS)
- Brain tumors
- Genetic conditions

  - Achromatopsia
  - Albinism
  - Cone-rod dystrophy
  - Marfan syndrome
  - Retinoschisis
  - Stargardt disease

- Traumatic brain injury
- Medications that may affect vision

  - Alpha-blockers
  - Anticonvulsants
  - Antihistamines
  - Antirheumatics
  - Beta-blockers
  - Corticosteroids (chronic use)
  - Diuretics
  - Erectile dysfunction (ED) drugs
  - Osteoporosis drugs

Role of OTP

The OTP will evaluate visual function through screening and functional observation to determine how visual impairment may be affecting performance and participation in desired occupations. This information will be incorporated into the occupational profile and be used to develop an appropriate intervention plan.

Occupational Impact

The impact of vision on occupational participation is significant. The degree to which an impairment limits functional performance is relative to factors such as the degree of vision loss, location in the visual field (central or peripheral), treatment options (medical or optical) and personal factors such as age of onset, level of support, and receptiveness to environmental modification and compensatory strategies. A person born with decreased vision may more readily utilize alternative strategies and technologies, while a person who has lived the majority of their life fully sighted may be less receptive to adaptation, but have a good visual memory on which to rely.

OT Areas of Emphasis

It is critical that the client be evaluated using their best-corrected vision, therefore the client should wear their eyeglasses and view through the appropriate area of the lenses for each task. If the OTP suspects a visual impairment, they should make or request a referral to an eye doctor for a comprehensive evaluation. In PC, the

OTP will focus on providing client education for evidence-based strategies to promote safety, participation, and maximal independence with desired occupations, including, but not limited to, environmental modifications, assistive technology, compensatory techniques, safe medication management, diabetes self-management education, alternative transportation resources, psychosocial support resources, and recommendations for community-based services such as vocational rehabilitation and referrals to vision rehabilitation specialists.

Evaluation

Suggested areas to assess:

- Visual Acuity
    - Distance Acuity (Adults)

        Snellen Eye Chart
        ETDRS Chart

    - Distance Acuity (Pediatrics)

        LEA Symbols Chart
        HOTV Pediatric Eye Chart

    - Near Visual Acuity (Adults)

        Sloan Letter Near Vision Card

    - Near Visual Acuity (Pediatrics)

        LEA Symbols Near Vison Card

- Visual Field
    - Confrontation testing (one person)
    - Simultaneous confrontation testing (two person)
    - Tangent screen
- ADL Assessment
    - Revised Self-Report Assessment of Functional Visual Performance (R-SRAFVP) (free, available online)
- Observation of functional visual performance
    - Read standard print from a book or newspaper
    - Fill out a check or other form
    - Narrated walk through a crowded or unfamiliar space
    - Measure water in a clear or Pyrex® measuring cup

- Environmental risk factors, including home safety and accessibility screening
- Fear of falling and falls efficacy

  – <u>Falls Efficacy Scale</u> (free, available online)
  – <u>Functional Reach Test</u> (free, available online)

- Psychosocial Assessment

  – <u>Geriatric Depression Scale</u> (free, available online)

- Special Tests (only when specific signs/symptoms are present; non-diagnostic)

  – Accommodation

    Near Point Convergence—Assesses ability to focus up close

  – Strabismus/Misalignment

    Cover Test—determines whether there is tropia
    Cover/Uncover Test—determines whether there is phoria

  – Eye Movements/Ocular Motility Deficiency

    Extraocular tracking assessment using moving visual target

  – Color Vison

    Ishihara Test

  – Contrast Sensitivity

    Pelli Robson Contrast Sensitivity Chart

  – Distortion/Missing Areas of Vision

    <u>Amsler grid</u>

  – Visual Neglect

    Cancellation tests
    Brain Injury Visual Assessment Battery for Adults (biVABA)

Intervention Strategies

Evidence-based interventions must be client-centered with the goal of maximizing safety and participation. In PC, the OTP will focus on education and training on environmental modifications, adaptive techniques, assistive technology, and community-based referrals. Interventions which include recommendations for optical devices, prescription changes, or those which seek to restore or correct vision problems (such as vision therapy) are strictly completed under the instruction and supervision of an ophthalmologist or optometrist. Clients requiring these services should be referred to the appropriate vision specialists.

- Environmental Modifications
  - Client education on environmental modifications to enhance visibility and safety awareness, including utilization of appropriate task and ambient room lighting, contrasting colors, glare reduction, high-contrast markings on steps and drop-offs, and removal of trip hazards.
- Medication and Health Management
  - Large print or talking glucometers, blood pressure monitors, and weight scales, large print or electronic schedules and reminders, talking medication bottles or RF label readers, large print prescription labels, prepackaged prescriptions, and readable educational handouts.
- Adaptive Techniques
  - Client education and training on organizational strategies, placement of tactile markers on appliances, enlarged print, bold writing tools, large button devices, and high-contrast cookware/drinkware.
- Assistive Technology
  - Client education and training on voice-activated technology, text-to-speech features, audiobooks, computer/smart phone modifications, online bill pay, online shopping/delivery, and transportation apps.
- Community-Based Referrals
  - Client education and referrals for access to alternative transportation, Meals on Wheels, vision support groups, vocational rehabilitation services, independent living services, and vision specialists including ophthalmology, optometry, and low vision OT specialists.

Other Considerations and Resources

Documentation and Billing

Medicare and most third-party payers provide reimbursement for OTPs to provide services related to low vision rehabilitation. It is important when submitting for prior authorization to be clear that services are related to rehabilitation and not vision therapy. Vision therapy is not traditionally under the scope of OT and is not currently reimbursable by Medicare or other payers. Most diagnoses related to vision, including codes for level of visual impairment, trigger reimbursement. Clients who require specialized training for use of prescription optical devices for reading and driving, eccentric viewing techniques, and visual scanning techniques should be referred to a low vision OT specialist. Note that low vision OT and traditional OT services may be reimbursed concurrently in certain cases, provided duplication of services does not occur.

References

1. Donahue SP, Nixon CN, Section on Ophthalmology, American Academy of Pediatrics, American Academy of Ophthalmology, American Association for Pediatric Ophthalmology and Strabismus, & American Association of Certified Orthoptists. Visual system assessments of infants, children, and young adults by pediatricians. Pediatrics. 2016;137(1):28–30. https://doi.org/10.1542/peds.2015-3596.
2. Klein R, Klein BE. The prevalence of age-related eye diseases and visual impairment in aging: current estimates. Investig Ophthalmol Vis Sci. 2013;54(14):ORSF5–ORSF13. https://doi.org/10.1167/iovs.13-12789.
3. Shimojo S, Paradiso M, Fujita I. What visual perception tells us about mind and brain. Proc Natl Acad Sci. 2001;98(22):12340–1. https://doi.org/10.1073/pnas.221383698.
4. International Council of Ophthalmology (ICO). Visual standards: aspects and ranges of vision loss with emphasis on population studies. 2002.
5. Leat SJ, Yadav NK, Irving EL. Development of visual acuity and contrast sensitivity in children. Aust J Optom. 2009;2(1):19–26. https://doi.org/10.3921/joptom.2009.19.
6. Spector RH. Visual Fields. In: Walker HK, Hall WD, Hurst JW, editors. Clinical methods: the history, physical, and laboratory examinations. 3rd ed. Boston: Butterworths; 1990.
7. Park UC, Kim SJ, Hwang JM, Yu YS. Clinical features and natural history of acquired third, fourth, and sixth cranial nerve palsy. Eye. 2008;22:691–6.
8. Shields SR. Managing eye disease in primary care: part 1. How to screen for occult disease. Postgrad Med. 2015;108(5):69–78. https://doi.org/10.3810/pgm.2000.10.1779.
9. Kaur S, Larsen H, Nattis A. Primary care approach to eye conditions. Osteopath Fam Phys. 2019;11(2):28–34.

Correction to: Nonprogressive Neurocognitive Disorders

Steven J. Taylor and Lydia Royeen

Correction to:
Chapter 17 in: Sue Dahl-Popolizio,
Primary Care Occupational Therapy, A Quick Reference Guide,
https://doi.org/10.1007/978-3-031-20882-9_17

The original version of the chapter has been revised. The chapter was previously published without the co-author. The author of chapter 17 was left out of the chapter. The necessary corrections have been made in both the Table of Contents and the chapter opener page to reflect the correction.

Steven J. Taylor is now added as a co-author to this chapter.

The updated version of the chapter can be found at https://doi.org/10.1007/978-3-031-20882-9_17

© Springer Nature Switzerland AG 2023   C1
S. Dahl-Popolizio et al. (eds.), *Primary Care Occupational Therapy*,
https://doi.org/10.1007/978-3-031-20882-9_37

Appendix

Common Orthoses in Primary Care

In primary care settings, time will be limited but you can make some common, basic orthoses if you have strong orthotic fabrication skills and basic supplies. If more involved orthotic fabrication is needed, the patient can be referred to an outpatient specialty clinic. If you need immediate guidance while fabricating any orthosis, there are many instructional videos available online with a quick Internet web search.

CMC Short Thumb Spica/Opponens

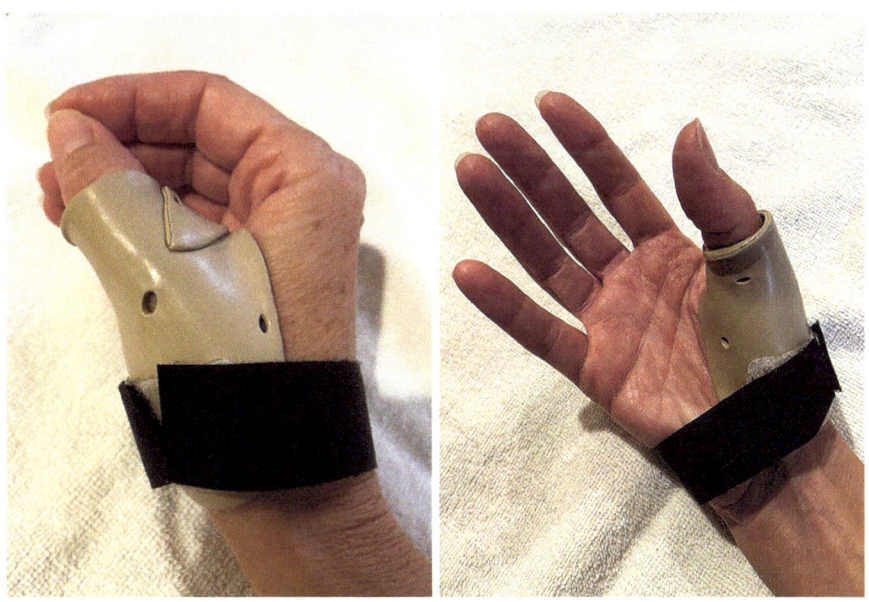

© Springer Nature Switzerland AG 2023
S. Dahl-Popolizio et al. (eds.), *Primary Care Occupational Therapy*,
https://doi.org/10.1007/978-3-031-20882-9

Pattern This half-circle shape allows you to quickly cut/wrap the material supporting the CMC and MCP joint, leaving the IP joint free. You can easily modify this pattern for size and to provide more support to the dorsal or volar aspects of the joint as needed. One long piece of Velcro is typically enough, but two pieces can be used (volar and dorsal aspects) if preferred.

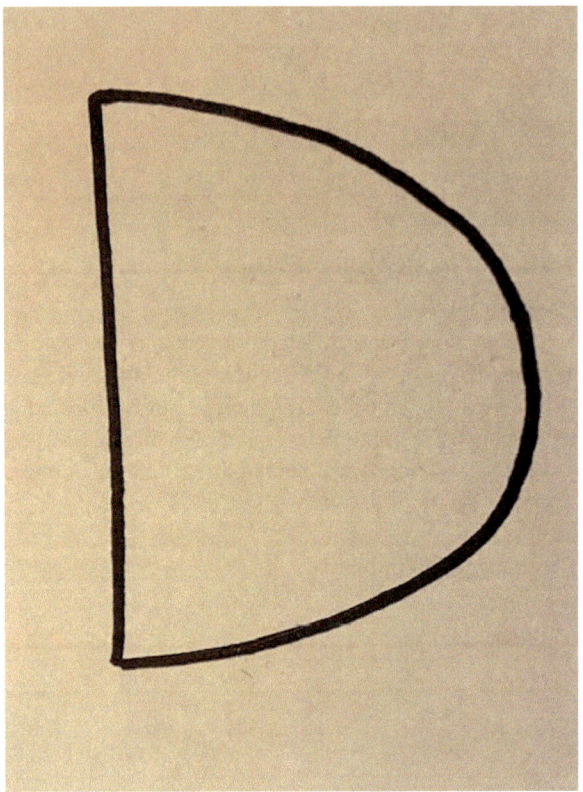

Trigger Finger (Stenosing Tenosynovitis)

The key to treating this condition effectively is reducing excursion of the tendon nodule through the A-1 pulley. This can be accomplished with various orthotic designs. The design we present is simple, easy to make/wear, and effective when PIP flexion is limited as the nodule does not pass through the A-1 pulley. This can be assessed immediately upon fabrication and fitting. Patient adherence and effectiveness of the orthosis have been very good.

Note PIP flexion is limited

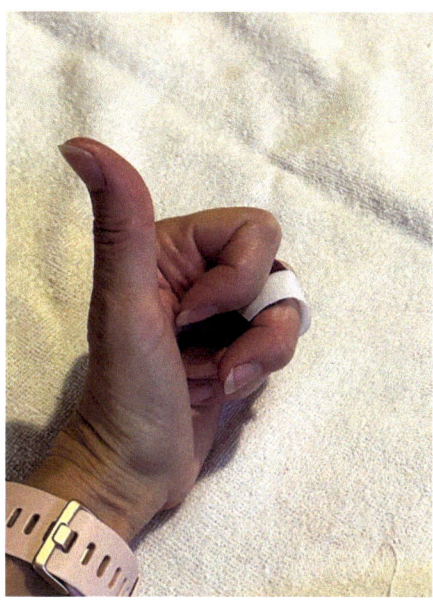

Straps do not significantly limit extension

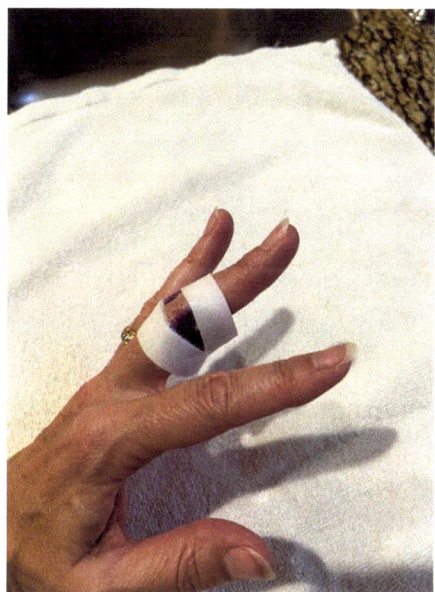

Pattern This is basically a rectangular pattern. The indentations at the waist help with Velcro placement and can help achieve smooth flexion with thicker orthotic material. Place one piece of Velcro just distal to the PIP, and one just volar to the PIP. This will secure the orthosis while allowing full to near full extension, while limiting flexion.

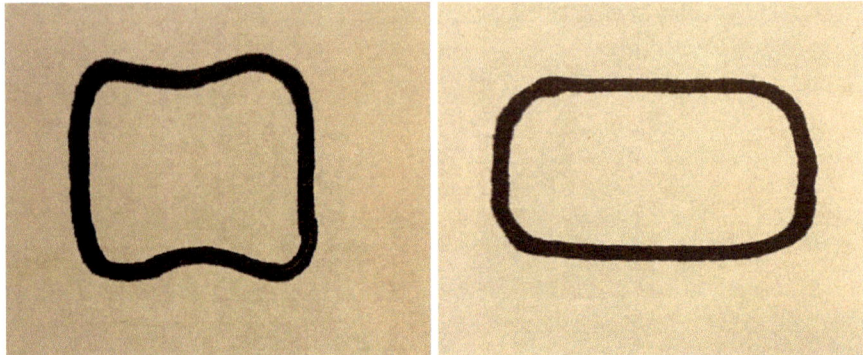

Trigger Thumb (Stenosing Tenosynovitis)

This orthosis does not require a formal pattern. It is simply a long strip of orthotic material formed into a figure-8, with the intersection at the dorsal IP joint. The volar segments are just distal and just proximal to the IP joint. This allows near full pad accessibility for sensation and pinch. As restriction is limited to IP flexion, nearly full function is available.

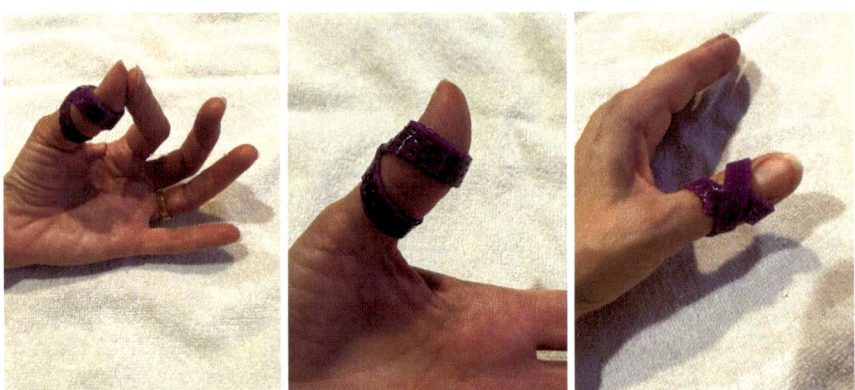

Volar Wrist Orthosis

This is the most common wrist orthosis and can be used for multiple diagnoses:

- Carpal tunnel syndrome
- General wrist strain/sprain
- Distal radius fracture (most common after ORIF)

- Lateral epicondylitis/epicondylosis
- Medial epicondylitis/epicondylosis
- Carpal ligament strain/pain
- Distal radio/ulnar joint pain
- Any wrist/forearm condition that will improve with wrist immobilization or general support

Note For most of these conditions, the wrist will be in neutral flexion/extension. For lateral epicondylitis/epicondylosis, the wrist will be in slight extension.

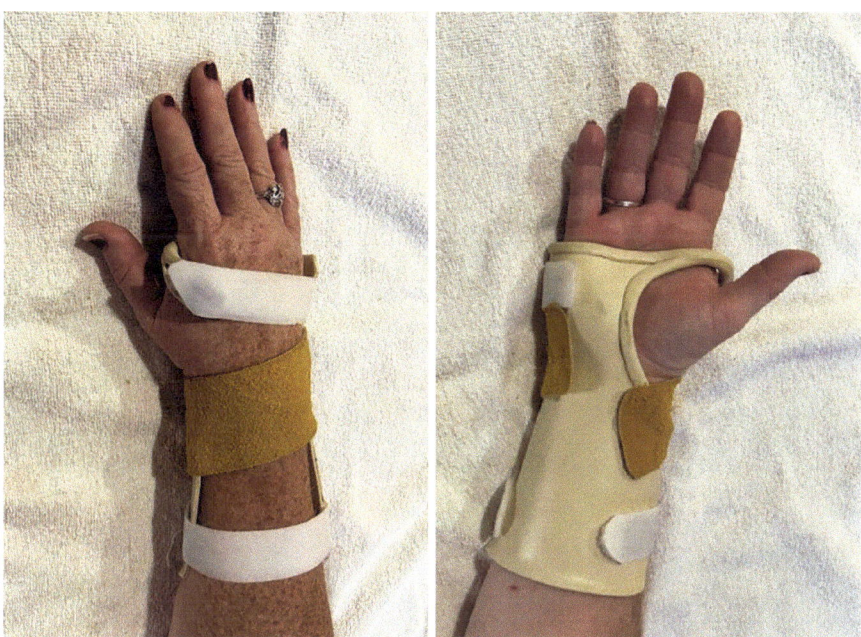

Pattern There are many patterns available. We included a common pattern that is quick and easy to cut and fit. Ensure the MP AROM is full and that the straps support the dorsal wrist, and are secure at the dorsum of the hand and proximal forearm. Orthosis should span approximately 2/3 the length of the forearm to reduce the risk of pressure at the volar forearm during functional activities.

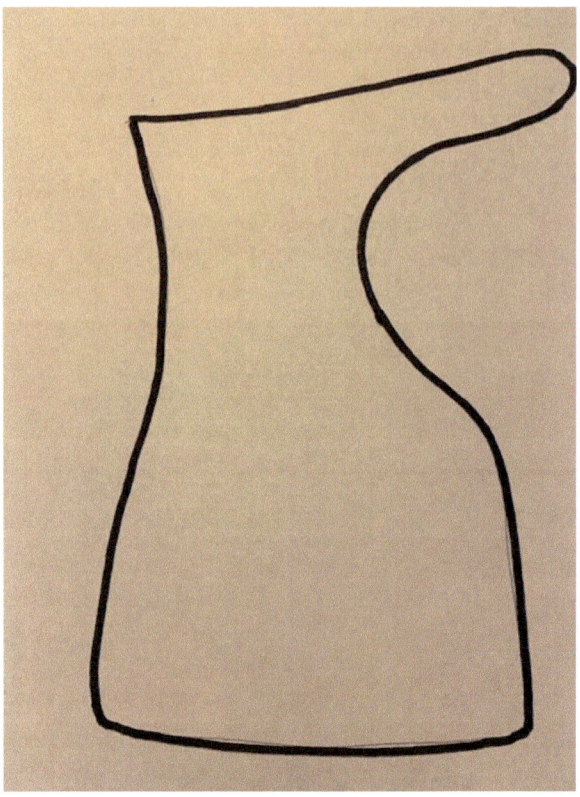

Joint Protection Techniques

To protect your joints—whenever possible:

- Use two hands when possible
- Use body or large muscle groups rather than small muscles to lift/support
- Keep joints in neutral position

Pick up bag–incorrect

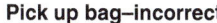

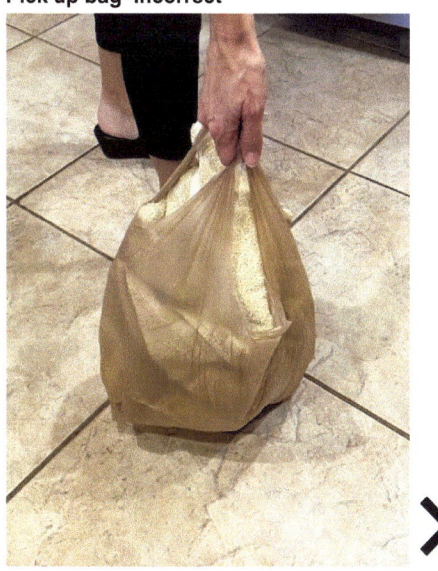

Pick up bag - correct

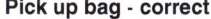

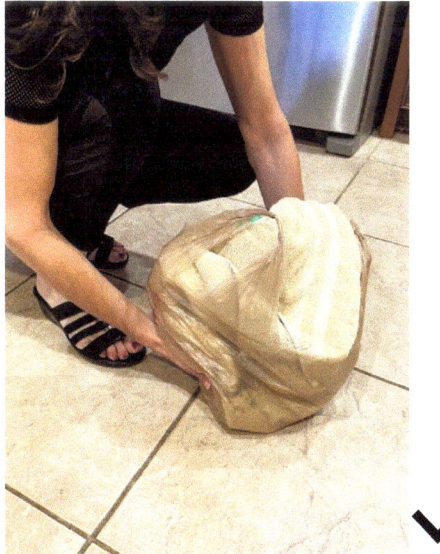

Carry bag – Incorrect

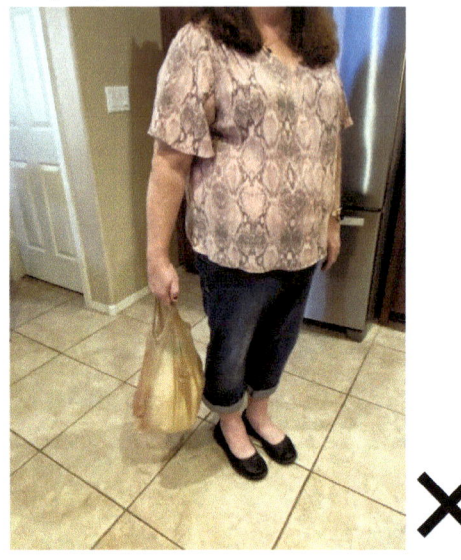

Carry bag - Correct

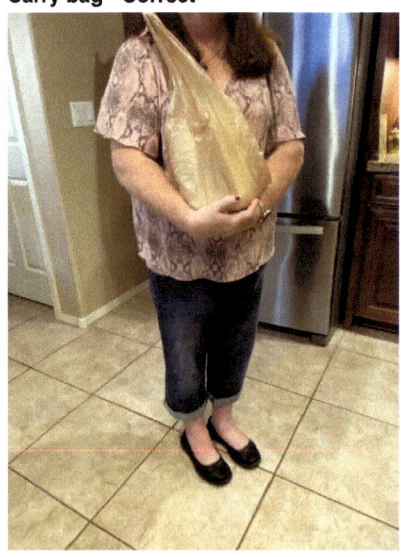

Pinch – Incorrect

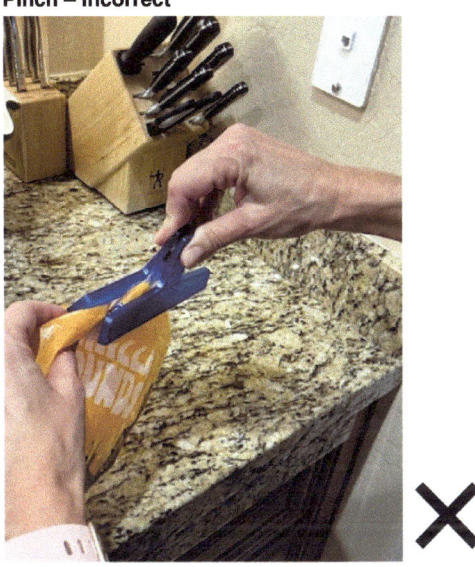

Pinch – Correct

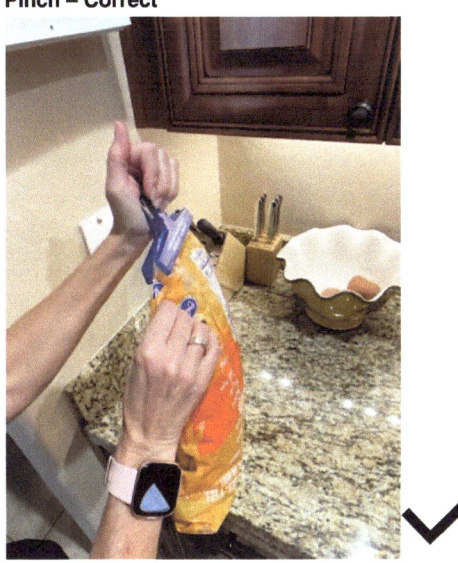

Note Use gross grasp rather than pinch.

Use Scissors – Incorrect

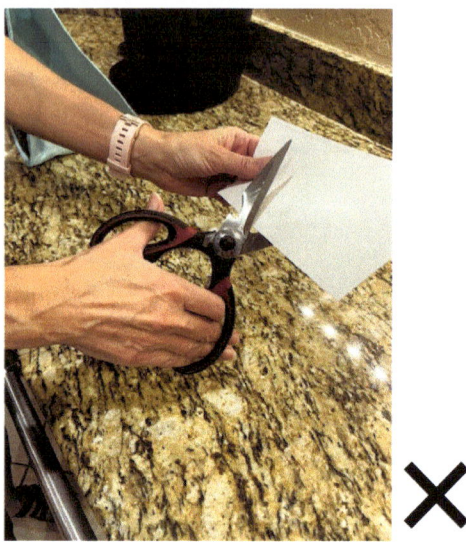

Use Scissors – Correct

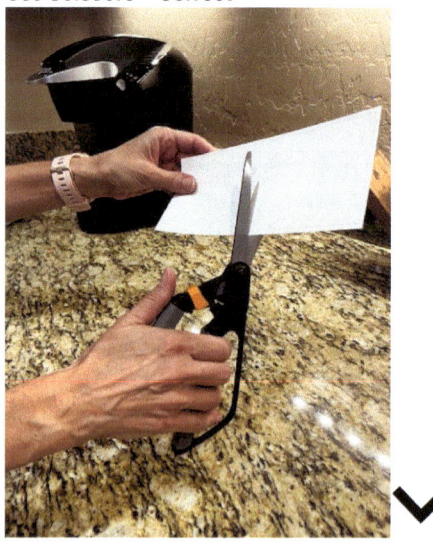

Note Use scissors that open for you (self-opening scissors) to avoid stress to thumb joints.

Stir – Incorrect

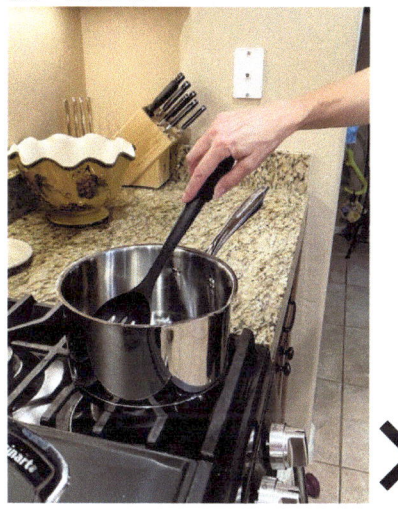

Stir – Correct

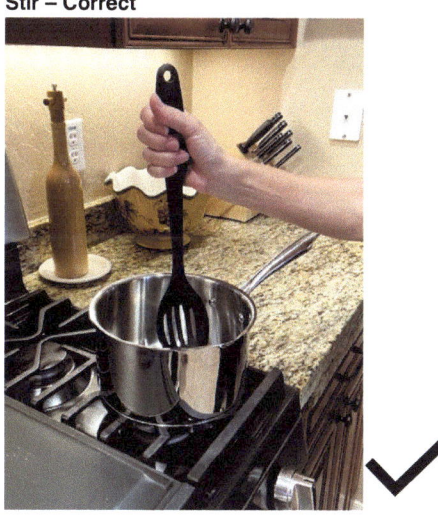

Note Use gross grasp with wrist neutral rather than pinch with wrist rotated/devi-
ated. Wider gripped tools are better for your joints.

Grasp Pan – Incorrect

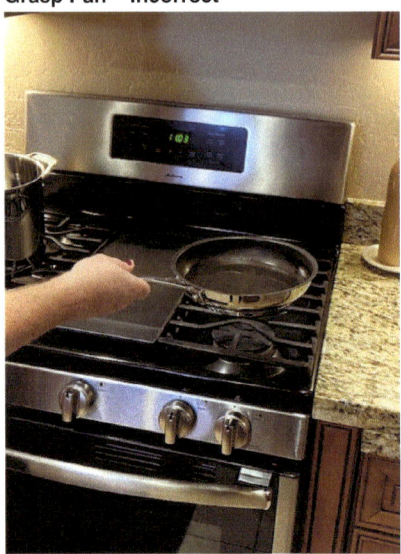

Grasp Pan – Correct

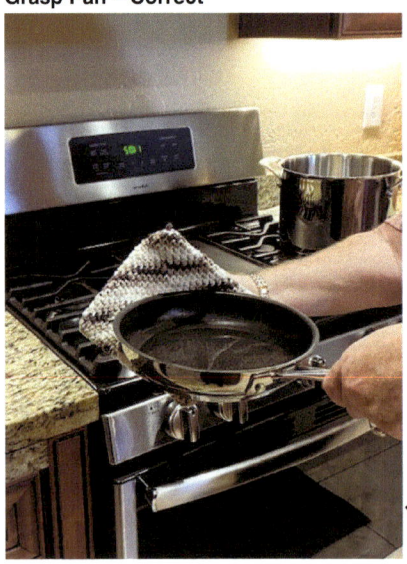

Mindfulness: Higher Literacy Level

What Is Mindfulness?

The practice of maintaining a non-judgemental state of heightened or complete awareness of one's thoughts, emotions, or experiences on a moment to moment basis.—Merriam Webster

How Can it Help?

- Reduce stress
- Increase positive feelings
- Reduce anxiety and depression
- Decrease blood pressure
- Improve digestion
- Improve sleep
- Improve mental functioning

What Can I Do?

- Daily mindfulness/meditation practice

  - Similar to a daily exercise routine, mindfulness can be practiced regularly and will get easier and more effective with practice. Choose any of the options listed here, or develop your own practice. In any mindfulness practice, the goal is never to do it "perfectly," because doing it "well" or "poorly" are judgments! Release your expectations or frustrations with yourself. Each time you find your mind wandering away from in-the-moment attention, simply notice the departure and gently bring it back to your practice.

- Mindful eating, bathing, stretching, etc.

  - As you engage in these or any other activity, practice being aware of each movement, each experience, and any emotions or thoughts that come up, without judging any part of it as "good" or "bad," or making up any meaning at all. Just notice and move on to the next moment in the activity.

- Deep Breathing

  - Notice your breath move in and out, like waves in the ocean. Slow down your breath, expanding the time you take for each inhale, and each exhale. This stimulates the vagus nerve which has a calming effect on the body and mind.

- Cycling 3's

  - Close your eyes and just breathe, noticing your breath, without trying to change it or decide that it is "good" or "bad." After a few moments, shift your attention to something that you can hear, and listen deeply to that sound. After a few moments, shift your attention to something that you can feel on your body, perhaps your feet on the floor, or the temperature on your skin, and really notice that sensation deeply. After a few moments, shift your attention back to your breath. Cycle through these three foci for several minutes.

- Visualizations
  - Close your eyes and imagine that you are in a space that is very soothing to you, perhaps a beach, a forest, a cathedral, or your childhood bedroom. Really notice every sight, sound, smell, and texture of the space that you are creating in your mind.

- Heart-centered breathing
  - Inhale, imagining the breath coming into your heart. Exhale, imagining the breath coming out from your heart. This improves the coordination of electrical signals between the heart and the brain and can reduce stress and improve your capacity to respond effectively in the face of a challenge.

- Loving kindness
  - Close your eyes and imagine someone who is easy for you to love. A friend, a spouse, a parent, or even a pet. Radiate love out to them with your whole being. Let that love expand to encompass other people in your family or community. Let the love expand to encompass you. Let the love expand to encompass even those who you disagree with, get angry with, or who you would judge as bad.

- Progressive muscle relaxation
  - Sit or lie comfortably and close your eyes. Tighten and relax each muscle group in your body, from head to toe. Notice the tension in the body without judging it, and notice as it releases. Notice how your breath moves with each progressive relaxation.

- Guided meditation via classes or Youtube or apps
  - If you would like support and guidance for mindfulness practice, look into classes through any of the local institutions listed below, type in "guided mindfulness" into Youtube, or download any of the apps listed below. Consult your healthcare provider to assess if what you discover is right for you.

Where Can I Find out More?

- Youtube.com
- Smartphone apps
  - Headspace, Aura, Breethe, Buddhify, Calm, iMindfulness, Insight Timer, Mindfulness Daily, Omvana, Sattva, Simply Being, Smiling Mind, Stop Breathe Think, The Mindfulness App
- Check out local yoga studios, churches, temples, or other spiritual or religious communities, senior centers, YMCA or community centers, or local colleges or universities

Mindfulness: Simplified

What Is Mindfulness?

Mindfulness is when I *pay attention* to:

- What I am experiencing
- What I am feeling
- What I am thinking

   I pay attention to these things in a *non-judgmental* way, which means:

- My experiences, feelings, and thoughts are not "good" or "bad," they just ARE.
- My experiences, feelings, and thoughts come and go, like clouds in the sky.
- As my experiences, feelings, and thoughts change, I let the change happen. I keep paying attention to what is happening NOW. I keep paying attention as each moment changes into the next.

How Can it Help?

- Reduce stress
- Increase positive feelings
- Reduce anxiety and depression
- Decrease blood pressure
- Improve digestion
- Improve sleep
- Improve mental functioning

What Can I Do?

- Daily mindfulness/meditation practice

   – Like daily exercise, mindfulness gets better with practice! Pick one of the ideas listed below and find time every day to work on it. Or, be mindful throughout your day, while eating, cooking, bathing, or walking!

- Cycling 3's

   – Close your eyes and just breathe, noticing your breath. Do not try to change it, or decide that it is "good" or "bad." After a few moments, shift your attention to something that you can hear. Listen deeply to that sound. After a few moments, shift your attention to something that you can feel on your body. Feel your feet on the floor, or the air on your skin, for example. Really notice that sensation deeply. After a few moments, shift your attention back to your breath. Cycle through these three attention points for several minutes.

- Heart-centered breathing

  – Breathe in, imagining the breath is coming in to your heart. Breathe out, imagining the breath coming out from your heart.

- Guided meditation via classes or Youtube or apps

  – You do not have to do mindfulness on your own. Look into classes at the places listed below. Type in "guided mindfulness" into Youtube for videos that can guide you. Or download any of the apps listed below. Check with your healthcare provider to see if what you discover is right for you.

Where Can I Find out More?

- Youtube.com
- Smartphone apps

  – Headspace, Aura, Breethe, Buddhify, Calm, iMindfulness, Insight Timer, Mindfulness Daily, Omvana, Sattva, Simply Being, Smiling Mind, Stop Breathe Think, The Mindfulness App

- Check out local yoga studios, churches, temples, or other spiritual or religious communities, senior centers, YMCA or community centers, or local colleges or universities

Motivational Interviewing
Created by Nicole Villegas

MI is a client-centered, collaborative conversation method to identify and strengthen your client's motivation and commitment to change.

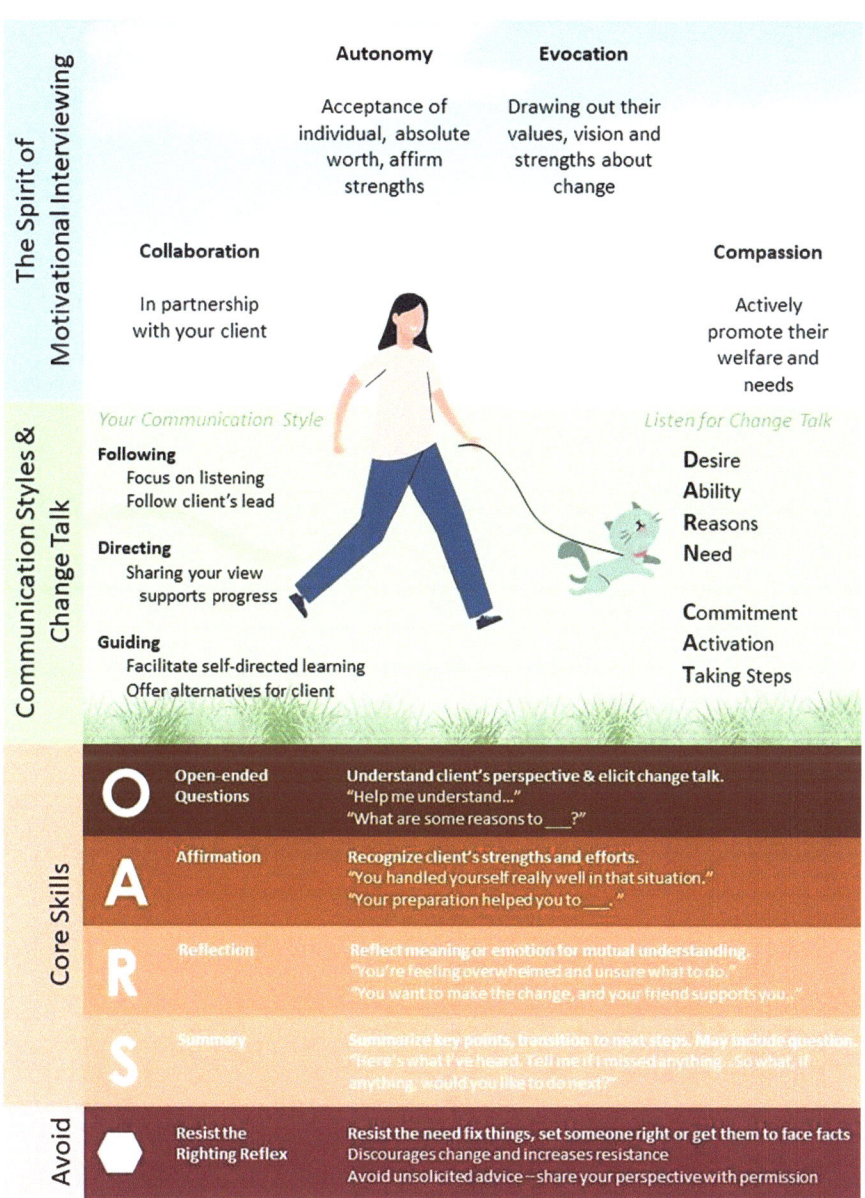

The Spirit of Motivational Interviewing

Autonomy
Acceptance of individual, absolute worth, affirm strengths

Evocation
Drawing out their values, vision and strengths about change

Collaboration
In partnership with your client

Compassion
Actively promote their welfare and needs

Communication Styles & Change Talk

Your Communication Style

Following
Focus on listening
Follow client's lead

Directing
Sharing your view supports progress

Guiding
Facilitate self-directed learning
Offer alternatives for client

Listen for Change Talk

Desire
Ability
Reasons
Need

Commitment
Activation
Taking Steps

Core Skills

O — Open-ended Questions — Understand client's perspective & elicit change talk. "Help me understand..." "What are some reasons to ___?"

A — Affirmation — Recognize client's strengths and efforts. "You handled yourself really well in that situation." "Your preparation helped you to ___."

R — Reflection — Reflect meaning or emotion for mutual understanding. "You're feeling overwhelmed and unsure what to do." "You want to make the change, and your friend supports you..."

S — Summary — Summarize key points, transition to next steps. May include question. "Here's what I've heard. Tell me if I missed anything. So what, if anything, would you like to do next?"

Avoid

⬡ — Resist the Righting Reflex — Resist the need fix things, set someone right or get them to face facts. Discourages change and increases resistance. Avoid unsolicited advice – share your perspective with permission

Conducting a Motivational Interview

Before	○ Review Client Profile ○ Review the Spirit of MI and reflect on your readiness to practice it today	
During	✓ **Learn more**	✓ **Elicit change talk**
	• Ask **O**pen-ended questions • **A**ffirm client's perspective • Listen **R**eflectively • **S**ummarize	• Use the rulers • Provide complex reflections • Ask evocative questions • Explore values
	✓ **Negotiate a plan for change**	
	• Discuss next steps • Engage in action planning/goal setting • Consider options, including scaffolding support • Arrive at a plan • Assess and elicit commitment	
After	○ Is the goal and plan aligned with your client's values? ○ What is your role and/or the role of the primary care team in following up to support your client? ○ Consider your role in the conversation. What went well? What would you like to improve next time?	

Rulers

Rating Scale for clients to rate level of Importance, Confidence, Commitment, etc.

Importance Ruler	*How important is it for you to _____? On a scale from 0 to 10 where 0 is not important at all and 10 is extremely important, where would you say you are?* 0 1 2 3 4 5 6 7 8 9 10 Not Important Very Important
Confidence ruler	*It sounds like you decided to make this change. How confident are you that you could do it? On a scale from 0 to 10 where 0 is not confident and 10 is extremely confident, where would you say you are?* 0 1 2 3 4 5 6 7 8 9 10 Not confident very confident
Follow up questions	*Why did you pick a __ and not zero?* *What would need to happen for you to get from a ___ to a [higher score]?*

Resources

Rollnick S, Butler CC, Kinnersley P, Gregory J, Mash B. Motivational interviewing. BMJ. 2010; 340: c1900.

Berger B, Villaume WA. Motivational interviewing for health care professionals: a sensible approach. 2nd ed. Washington, District of Columbia: American Pharmacists Association; 2020.

Motivational Interviewing Network of Trainers (MINT) free training resources. https://motivationalinterviewing.org/library/training.

Nerve Glides

Median Nerve Glides—Distal Glide

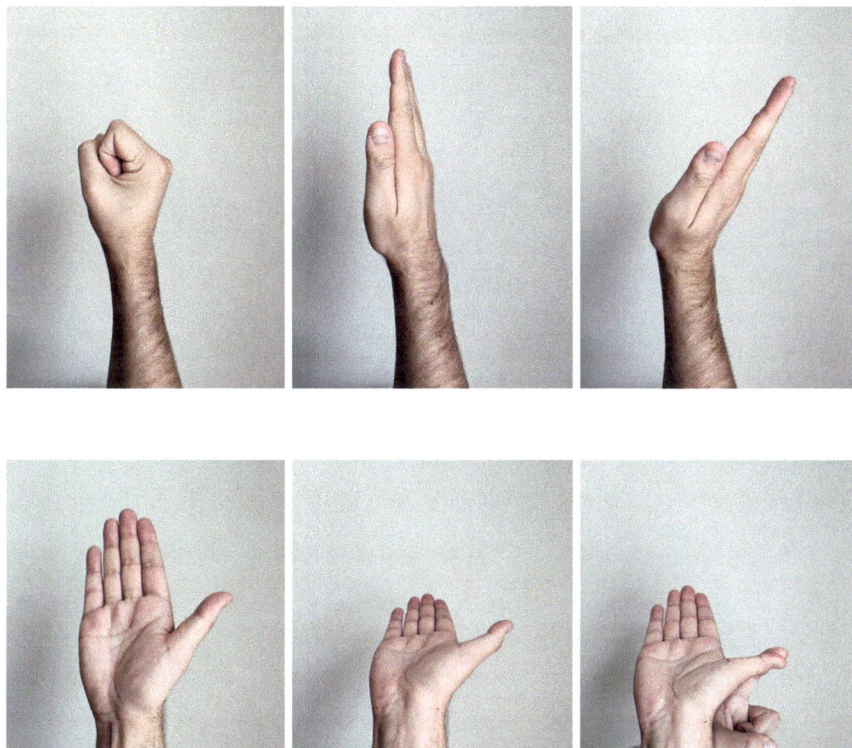

Median Nerve Glides—Proximal Glide

Note Use the hand of the arm you are not stretching to help keep your shoulder down.

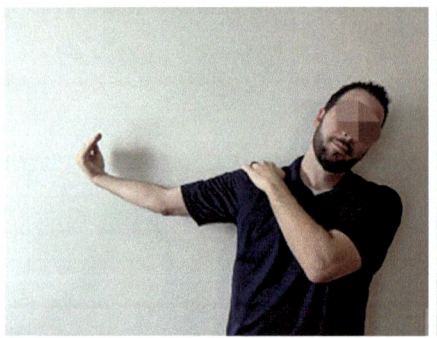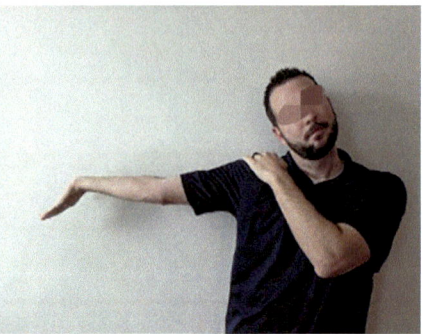

Note These images are for demonstration purposes only. To avoid injury you should only do the exercises as instructed by your therapist for your specific condition. You should feel a gentle stretch only. Stop the nerve glide and tell your therapist if pain occurs.

Ulnar Nerve Glides—Version 1

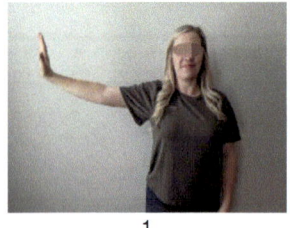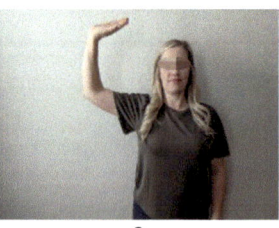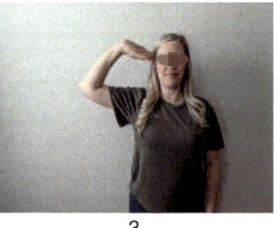

1	2	3

Gradually move through all three positions, hold at the last position (3).

Ulnar Nerve Glide—Version 2

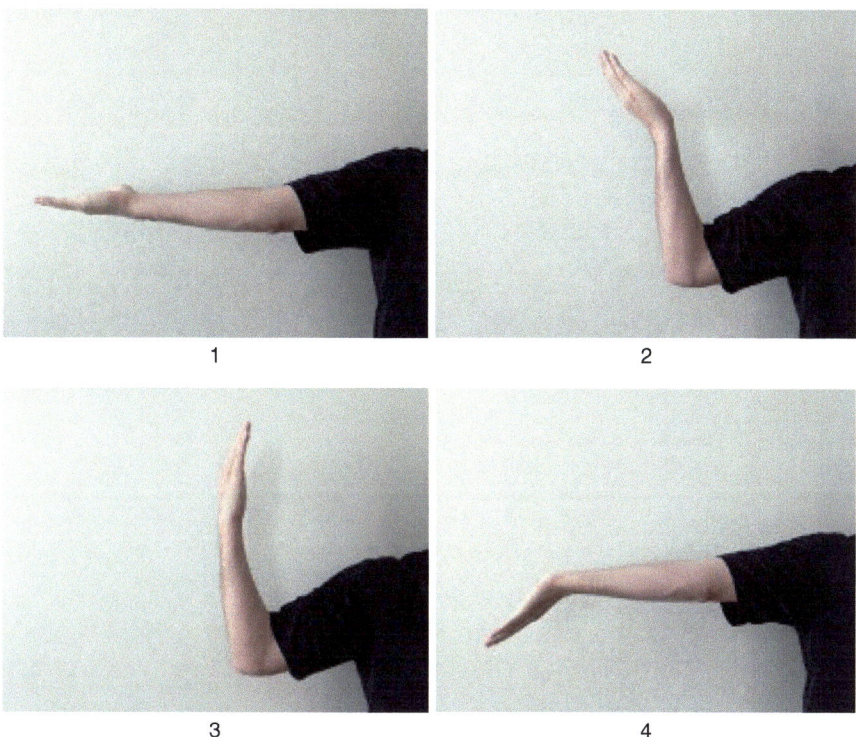

With arm out and elbow straight (1), gently bend (flex) elbow and extend your wrist back (2), then bring wrist back straight (neutral position) (3), and then straighten elbow and extend wrist back again (4).

Note These images are for demonstration purposes only. To avoid injury you should only do the exercises as instructed by your therapist for your specific condition. You should feel a gentle stretch only. Stop the nerve glide and tell your therapist if pain occurs.

Radial Nerve Glide

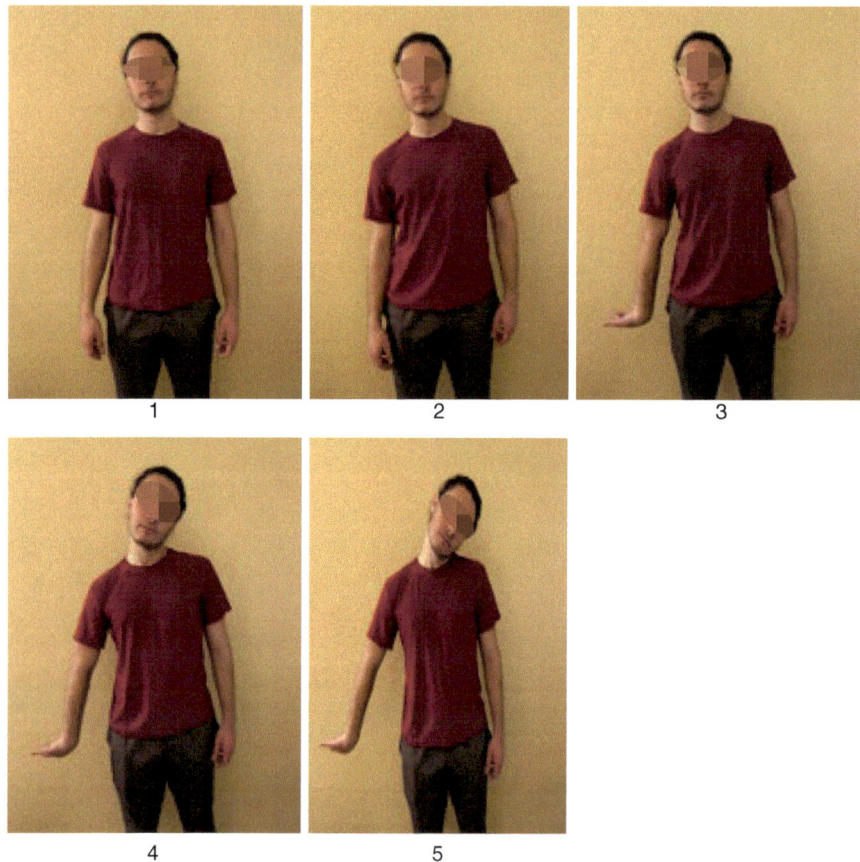

While standing (1), press the affected shoulder down (2), rotate your palm away from the body and bend (flex) the wrist (3), gradually bend (flex) your head/neck away from the affected arm (4), then gradually push your arm out/away from your body (5)—you will feel a gradual stretch along your radial nerve.

Brachial Plexus Glide

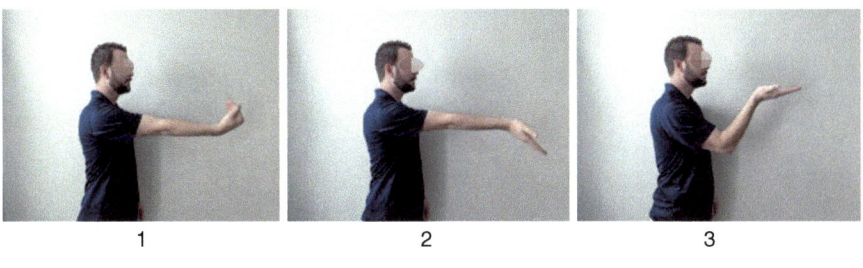

1   2   3

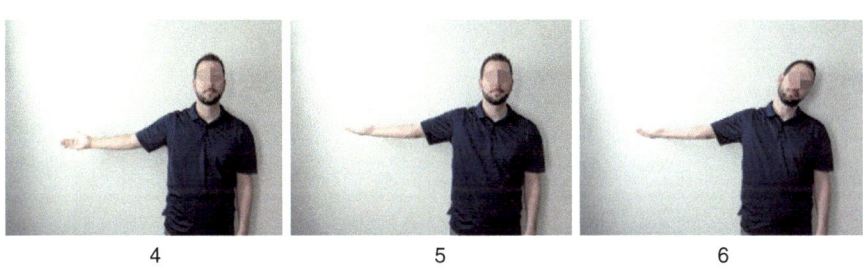

4   5   6

Move through these positions to gradually end with your arm out to the side, neck bent (flexed) away from your arm. To increase this stretch at the end, with the palm up, gradually bend (extend) your wrist by pointing your fingers gradually towards the ground.

Note These images are for demonstration purposes only. To avoid injury you should only do the exercises as instructed by your therapist for your specific condition. You should feel a gentle stretch only. Stop the nerve glide and tell your therapist if pain occurs.

Occupational Balance

Daily Occupational Balance

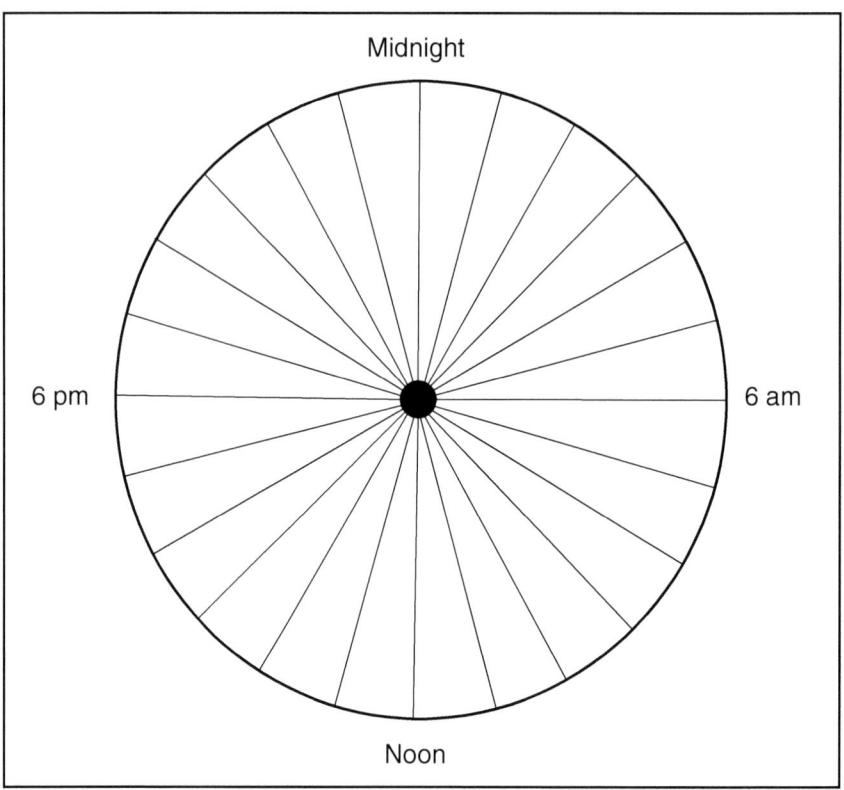

Self-Care/ADL =   Sleep =

IADL =   Leisure =

Work/Productivity =   Social =

Pediatric Primary Care: Caregiver Education (Newborn to 21 Years)

Newborn

Caregiver Education

Caregiver education and understanding is essential in all pediatric primary care, especially with infants. Caregivers may feel overwhelmed or anxious when caring for a new infant. It is therefore essential for educational materials to be given in a variety of ways including written, verbal, and even video instruction, encouraging the parent to video the exercise on their phone to watch again for guidance. If an infant needs occupational therapy, it is important to encourage the family to seek an early intervention evaluation program from their state. It is critical caregivers understand that as an infant grows and develops, the appropriate therapy interventions to complete at home will also change and develop.

Caregiver Considerations
- Parent–infant bonding (holding, carrying, rocking)
- Never shake a baby
- Discuss feeding
- Car seat safety
- Safe sleep
- Safe home environment
- Family routine
- Read, sing, and talk to the infant

Infants

Caregiver Education

Caregiver education and understanding is essential in all pediatric primary care, but especially with infants. Caregivers may feel overwhelmed or anxious with caring for a new infant. It is therefore essential for educational materials to be given in a variety of ways including written, verbal, and even video instruction, encouraging the parent to video the exercise on their phone to watch back for guidance. If an infant needs occupational therapy, it is important to encourage the family to seek an early intervention evaluation program from their state. It is critical caregivers understand that as an infant grows and develops, the appropriate therapy interventions to complete at home will also change and develop. The primary care occupational therapist may find it beneficial to have caregiver education handouts on the following topics readily available.

- Parent–infant bonding (holding, carrying, rocking)
- Alertness and self-regulation
- Never shake a baby
- Car seat safety
- Tummy time
- Create a routine for feedings, nap, bedtime
- Communication and early literacy
- Limit media
- Putting self to sleep, self-calming
- Safe sleep and naptime
- Safe home environment (water, outlets, stairs, cleaning products/poisoning, etc.)
- Keep consistent daily routines
- Separation anxiety
- Play
- Nutrition and feeding (self-feeding, mealtime routines, the transition to solid foods, cup drinking)

Toddlers

Caregiver Education

Caregiver education should be presented in a variety of formats using ordinary language, not medical jargon, and consider the family contexts and environment. Written materials should be at a fifth grade reading level to address the literacy needs of all caregivers. Education should help promote healthy development by establishing rules and routines around behavior, activities of daily living, sleep, physical activity, and social media use. Safety about harmful environmental exposures, car seats, and falls should be reviewed.

Caregiver Considerations

- Sleep routines
- Discipline/behavior management
- Brushing teeth
- Safety

Two to Five Years of Age

Caregiver Education

Caregiver education should be presented in a variety of formats using ordinary language, not medical jargon and consider the family contexts and environment. Written materials should be at a fifth grade reading level to address the literacy needs of all caregivers. Education should help promote healthy development by establishing rules and routines around behavior, activities of daily living, sleep, physical activity, and social media use. Safety about harmful environmental exposures, car seats, and falls should be reviewed.

School-Aged Children (6–14 Years of Age)

Caregiver Education

Caregiver education is essential to ensure skilled intervention is delivered appropriately. The primary care occupational therapist may find it beneficial to have caregiver education handouts on the following topics readily available.

Caregiver Considerations

- Teach nonviolent conflict-resolution techniques
- Bullies and Bully prevention
- Family rules and routines
- School
- Oral health
- Nutrition
- Physical activity
- Media use
- Safety
- Rules and consequences
- Puberty and personal hygiene
- Sexuality
- Dating
- Tobacco/cigarettes/alcohol use
- Sports
- Emotional well-being
- Sleep

Adolescence (15–21 Years)

Patient and Caregiver Education

Caregiver education is essential to ensure skilled intervention is delivered appropriately. The primary care occupational therapist may find it beneficial to have caregiver education handouts on the following topics readily available.

- Teach nonviolent conflict-resolution
- Bully prevention
- Rules and consequences
- Puberty and personal hygiene
- Sexuality/dating

- School
- Oral health
- Physical activity
- Nutrition
- Safety
- Tobacco/cigarettes/alcohol use
- Sports
- Emotional well-being
- Sleep
- Teach nonviolent conflict-resolution

Pediatric: Fine Motor, Bilateral Coordination, and Hand Strengthening Activities

Pediatric Primary Care Occupational Therapy

- Squirt water from a plastic bottle or spray bottle
- Play table hockey with a cotton ball while squirting air from a squirt bottle or ear bulb
- Hide small beans or beads in playdough, resistive putty, or clay
- Paper punch around a picture
- Use a sponge to squeeze out water while filling different containers
- Tear sheets of newspaper and crumble in hands
- Assemble pop beads, Legos, Tinker Toys, bristle blocks, or other construction toys
- Pop packaging bubbles using isolated fingers
- Place clothespins around a container or on a popsicle stick (match letters or pictures)
- Place coins, buttons, or beads in the palm of hand and work to fingertips
- Pick up items (pom-poms, cotton balls) using tongs or tweezers
- Make rubbings of textured surfaces
- Snip or cut playdough, index cards, old holiday (birthday) cards, or straws
- Mix colors or paint using an eyedropper with water and food coloring
- Play with windup toys
- Put modeling clay in a tray, use the index finger, a writing stylus, or a popsicle stick to draw or make shapes
- Play with Wikki Stix (thin, moldable wax sticks)
- Squeeze hand rockets (foam rocket blasters or launchers)
- Pull apart and push together rapper snappers (corrugated tubes)
- Put on a puppet show with finger puppets
- Engage in fingerplay songs, games, or rhymes (Where is Thumbkin, The Itsy-Bitsy Spider)
- String cereal (Cheerios, Fruit Loops) or macaroni

Pediatric: Getting Dressed

Pediatric Primary Care Occupational Therapy

- Children at a young age usually want to dress themselves. Self-help toys, books, or adult clothes (for dress-up) may aid you in teaching some of the basic dressing skills such as buttoning, zipping, lacing, snapping, and tying bows. Dressing is a slow process for young children, so allow plenty of time and select clothing that will present a minimum of frustration:
  - A minimum of closures
  - Large buttons and buttonholes
  - Large tabs on zippers (zipper pulls)
  - Large neck and armholes
  - Pull-on shirts
  - Pants with an elastic waist
  - Shoes with Velcro closures or elastic shoestrings
- Your child may have difficulty telling the front from the back. If the garment does not have labels, put an identifying mark with a laundry pen or iron-on patch, and then teach your child that the mark goes in the back.
- Deciding which shoe goes on which foot can be complex. Marking the shoes can help. Use a felt-tip pen to make arrows inside the shoes. When the shoes are placed side by side on the floor, the arrows should point to one another.
- The order of dressing can be confusing as well. It may help to lay out clothes in the order in which they are put on the body. Remember that undressing is learned before dressing.

Pediatric: Regulating Activities

Pediatric Primary Care Occupational Therapy

- Hang from monkey bars or pull-up bars
- Climb up a slide from the bottom
- Rock in a rocking chair
- Give bear hugs
- Ride a scooter board on stomach and push with arms and hands
- Jump on a mini trampoline
- Pull/push a wagon with someone or something inside
- Play "Row, Row, Row Your Boat" sitting on floor, pushing/pulling each other
- Play magic carpet (pull someone on a sheet, blanket, or small rug)
- Bounce on a bouncy ball with a handle
- Play sandwich games (between two couch cushions, pillows, or blankets)
- Push on walls and pretend that you are trying to move them
- Carry a heavy box (laundry basket) around the house
- Sweep floor, vacuum, wash table, or dust furniture
- Animal walks (bear, crab, dog) and wheelbarrow walks
- Play tug-of-war with a jump rope
- Dig in dirt or sand with hands, shovel, or containers
- Squeeze silly putty or clay
- Sip applesauce or thick milkshake through straw
- Chew gum, eat chewy or crunchy foods
- Blow bubbles, whistles, party blowers
- Practice deep breathing

Pediatric: Self-Care Skills

Pediatric Primary Care Occupational Therapy

2 Years

- Remains dry for 2 h
- Fusses to be changed
- Discriminates between edibles/non-edibles
- Eats using a spoon with some spillage
- Drinks from an open cup without assistance
- Cooperates with toothbrushing
- Takes unfastened coat off

2 ½ Years

- Tries to put on socks
- Removes shoes and socks
- Removes pants
- Unzips large zipper
- Drinks from a cup, one hand, unassisted
- Unbuttons and unsnaps

3 Years

- Puts on socks with difficulty in heel placement
- Puts on shoes (maybe wrong feet)
- Puts on a coat with assistance
- Puts on a shirt with some assistance
- Zips and unzips non-separating zipper
- Buttons one large button
- Urinates without toileting assistance
- Washes/dries hands with assistance
- Turns faucet on/off
- Brushes teeth with assistance
- Uses spoon, minimal spillage
- Opens door by turning the handle

3½ Years

– Unzips a separating zipper
– Buttons 3–4 buttons
– Wipes nose when requested to do so

4 Years

– Pours from a small pitcher
– Holds spoon with fingers
– Uses napkin
– Puts on socks with correct heel placement
– Puts shoes on correct feet
– Dresses with minimal supervision other than help with fasteners
– Inserts shank in zipper
– Buttons/unbuttons

5 Years

– Attempts to tie shoes
– Brushes teeth without assistance
– Uses fork and spoon with no spillage
– Spreads with a knife.

Patient Health QUESTIONNAIRE-9

Patient Health Questionnaire-9
(PHQ-9)

Over the last 2 weeks, how often have you been bothered by any of the following problems *(use ✓ to indicate your answer)*	Not at all	Several days	More than half the days	Nearly every day
1. Little interest or pleasure in doing things	0	1	2	3
2. Feeling down, depressed, or hopeless	0	1	2	3
3. Trouble falling or staying asleep, or sleeping too much	0	1	2	3
4. Feeling tired or having little energy	0	1	2	3
5. Poor appetite or overeating	0	1	2	3
6. Feeling bad about yourself—or that you are a failure or have let yourself or your family down	0	1	2	3
7. Trouble concentrating on things, such as reading the newspaper or watching television	0	1	2	3
8. Moving or speaking so slowly that other people could have noticed? Or the opposite—being so fidgety or restless that you have been moving around a lot more than usual	0	1	2	3
9. Thoughts that you would be better off dead or hurting yourself in some way	0	1	2	3

FOR OFFICE CODING ___0___ + _____ + _____ + _____
= Total score_____

If you checked off <u>any</u> problems, how <u>difficult</u> have these problems made it for you to do your work, take care of things at home, or get along with other people?

Not at all Difficult	Somewhat Difficult	Very Difficult	Extremely Difficult
☐	☐	☐	☐

Developed by Drs. Robert L. Spitzer, Janet B.W. Williams, Kurt Kroenke and colleagues, with an educational grant from Pfizer Inc. no permission required to reproduce, translate, display, or distribute

Progressive Muscle Relaxation (PMR)

The body responds to a perceived threat in a variety of ways, including muscle tension. This body strategy to guard against a potential threat can be helpful in some circumstances however in the face of many stressors, muscle tension can contribute to aches and pains, fatigue, and reduced mental and physical flexibility which can reduce our ability to navigate a challenge. Think about how you respond to anxiety. Do you "tense up" when you are feeling anxious? Intentionally relaxing muscles can deliver a signal of calm and safety from the body to the brain, which helps reduce anxiety and can improve our capacity to handle a challenging situation. In PMR exercises, you tense up particular muscles and then relax them.

Preparation

Keep in Mind the Following:

- Physical injuries. Consult your doctor before you begin PMR if you have any injuries.
- Environment. Reduce input to all five senses. Seek a quiet, calm place.
- Position. Support your body in a relaxed position, sitting or lying down, and consider removing uncomfortable clothing or shoes.
- Body. Avoid practicing PMR after a large meal or if consuming any intoxicants, such as alcohol.

Process

- Breathe slowly and give yourself permission to relax.
- Tense the muscle group so that you can feel the tension but without creating discomfort. Hold tension for ~5 s.
- Relax the muscle group and keep it relaxed for ~10 s. It may be helpful to exhale or say something like "Relax" as you relax the muscle.
- After tightening and relaxing each muscle group, allow the body to feel completely relaxed, melting into whatever supportive surface you are sitting or lying on. Sustain this relaxed state for several minutes if possible.

Sequence

- Right hand and forearm. Squeeze hand into fist
- Right upper arm. Pull arm in tight to your body
- Left hand and forearm
- Left upper arm

- Face and neck. Scrunch up mouth and eyebrows
- Shoulders. Squeeze your shoulders up towards your ears
- Shoulder blades/Back. Squeeze shoulder blades together
- Chest and stomach. Breathe in deeply, filling up your lungs and chest with air
- Hips and buttocks. Squeeze your buttock muscles and press hips forward
- Right upper leg. Tighten your right thigh
- Right lower leg. Tighten your calf
- Right foot. Curl your toes
- Left upper leg
- Left lower leg
- Left foot

Practice

With continued practice of PMR, awareness of the muscles of the body increases, and tension can be more easily recognized and addressed. This trains the body and brain to work together to handle stress in a new way!

Reference

Center for Clinical Intervention. Progressive muscle relaxation. Available from https://www.cci.health.wa.gov.au/~/media/CCI/Mental%20Health%20Profes-sionals/Panic/Panic%20-%20Information%20Sheets/Panic%20Information%20Sheet%20-%2005%20-%20Progressive%20Muscle%20Relaxation.pdf.

Provocative Tests for Distal Nerve Compression

Carpal Tunnel

Phalen's Test A provocative test for Carpal Tunnel Syndrome. As demonstrated in the picture below, the patient performs maximum wrist flexion for 60 s. Carpal Tunnel Syndrome is suspected if the patient's symptoms are reproduced including paresthesias in the thumb, index, middle, and/or medial half of the ring finger. If these symptoms occur in the small finger (pinky) or the ulnar half of the ring finger, carpal tunnel is not the source of the symptoms or is not the only source of the patient's complaints.

Tinel's Sign The OT can also tap on the volar aspect of the wrist over the carpal tunnel. The test is positive if paresthesias occur in the median nerve distribution.

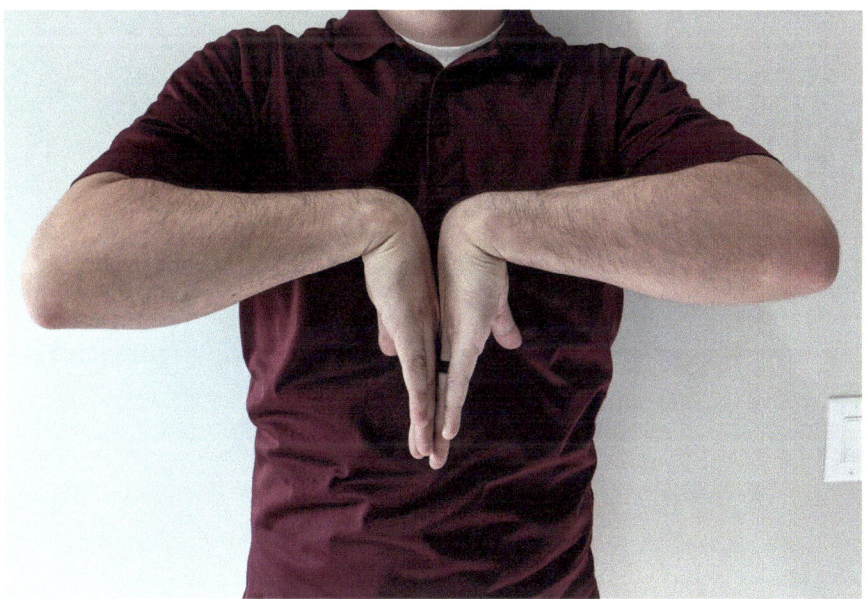

Cubital Tunnel Syndrome

Elbow Flexion Test A provocative test for Cubital Tunnel Syndrome. The patient performs shoulder external rotation, maximum elbow flexion, and wrist extension for 60 s. Cubital Tunnel Syndrome is suspected if symptoms are reproduced (e.g., paresthesias in the distribution of the ulnar nerve). The OT can also tap over the ulnar nerve distribution on the posterior elbow (**Tinel's sign**). The test is positive if paresthesias occur in the ulnar nerve distribution.

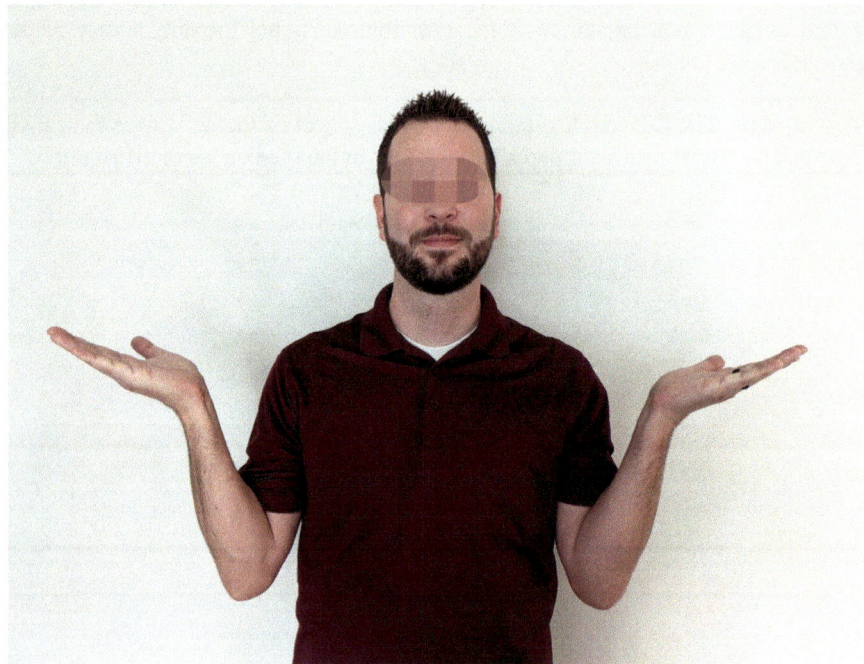

Radial Tunnel Syndrome

Resisted Middle Finger Extension Test A provocative test for Radial Tunnel Syndrome. The OT provides resistance against extension of the patient's middle finger/third digit. Radial Tunnel Syndrome is suspected if this resistance produces pain. Two additional tests for Radial Tunnel Syndrome include resisted supination and resisted wrist extension. Pain with either of these tests can also indicate Radial Tunnel Syndrome.

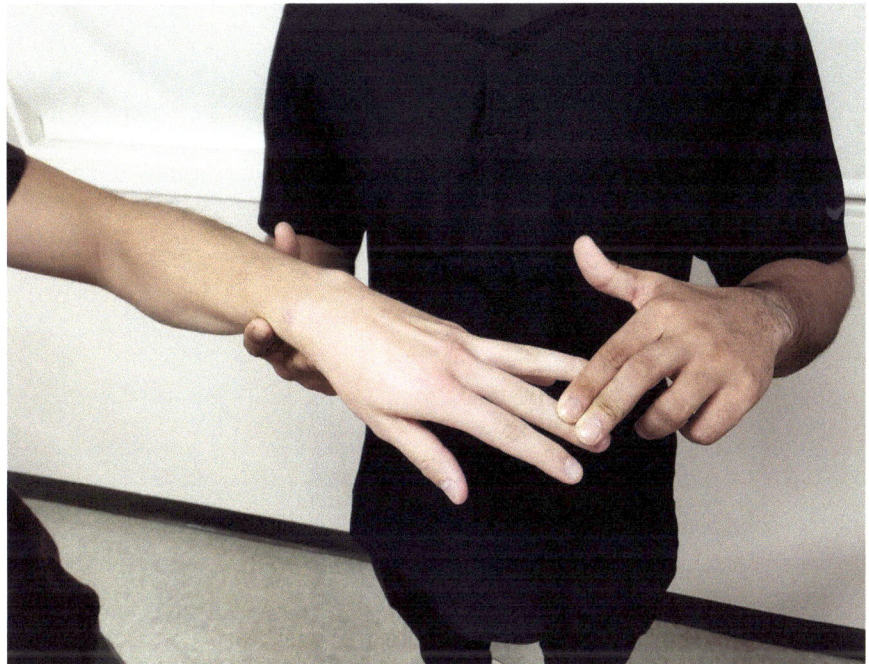

Provocative Tests for Proximal Nerve Involvement

Spurling's Test A provocative test for cervical radiculopathy from nerve root compression. Place the patient in cervical extension and rotation towards the side of the suspected nerve root compression. Provide axial compression and note any symptoms. Nerve root compression is suspected if the patient complains of pain that radiates to the shoulder or the upper extremity on the same side the head is rotated towards with axial compression.

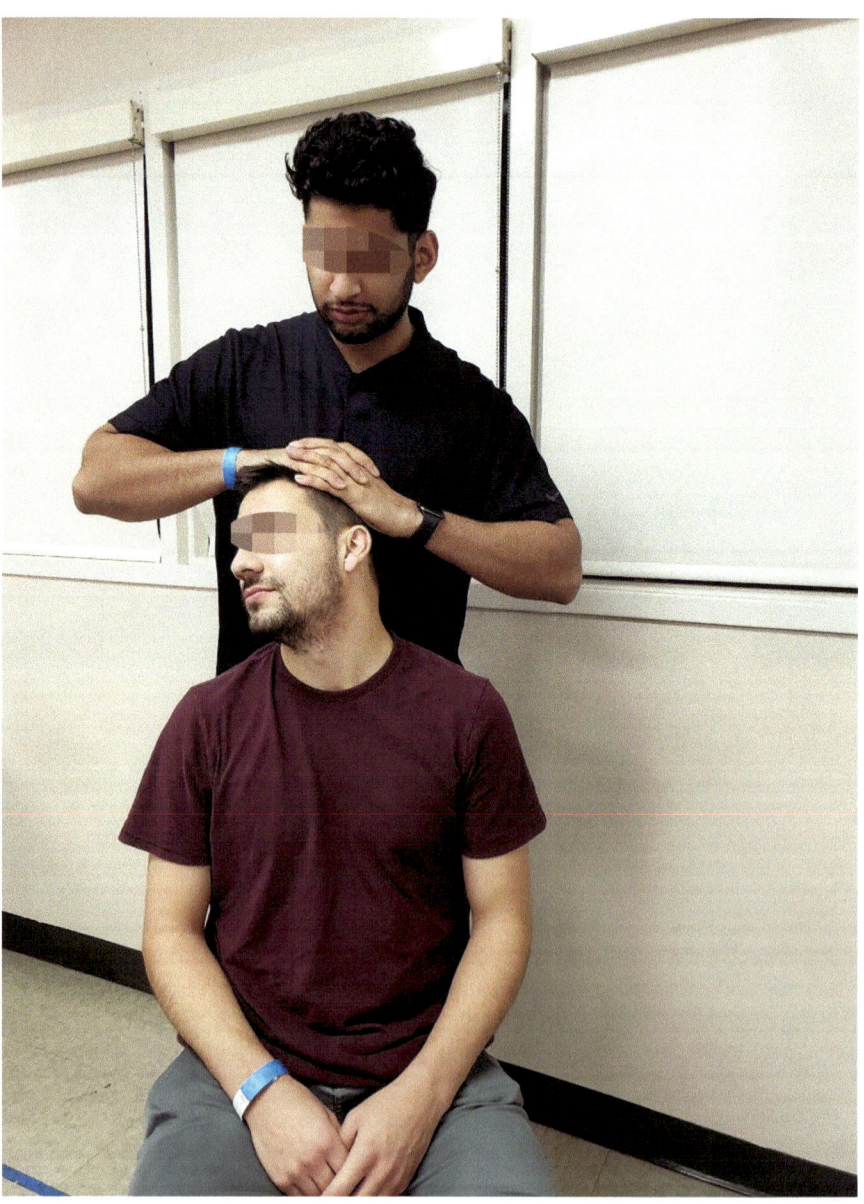

Adson's Test   A provocative test for Thoracic Outlet Syndrome (TOS). The patient's arm on the suspected side is abducted to 30° at the shoulder and extended. The OT palpates the radial artery and asks the patient to extend their neck, turn towards the symptomatic shoulder and take a deep breath and hold it. The OT evaluates the quality of the radial pulse in this position compared to when the arm was resting at the patient's side. TOS is suspected if there is a marked decrease or disappearance of the radial pulse or a significant difference compared to the unaffected arm. A modified version of this test is also used by many clinicians where the only difference is the patient is asked to turn their head away from the symptomatic shoulder.

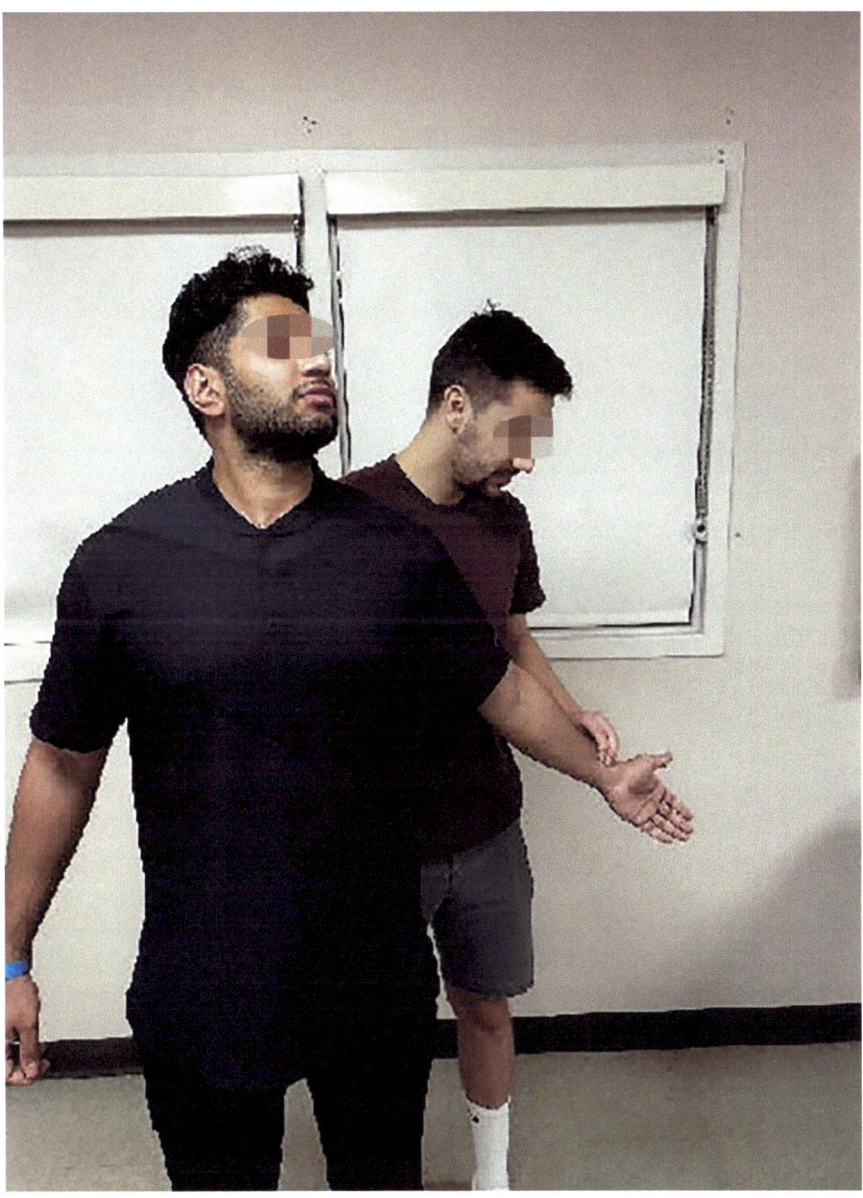

Roos Test A provocative test for TOS and is also known as the Elevated Arm Stress Test (EAST). The patient places both arms in the 90° abduction-external rotation position with the shoulder and elbows in the same plane as the chest. The patient is asked to open and close their hands slowly over a 3-min period while maintaining this position. TOS is suspected if the patient reports a gradual increase in pain at the neck, shoulder, and progressing down the arm; paresthesias in the upper extremity; reproduction of reported symptoms; inability to complete the test; or changes due to arterial or venous compression.

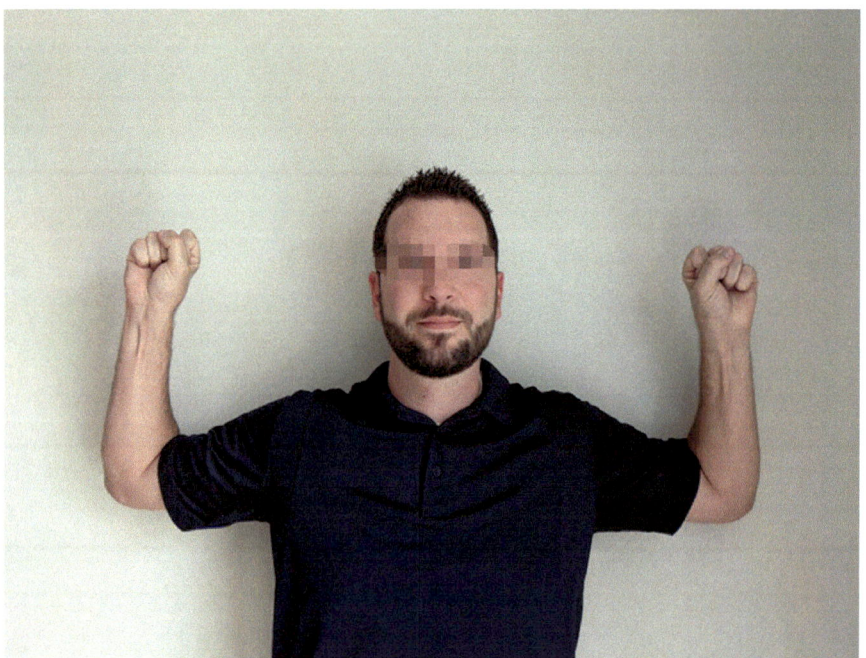

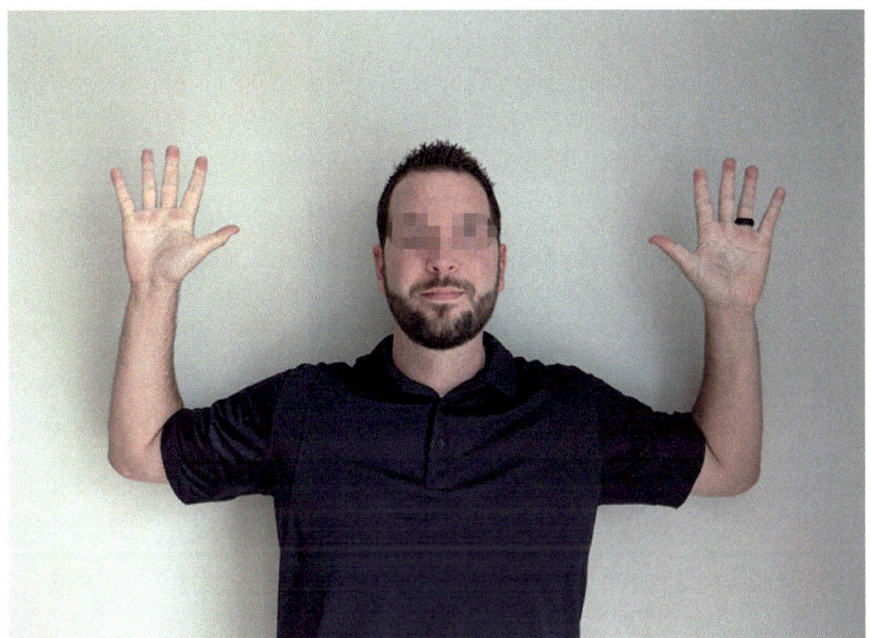

Sleep Hygiene

Sleep hygiene is a term that describes habits that can support restful sleep. If you experience difficulty falling asleep or staying asleep, try out some of these tips:

- Keep a consistent sleep schedule. Get up at the same time every day, even on weekends or during vacations.
- Do not go to bed unless you are sleepy.
- Follow the 20/20 rule. If you do not fall asleep after 20 min, get out of bed. Go do a quiet activity without a lot of light exposure for 20 min, and do not go back to bed until you are feeling sleepy. Follow this same process for wake-ups during the night.
- Establish a relaxing bedtime routine. Consider ideas such as a warm bath or shower, soothing music, comfortable pajamas, a light snack, stretching, or a cup of uncaffeinated herbal tea.
- Use your bed only for sleep and intimacy. This trains your brain for sleeping in that distinct environment, instead of gearing up for a different activity while you are attempting to sleep. Do not use your bedroom for watching TV, working, reading, etc.
- Cultivate a pro-sleep environment. Make your bedroom quiet, dark, and cool. Limit all light exposure and use room-darkening blinds, and have a lamp or flashlight accessible to you from your bed, for a safe path to the bathroom when needed.
- Try wearing earplugs and an eye mask to further limit sensory input. The brain is always seeking to make sense of sensory input. The less input it gets, the less it has to work with, which will support it "turning off" and drifting to sleep.
- If total silence is impossible or uncomfortable, consider a white noise machine. It is better to have constant and indistinct sound rather than sounds that the brain will try to interpret (like a fan, as opposed to the radio).
- Limit exposure to bright light in the evenings, including TV, computer, cellphone, kindle, and any kind of light from electronics.
- If using electronics before bed is necessary, consider wearing blue light blocking glasses, to reduce the stimulating effect of blue light from screens.
- Avoid eating a large meal before bedtime, because then the body will be working on digesting instead of focusing on rest and recovery.
- Consider a light, healthy snack before bed to stabilize blood sugar overnight.
- Exercise regularly and maintain a healthy diet.
- Avoid consuming caffeine in the afternoon or evening.
- Avoid consuming alcohol in the evening.
- Reduce your fluid intake before bedtime if waking up to urinate is disturbing sleep.

Sweet Dreams!

Schedule

SCHEDULE

TIME	MON	TUES	WED	THUR	FRI	SAT	SUN

Weekly Sleep Log

Instructions   List the dates for this week on the line below the corresponding days of the week. Before going to bed, list any naps you took during the day, and any sleep medications you took before going to sleep, in the bottom two rows. After you wake up the next day, answer the questions from the night before. For example, when you wake up on Tuesday, write in the answers for the Monday column for the sleep you just woke up from. Keep time estimates APPROXIMATE! Do not use timers or clocks to get more specific! Round to 15 min increments. See the asterisk below for the total hours of sleep calculation.

Date:	Mon	Tue	Wed	Thur	Fri	Sat	Sun
What time did you go to bed?							
What time did you turn the lights out to go to sleep?							
About how long did it take you to fall asleep?							
How many times did you wake up last night?							
About how long were you awake in total during the night?							
What was your final wake up time?							
What time did you get out of bed?							
About how many hours did you sleep last night? *							
If you took sleep medications, list the med and the dose							
If you took any naps, list the time of day and durations							

* Take the amount of time between your lights out time and your wake up time. Subtract the amount of time it took you to fall asleep. Subtract the total amount of time you were awake during the night.

Write down your NSTs and PSTs. NSTs are any negative thoughts related to your sleep, for example, "I'll be exhausted tomorrow if i don't fall asleep now," or "I'll never be able to sleep tonight." PSTs are any positive thoughts related to your sleep, for example, "I love getting into my cozy bed," or "I feel so relaxed and rested."

	Negative Sleep Thoughts (NSTs)	Positive Sleep Thoughts (PSTs)
Monday		
Tuesday		
Wednesday		
Thursday		
Friday		
Saturday		
Sunday		

Weekly Sleep Goals:

1.
2.
3.
4.

SMART Goals and Monthly Tracker

Instructions   Write out goals below, making sure that they meet all of the qualities of SMART goals. Use the Monthly Tracker to monitor your daily adherence to your goals. Update your goals as you progress!

S	Specific	When we create specificity in a goal, we are more likely to achieve it. Visualize the goal actually happening. What does it look like? Where does it happen? Get specific
M	Measurable	Ensure that your goal is detailed enough so that you can clearly tell if it has been achieved. For example, "being more physically active" is vague, whereas "walk to the tree and back every day" is measurable
A	Achievable	The best goal is the goal that can be met! Start with goals that you can more easily achieve, and build up to the bigger goals as you develop your capacity to make and achieve goals
R	Relevant	If a goal is not in line with what is truly important to you, it is less likely that it will be met. Spend some time digging into what matters most to you in your life, and see how your goals and plans can work to further your investment in your own values
T	Time-bound	Set a deadline, e.g., "By the first of the month …". Clarify when you will begin taking action, e.g., "Beginning tomorrow …". Clarify when the actions will happen, for example, "go for a walk for 15 min, at 10 am …"

  Goal 1:
  Goal 2:
  Goal 3:
  Goal 4:

	DAYS OF THE MONTH:																														
	1	2	3	4	5	6	7	8	9	10	11	12	13	14	15	16	17	18	19	20	21	22	23	24	25	26	27	28	29	30	31
Goal 1:																															
Goal 2:																															
Goal 3:																															
Goal 4:																															

Spoon Tracking Sheet

INSTRUCTION AND EXAMPLE		Monday
AM self-assessment: *Write down the number of spoons it feels like you have when you wake up in the morning.*	##	AM self-assessment:

INSTRUCTION AND EXAMPLE		**Monday**	
Tasks:	Spoons:	Tasks:	Spoons:
Write down tasks that you do throughout the day. *Try to get a distribution of AM and PM, and routine and novel tasks.*	***BEFORE*** *the activity, write down how many spoons you ESTIMATE it will cost to do the activity*	##	
	AFTER *the activity, write down how many spoons it feels like it ACTUALLY cost to do the activity*	##	
Make and eat breakfast		##	
		##	
Walk the dog		##	
		##	
Go to doctor appointment		##	
		##	
Pay phone bill		##	
		##	
Watch TV		##	
		##	
PM self-assessment: *Write down the number of spoons it feels like you have left as you get into bed, at that moment. This is **NOT** a tally!*	##	PM self-assessment:	

Tuesday		**Wednesday**		**Thursday**	
AM Self-Assessment:		AM Self-Assessment:		AM Self-Assessment:	
Tasks:	Spoons:	Tasks:	Spoons:	Tasks:	Spoons:
PMSelf-Assessment:		PM Self-Assessment:		PM Self-Assessment:	

Friday		Saturday		Sunday	
AM Self-Assessment:		AM Self-Assessment:		AM Self-Assessment:	
Tasks:	Spoons:	Tasks:	Spoons:		

Transtheoretical Model (TTM)|Stages of Change

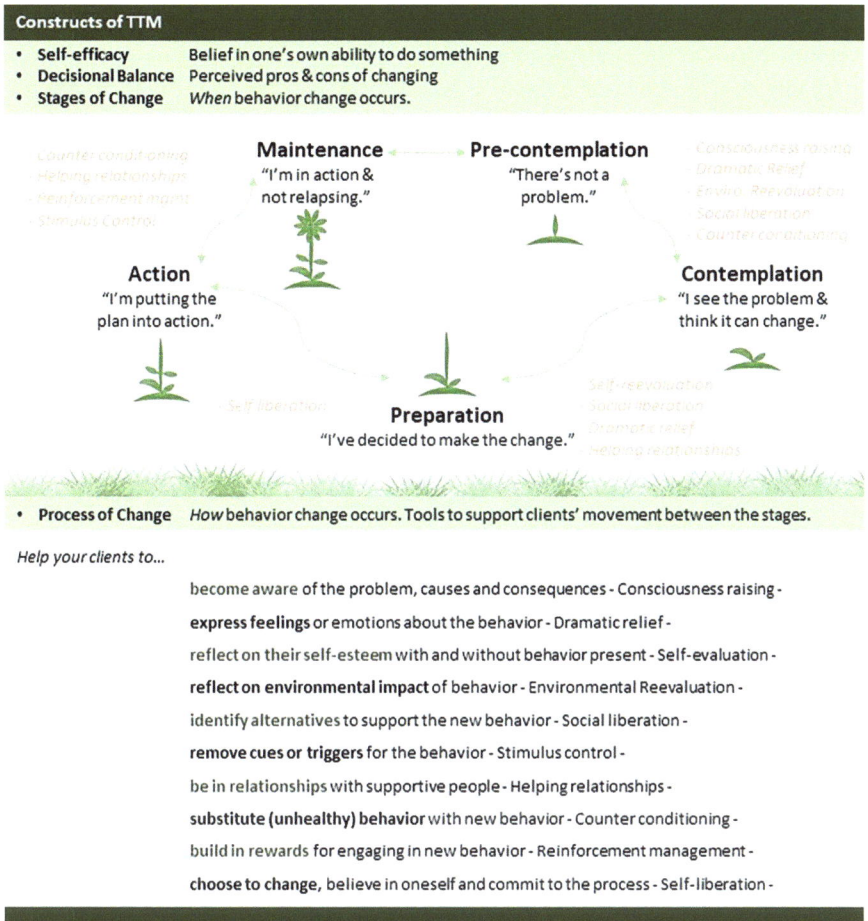

Constructs of TTM

- **Self-efficacy**   Belief in one's own ability to do something
- **Decisional Balance**   Perceived pros & cons of changing
- **Stages of Change**   *When* behavior change occurs.

Maintenance → **Pre-contemplation**
"I'm in action & not relapsing."   "There's not a problem."

Action
"I'm putting the plan into action."

Contemplation
"I see the problem & think it can change."

Preparation
"I've decided to make the change."

- **Process of Change**   *How* behavior change occurs. Tools to support clients' movement between the stages.

Help your clients to...

become aware of the problem, causes and consequences - Consciousness raising -

express feelings or emotions about the behavior - Dramatic relief -

reflect on their self-esteem with and without behavior present - Self-evaluation -

reflect on environmental impact of behavior - Environmental Reevaluation -

identify alternatives to support the new behavior - Social liberation -

remove cues or triggers for the behavior - Stimulus control -

be in relationships with supportive people - Helping relationships -

substitute (unhealthy) behavior with new behavior - Counter conditioning -

build in rewards for engaging in new behavior - Reinforcement management -

choose to change, believe in oneself and commit to the process - Self-liberation -

Created by Nicole Villegas, OTD, OTR/L

References and Resources

Hilliard ME, Riekert KA, Ockene JK, and Pbert L. The handbook of health behavior change, vol. fifth ed. Cham: Springer; 2018.

Norcross JC, Krebs PM, Prochaska JO. Stages of change. J Clin Psychol. 2011; 67(2):143–54.

Raihan N, Cogburn M. Stages of change theory. In: StatPearls. Treasure Island (FL): StatPearls Publishing; 2020. Available from: https://www.ncbi.nlm.nih.gov/books/NBK556005/.

Vanbuskirk KA, and Wetherell JL. Motivational interviewing with primary care populations: a systematic review and meta-analysis. J Behav Med. 2014; 37(4):768–80. https://doi.org/10.1007/s10865-013-9527-4.

Strength, Weaknesses, Opportunities, and Threats (SWOT) Analysis

SWOT Analysis is a tool that facilitates the examination of an organization's strengths, weaknesses, opportunities, and threats. The purpose of this tool is to allow for a full analysis of the position of the organization. It may help with decision-making, identification of potential risks (Weaknesses and Threats), and leveraging of strengths and opportunities.

Internal Factors: Strengths and Weaknesses are *internal* factors of the organization. Common considerations are financial resources (funding, income sources), physical resources (space, location, equipment), human resources (employees, skills, volunteers), and current processes.

External Factors: Opportunities and Threats are *external* factors. Examples include marketing trends, economic trends, funding, demographics, relationships with other organizations, political, and economic regulations.

Utilize the below chart to begin brainstorming.

STRENGTHS	WEAKNESSES
What do you do well?	*What could you do better?*
What do others consider your strengths?	*What resources are you lacking?*
What resources do you have access to?	*What do others consider your weaknesses?*
OPPORTUNITIES	**THREATS**
What can you take advantage of?	*What could potentially harm your organization?*
	What are other organizations doing?

Stressors

Can Control

Can Not Control

Theraputty Exercises

Finger Abduction/Adduction Make cylinder with the putty, place fingers on putty—abduct and adduct fingers, reforming cylinder as needed to keep resistance.

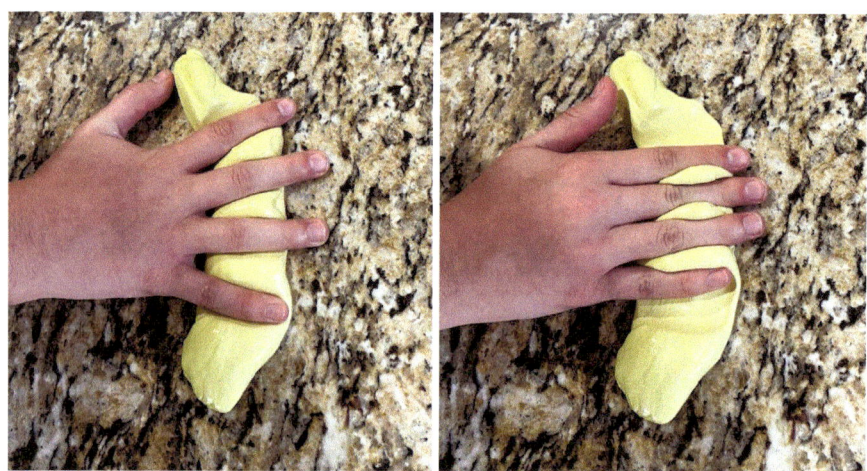

Finger Extension Make a pancake with the putty. Place pancake over fingertips— open fingers. Reform pancake with each repetition.

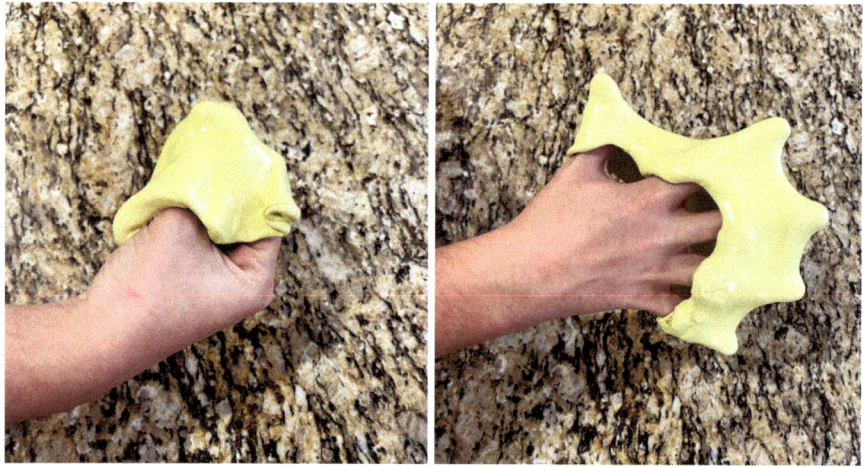

Finger Flexion/Lateral (Key) Pinch/Three Point Pinch Roll putty into a ball— squeeze putty with full finger flexion/Key Pinch/Lateral Pinch. Reform ball with each repetition.

Flexion

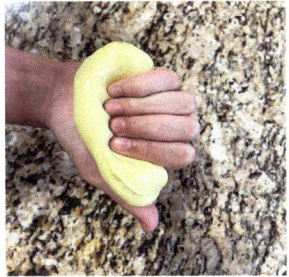

Lateral (Key) Pinch

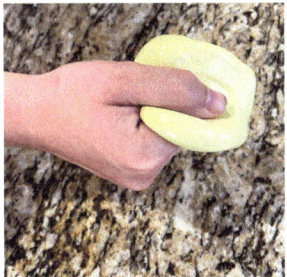

3 Point Pinch

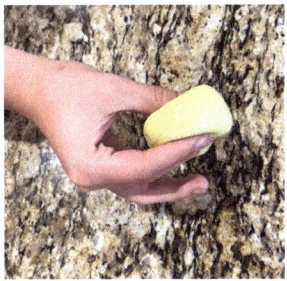

Instructions Complete each motion slowly, 5×—2–3×/day.

Caution Do not do more than this until you have completed putty successfully for a few days as you can cause further injury if you overdo it, and you will not know until a while later.

Do not hold putty for prolonged periods as it tends to become "drippy" when it is warm, and it can stain.

Walk to Run Program

Following this program can help to increase running endurance over time. Always warm up before exercising, wear comfortable shoes, and drink water to prevent dehydration. This program can be modified to meet your needs and abilities. Talk to your provider about safety and precautions prior to starting this program.
    Alternate walking and running for a total of 30 min each day.

Week	Walk	Run	Walk	Run	Walk	Run	Walk	Run	Walk	Run
1	4 min	2 min	4 min	2 min	4 min	2 min	4 min	2 min	4 min	2 min
2	3 min	3 min	3 min	3 min	3 min	3 min	3 min	3 min	3 min	3 min
3	2 min	4 min	2 min	4 min	2 min	4 min	2 min	4 min	2 min	4 min
4	3 min	5 min	3 min	5 min	3 min	5 min	3 min	3 min		
5	3 min	7 min	3 min	7 min	3 min	7 min				
6	2 min	8 min	2 min	8 min	2 min	8 min				
7	1 min	9 min	1 min	9 min	1 min	9 min				
8	2 min	13 min	2 min	13 min	2 min					
9	1 min	14 min	1 min	14 min						
10		30 min								

Water Tracker

Instructions Color in a drop for each glass of water you drink.

Goal Color in the whole sheet each week!

MONDAY

TUESDAY

WEDNESDAY

THURSDAY

FRIDAY

SATURDAY

SUNDAY

Index

© Springer Nature Switzerland AG 2023
S. Dahl-Popolizio et al. (eds.), *Primary Care Occupational Therapy*,
https://doi.org/10.1007/978-3-031-20882-9